Fundamentals of
MEDICAL VIROLOGY

for Students of Medicine and Related Sciences

Fundamentals of
MEDICAL VIROLOGY

for Students of Medicine and Related Sciences

JEAN D. ACTON, Ph.D.
Associate Professor of Microbiology
Department of Microbiology
The Bowman Gray School
  of Medicine
Wake Forest University
Winston-Salem, North Carolina

LOUIS S. KUCERA, Ph.D.
Associate Professor of Microbiology
Department of Microbiology
The Bowman Gray School
  of Medicine
Wake Forest University
Winston-Salem, North Carolina

QUENTIN N. MYRVIK, Ph.D.
Professor and Chairman
Department of Microbiology
The Bowman Gray School
  of Medicine
Wake Forest University
Winston-Salem, North Carolina

RUSSELL S. WEISER, Ph.D.
Professor of Immunology
Department of Microbiology
University of Washington School
  of Medicine
Seattle, Washington

LEA & FEBIGER   *Philadelphia · 1974*

576.64
F 981

Cover illustration: A thin section of a herpesvirus-infected *Rana pipiens* embryo cell containing a nuclear crystalline array of typical herpesvirus in various stages of development. X39500. From A. Granoff: Lucke tumor-associated viruses—A review. In Oncogenesis and Herpesviruses, 1972. Biggs, P. M., de-The, G. and Payne, L. N. (eds.), Lyon, France, International Agency for Research on Cancer, pp. 171-182.

Library of Congress Cataloging in Publication Data

Main entry under title;

Fundamentals of medical virology for students of medicine and related sciences.

Includes bibliographies.

1. Virology. 2. Virus diseases. I. Acton, Jean D. [DNLM: 1. Virus diseases—Viruses. WC500 F981 1974] QR360.F85 1974 576'.64 74-5257 ISBN 0-8121-0433-1

Published in Great Britain by Henry Kimpton Publishers, London

PRINTED IN THE UNITED STATES OF AMERICA

Preface

The ever-accelerating rate at which new information is being added to the enormous body of existing knowledge in medicine and allied sciences poses serious difficulties for both medical students and medical educators. The problem of recognizing and selecting study material that is most relevant to the student's education is formidable since there are no reliable criteria for objective judgment. Nevertheless, selection is necessary to avoid overburdening the student.

Although educators continue to experiment with revolutionary changes in curricula and teaching methods, uncertainty persists concerning what should be taught to best prepare the student for delivering optimal patient care.

This uncertainty in turn makes it difficult to compile suitable texts to serve the needs of the majority of instructors in any medical science.

The intent of this book is to present the student with the fundamentals and principles of both basic and applied virology. The first half of the book includes the current classification scheme, molecular biology, and genetics of animal viruses, mechanisms of pathogenesis, chemotherapy, and laboratory methods used in diagnosis of viral infections. In the latter half of the book, the viral diseases involving each of the major organ systems are discussed. We have used the "organ systems approach," rather than the conventional presentation of the viruses by major groups in order to develop the student's acumen for differential diagnosis of infectious diseases. Special emphasis is placed on clinical symptoms, the mechanisms of pathogenesis, host resistance, and chemoprophylaxis of viral infections, as well as on laboratory diagnoses and epidemiology. Knowledge in these areas should aid the student in predicting the outcome of the disease and provide an introduction to clinical research problems. The final chapters on "slow" viruses and oncogenic viruses were written with the intent of presenting the student with the current "state-of-the-art" of virus research and the probable role of viruses in the etiology of persistent neurologic diseases and cancer in humans.

Selected references are included at the end of each chapter to introduce the reader to the literature and to provide a mechanism for obtaining further information on a given topic. They consist of recent reviews and current journal articles as well as occasional historical references. The book is especially designed for students of medicine, upper division biology students, and animal virologists. It is our sincere hope that it also will be of value to practicing physicians, public health personnel and to persons working in viral diagnostic and research laboratories.

JEAN D. ACTON
LOUIS S. KUCERA

Winston-Salem, North Carolina   QUENTIN N. MYRVIK
Seattle, Washington   RUSSELL S. WEISER

Contents

Fundamentals of
MEDICAL VIROLOGY

for Students of Medicine and Related Sciences

Characterization of Viruses

A. History

The word *virus* is of Latin origin and was used in ancient times to denote a noxious agent or poison. Before the discovery of filterable viruses, the word *virus* was frequently used to designate any infectious microbe irrespective of its nature. Certain infectious diseases, later shown to be caused by viruses, were recognized long before the nature of the etiologic agents was understood. It is noteworthy that in 1798 Jenner introduced the practice of vaccination against smallpox with exudate from cowpox lesions without recognizing that he was dealing with a viral agent. In 1884, 14 years before the isolation of the first animal virus, Pasteur developed a vaccine for rabies. By the middle of the last century, scientists were making major efforts to determine the cause and effect of many biological phenomena, including disease. It was evident to those pioneer investigators that disease could be caused by several different classes of harmful agents including poisons, toxins, and pathogenic bacteria. By the 1880s Koch, Pasteur, Ehrlich, and others had made great progress in describing, isolating, and culturing pathogenic bacteria and relating them to specific diseases. However, it soon became obvious that there were many infectious diseases which were not caused by bacteria, toxins, or poisons. Bacteria could not be cultured from specimens obtained from the lesions of some diseases that could be serially passed from one animal to another and were, therefore, infectious. Furthermore, such material remained infectious after passage through bacteriological filters. Eventually agents of this type were given the name *filterable viruses* and later, simply *viruses*.

Iwanowski is generally recognized as the "father" of the science of
virology because of his discovery of the tobacco mosaic virus (TMV) in
1892. He reported that the agent which produced the mosaic disease of
tobacco plants passed freely through "bacteriological filters." However,
his conclusions concerning the nature of the etiological agent of the disease
were erroneous. He suggested that the disease was caused either by a
toxin elaborated by some bacterial agent or by a bacterium which passed
through the filters he used. The significance of Iwanowski's findings was
not recognized until other viruses were described.

The introduction of the chick embryo for virus propagation (1928–
1930), followed by improvements in existing cell-culture techniques for
growing viruses (1945–1950), marked the beginning of the highly productive era of modern virology. A list of discoveries which have contributed
most importantly to the development of virology is presented in Table 1–1.

TABLE 1–1

Some Important Milestones in the Development of Medical Virology

Approximate Date	Principal Contributor(s)	Contribution(s)
1892	Iwanowski	Recognized that a "filterable agent" was responsible for mosaic disease in tobacco plants.
1898	Löffler and Frosch	Discovered the foot-and-mouth disease virus, the first animal virus to be described.
1898	Beijerinck	"Rediscovered" tobacco mosaic virus and called it *contagium vivum fluidum*.
1902	Reed	Discovered the cause of yellow fever, the first human virus to be described.
1907	von Prowazek	Described the first insect virus.
1908	Ellerman and Bang	Demonstrated that chicken leukemia could be transferred with cell-free extracts.
1911	Rous	Described the transmission of Rous sarcoma virus in chickens.
1915	Twort	Discovered bacteriophage.
1917	D'Herelle	"Rediscovered" bacteriophage and developed the plaque assay for quantifying infectious virus; coined the term *bacteriophage*.
1931	Woodruff and Goodpasture	Introduced embryonated eggs for propagating viruses.
1933	Shope	Described papilloma virus of rabbits.
1934	Lucké	Described a renal carcinoma with a suspected herpes-type virus etiology in frogs.

Table 1—1 (continued)

Approximate Date	Principal Contributor(s)	Contribution(s)
1935	Stanley	Obtained tobacco mosaic virus in crystalline form.
1936	Bittner	Described mouse mammary tumor virus and its transmission by milk.
1939	Delbrück	Began systematic studies of bacteriophage.
1941	Hirst	Demonstrated that influenza virus would agglutinate red blood cells (hemagglutination test).
1949	Enders	Showed that poliovirus multiplies in and destroys nonneural tissue in culture.
1951	Gross	Induced lymphoid leukemia in mice with a cell-free extract of tumors from leukemic mice.
1952	Dulbecco	Developed the plaque technique for assaying animal viruses.
1952	Hershey and Chase	Showed that only the DNA of bacteriophage is required for replication.
1953	Salk	Developed inactivated poliovirus vaccine.
1955	Sabin	Developed an active, attenuated poliovirus vaccine.
1957	Colter	Extracted infectious nucleic acid from animal viruses.
1957	Stewart, Eddy, Gochenour, Borgese, and Grubbs	Isolated polyoma virus in tissue culture.
1959	Friend	Reported cell-free transmission of reticulum cell leukemia in mice.
1958	Burkitt	Reported on a lymphoma involving the jaw in African children.
1960	Enders	Developed an active, attenuated measles virus vaccine.
1962	Rauscher	Described a virus-induced lymphoid leukemia in mice.
1962	Trentin, Yabe, and Taylor	Reported that adenoviruses of human origin induced tumors in newborn hamsters.
1964	Temin	Postulated that viral RNA can direct the synthesis of DNA provirus.
1964	Epstein and Barr	Described the presence of a herpes-type virus associated with Burkitt lymphoma.

Table 1—1 (continued)

Approximate Date	Principal Contributor(s)	Contribution(s)
1969	Huebner and Todaro	Presented the viral oncogene hypothesis that most or all vertebrate species contain genomes of RNA tumor viruses that are vertically transmitted from parent to off-spring.
1970	Baltimore; Temin	Independently found evidence of RNA-directed DNA polymerase (reverse transcriptase) in virions of RNA tumor viruses.
1970	Spiegelman	Established that the RNA-directed DNA polymerase in oncogenic RNA viruses catalyzes the synthesis of an RNA:DNA hybrid.
1971	Kufe, Hehlmann, and Spiegelman	Reported that human sarcomas contain RNA sequences homologous to those found in a virus known to cause sarcoma in mice.
1972	Hehlmann, Kufe, and Spiegelman	Demonstrated that human leukemic cells, but not normal cells, contain RNA sequences homologous to those found in Rauscher leukemia virus.

B.   Definition and Origin

Because of the many specialized virus-host cell relationships which have been discovered, there is no completely satisfactory definition of a virus. The following definition is presented in an attempt to differentiate viruses from rickettsia, chlamydia, and cell organelles which contain nucleic acid. *Viruses are obligate intracellular parasites that contain either DNA or RNA; they depend on the synthetic machinery of the cell for replication of the infectious particle, the virion.*

How viruses reached the state of obligate intracellular parasitism poses an interesting, if presently unanswerable, question. Probably, the various groups of viruses arose by parallel evolution rather than by degeneration of a complex common ancestor. The fact that a number of cytoplasmic organelles contain functional DNA which serves as template for synthesis of messenger RNA (mRNA) and codes for protein suggests that the DNA in these organelles was originally derived from nuclear DNA and acquired the capability of autonomous replication. It is conceivable that a further step in evolution gave rise to progenitors of the various groups of DNA viruses.

Concomitantly, the RNA viruses may have evolved from cellular RNA-replicating systems. Cellular mRNA could have acquired the ability to initiate its own replication. In this regard, double-stranded RNA has been detected in a number of species of uninfected animal cells. However, the presence of a latent RNA virus in these cells has not been ruled out. Another alternative is that RNA viruses were derived from DNA viruses whose mRNA acquired the attribute of self-replication thus eliminating the requirement for transcription from DNA.

The development of experimental procedures for determining the "relatedness" of species of DNA and RNA by complementation or hybridization, "nearest neighbor" base sequence frequencies, and base ratios has provided approaches for studying the origin of viruses. Nearest neighbor base sequence analysis between the nucleic acids of certain viruses and the DNA of mammalian cells or of bacteria is compatible with the hypothesis that some viruses arose from the DNA of animal cells and others from bacteria. Although the viruses within a given major group, such as the adenoviruses, appear to have only small regions of viral genome which are homologous, they probably evolved from a common ancestor. Refinement and extension of existing analytical procedures may yield information about the phylogenetic relationship of the various groups of viruses.

C. Composition and Structure of the Virion

All virions are composed of nucleic acid, either single- or double-stranded RNA or DNA, enclosed in a protein coat, the *capsid*. The capsid is composed either of similar repeating protein molecules called *structural units* or of *capsomeres* (aggregates of structural units). The structure composed of the nucleic acid surrounded by the capsid is the *nucleocapsid*. Some viruses are naked nucleocapsids, whereas others are enclosed in an *envelope* or *peplos* of cellular membrane origin and, thus, are said to be "enveloped" (Fig. 1–1). Some envelopes are covered with "spikes" or surface projections of varying lengths spaced at regular intervals. The spikes are presumably viral coded and are incorporated into the host cell membrane prior to virion maturation and release by a budding process.

Initial observations with the electron microscope have indicated that viruses can be classified into one of three broad structural groups: spherical, rod shaped, or tadpole shaped. The viruses infecting animals belong to one of the first two structural groups, whereas those infecting bacteria (bacteriophage) belong in the third category (Chapter 3, *Fundamentals of Bacteriology and Mycology*). Refinement of techniques for negative staining of purified virus preparations and for fixing and staining virus-infected cells for electron microscopy has permitted a more precise visualization of virus symmetry and structure.

All of the virions which originally appeared to be spherical have been shown to have nucleocapsids with either icosahedral or helical symmetry.

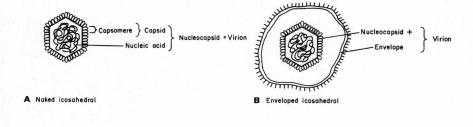

A Naked icosahedral   **B** Enveloped icosahedral

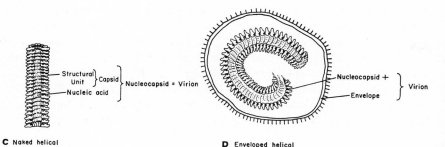

C Naked helical   **D** Enveloped helical

Figure 1—1. Schematic representation of the structure and symmetry of four types of virions. The capsids of icosahedral viruses are composed of aggregates of structural units called *capsomeres*. The capsids of helical viruses are composed of identical repeating structural units. The capsid plus the nucleic acid comprises the nucleocapsid.

Viruses with icosahedral symmetry contain capsomeres which may be round or prismatic in shape and are arranged in equilateral triangles. The icosahedron has 12 vertices, 20 triangular faces, and 30 edges (Fig. 1–2). Diagrams of viruses with icosahedral symmetry are shown in Figures

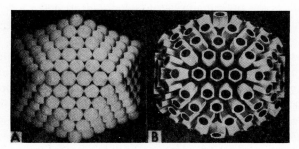

Figure 1—2. Models of icosahedral viruses showing (A) round and (B) prismatic capsomeres arranged in equilateral triangular faces. (Reproduced with permission from Wildy, P., and Watson, D. H.: Electron microscopic studies on the architecture of animal viruses. *In:* Symposia on Quantitative Biology. Vol. 27. Cold Spring Harbor, N. Y.: The Biological Laboratory, Long Island Biological Association, 1962.)

1–1A and 1–1B. It is apparent from Figure 1–1B and 1–1D that an enveloped icosahedral or helical virus can appear as a spherical particle.

The elucidation of the structure of rod-shaped viruses indicates that they all possess helical symmetry and may be rigid or flexible. The helical viruses which infect vertebrates all appear to be flexible and to be surrounded by an envelope (Fig. 1–1D). When the helical nucleocapsid is coiled in an envelope, the virion may assume the shape of either a rod or a sphere. Some viruses, such as influenza virus, possess virions of both shapes and, therefore, are said to be pleomorphic.

The best-studied helical virus is tobacco mosaic virus, a non-enveloped rigid RNA plant virus (Fig. 1–1C). Fragments of TMV rods observed in the direction of the virion axis have a central channel readily observed in electron micrographs of negatively stained preparations. The nucleocapsid is composed of identical structural units arranged in a helix with the nucleic acid coiled between the turns of the helix.

The nucleocapsids of the enveloped animal viruses with helical symmetry have been observed following treatment with ether or with other substances which disrupt the lipid-containing envelope. The internal components of the animal viruses with helical symmetry resemble TMV in that the structural units of most, if not all, are arranged in a single helix. It has been suggested that the pleomorphism of some viruses (such as parainfluenza virus type 1) is, in part, a consequence of envelope and nucleocapsid flexibility which permits considerable variability in their configuration. It is also possible that pleomorphism may result from the incorporation of multiple nucleocapsids into a single envelope.

Not all viruses exhibit classical icosahedral or helical symmetry. Those which do not fit into these two categories, because of their unusual complexity, have been arbitrarily classified as *complex* or *binal* viruses. The symmetry of the poxviruses, the largest and most complex viruses which infect vertebrates, has not been determined with certainty; it has been suggested that the internal component be called a "core" until agreement can be reached on the question of what constitutes the nucleocapsid.

Although members of the poxvirus group vary with respect to size and morphology, vaccinia virus can be considered to be representative of this group. Electron microscopic examinations of shadowed preparations and thin sections of the mature vaccinia virion have shown it to be a brick-shaped particle with an outer multilayered membrane surrounding a biconcave core (Fig. 1–3). A pair of lens-shaped lateral bodies lie in the concavities of the core and are responsible for the central thickening of the particle.

In contrast to enveloped viruses which derive their envelope from the cell membrane, the outer coat of the vaccinia virus is acquired while the virus is within the cytoplasm of the host cell. Occasionally, a surface membrane is acquired by vaccinia virus upon release from the cell; however, this membrane does not appear to be an integral component of the virion; i.e., a true envelope. The poxviruses are not considered to be true enveloped viruses because (1) most poxviruses do not possess an envelope, (2) the envelope is not required for infectivity, and (3) the envelope, when present, may not contain virus-specific antigen.

D.   Classification Schemes

Ideally a classification scheme should reflect the evolutionary and phylogenetic relationships between groups of organisms. Since such relationships have not been established between the major virus groups, the existing classification schemes have evolved primarily to serve as useful keys for identifying and classifying viral isolates.

Unfortunately, the viral nomenclature in current use is the result of free-lance labeling of viruses by investigators often with disregard for developing a systematic approach to classification. For example, many viruses were named for the geographical location from which they were first isolated or where the first case of a disease occurred; for example, O'nyong-nyong virus initially was isolated in Africa, and the first diagnosed coxsackievirus infection occurred in Coxsackie, New York. The practice of incorporating into the virus name the disease associated with it has some value because it relates significant information about the virus; for example, poliovirus causes poliomyelitis. However, the discovery of increasing numbers of viruses posed the need for grouping them in some logical taxonomic order.

Among the criteria which have been used to classify viruses into groups are the nature of the disease and the organ system most frequently involved. Thus the dermatropic viruses included the measles, smallpox, and herpes agents, whereas poliovirus and the equine encephalitis agents were classified as neurotropic viruses. Other schemes were based on the mode or route of transmission. Whereas such systems are useful for associating certain viruses with specific syndromes, they fail to take into account the wide variability in the characteristics of individual viruses within a given group and the fact that viruses can replicate in many different tissues without producing clinical disease.

Despite the efforts of international committees, no "official" system of classification has been adopted. A subcommittee on the nomenclature of viruses recommended that virus groups, based on the characteristics of the virion, be given latinized binomial names. However, this proposal has not gained wide acceptance, and most of the systems in use today retain only the group names. In the most generally accepted scheme of classification, the viruses are divided into two major divisions: the *riboviruses* and the *deoxyriboviruses,* based on the type of nucleic acid present in the virion. Criteria used for subdividing these two divisions into the major virus groups include (1) symmetry of the nucleocapsid, (2) presence or absence of an envelope, (3) number of strands of nucleic acid, (4) size and shape of the virion, and (5) number of capsomeres of icosahedral viruses or the diameter of the helix in helical viruses. A simplified classification, based on Melnick's system, is presented in Table 1–2. Diagrams of viruses representing the major virus groups are illustrated in Figure 1–3.

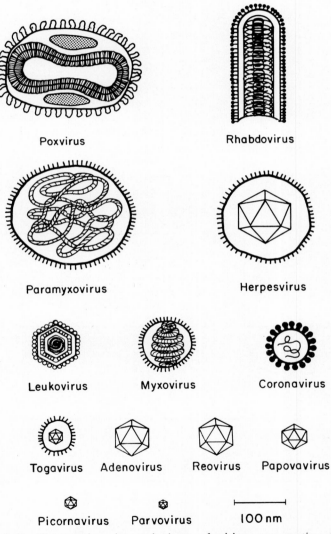

Figure 1–3. Comparative size and shape of virions representing the major virus groups.

TABLE 1—2

General Properties of Major Virus Groups

Nucleic Acid Type	No. Strands Nucleic Acid	Nucleocapsid Symmetry	Virion Naked or Enveloped	Shape of Virion	Size of Virion (nm)	Group
DNA	1	Icosahedral	Naked	Spherical	18-24	Parvovirus
	2	Icosahedral	Naked	Spherical	40-55	Papovavirus
				Spherical	70-80	Adenovirus
			Enveloped	Roughly Spherical	110	Herpesvirus
		Complex	Naked	Brick Shaped	230 × 300	Poxvirus
RNA	2	Icosahedral	Naked	Spherical	54-75	Diplornavirus (Reovirus)
	1	Icosahedral	Naked	Spherical	18-30	Picornavirus
			Enveloped	Spherical	35-40	Togavirus (Arbovirus)
				Roughly Spherical	100	Leukovirus (Oncornavirus)
		Helical	Enveloped	Roughly Spherical	80-120	Orthomyxovirus (Myxovirus)
				Pleomorphic	100 × 300	Paramyxovirus
				Bullet Shaped	60 × 225	Rhabdovirus
		Unknown	Enveloped	Oval or Pleomorphic	110-130	Arenavirus
				Roughly Spherical	80-160	Coronavirus

E. Characterization of Major Groups of Viruses

Usually more than one type of disease entity can be caused by viruses within each major group. Conversely, the same clinical picture often can be caused by different viruses or by other microorganisms. For example, meningitis can be a consequence of infection with picornaviruses, togaviruses, herpesviruses, as well as a number of species of bacteria. The clinical symptoms produced by a given agent also can vary. For example, poliovirus infection can be inapparent or it can result in mild illness, aseptic meningitis, or paralytic poliomyelitis. The virus groups and important viral agents, together with the common diseases they cause, are summarized in Table 1–3. This list serves to introduce the major viral diseases of man which will be discussed in subsequent chapters.

TABLE 1—3

Selected Viruses Associated with Major Virus Groups

1. PAPOVAVIRUS—cyclic, double-stranded DNA; replicate in nucleus.
   Papillomavirus: *Warts*
   Polyomavirus: *No disease in man*
   Simian vacuolating virus (SV40): *Progressive multifocal leukoencephalopathy*

2. ADENOVIRUS—linear, double-stranded DNA; replicate in nucleus.
   Adenoviruses: *Respiratory tract, eye infections*

3. PARVOVIRUS—linear, single-stranded DNA; replicate in nucleus.
   Adeno-associated (satellite) viruses: *No disease in man*
   H1 and H3 viruses: *Isolated from human malignancy; significance unknown*

4. HERPESVIRUS—linear, double-stranded DNA; replicate in nucleus; acquire envelope by budding from nucleus into cytoplasm.
   Herpes simplex: *"Fever blisters," cervical cancer*
   Varicella-zoster: *Chickenpox, shingles*
   Cytomegalovirus: *Cytomegalic inclusion disease*
   Epstein Barr (EB): *Burkitt's lymphoma, mononucleosis*
   B virus: *Ascending myelitis*

5. POXVIRUS—linear, double-stranded DNA; replicate in cytoplasm; membrane is viral coded, is acquired within cytoplasm and is not considered to be an "envelope." DNA-dependent RNA polymerase and DNA-dependent DNA polymerase associated with virion.
   Variola: *Smallpox*
   Vaccinia: *Complications following vaccination*
   Molluscum contagiosum: *Benign skin nodules*
   Orf: *Milkers' nodules*

6. PICORNAVIRUS—linear, single-stranded RNA; replicate in cytoplasm.
   A. Enterovirus
      1. Poliovirus: *Poliomyelitis*
      2. Coxsackieviruses: *Aseptic meningitis, herpangina, pleurodynia, myo- and pericarditis, common cold*
      3. Echoviruses: *Aseptic meningitis, febrile illness with or without rash, common cold*
   B. Rhinoviruses: *Common cold*

Table 1—3 (continued)

Selected Viruses Associated with Major Virus Groups

7. DIPLORNAVIRUS (REOVIRUS)—linear, double-stranded RNA; RNA in segments; replicate in cytoplasm; virion contains RNA polymerase which transcribes mRNA from the double-stranded genome.

> Reovirus: May cause *minor febrile illness, diarrhea,* and *upper respiratory disease,* but relationship to clinical disease in man is not clear.
> Orbivirus: *Colorado tick fever*

8. TOGAVIRUS (ARBOVIRUS)—linear, single-stranded RNA; replicate in cytoplasm; acquire envelope by budding from plasma membrane. Many transmitted by arthropod vectors.

> Group A. Eastern and Western encephalitis viruses (equine encephalitis viruses): *Encephalitis*
> Group B. St. Louis encephalitis virus: *Encephalitis*
> Yellow fever virus: *Yellow fever*
> California Group. California encephalitis viruses: *Encephalitis*
> Ungrouped. Rubella virus: *German measles*

9. ORTHOMYXOVIRUS (MYXOVIRUS)—linear, single-stranded RNA; phases of replicative cycle in nucleus and cytoplasm; envelope acquired by budding from plasma membrane. RNA-dependent RNA polymerase associated with virion.

> Influenza viruses: *Influenza*

10. PARAMYXOVIRUS—linear, single-stranded RNA; some may have phases of replicative cycle in nucleus and cytoplasm; "negative" strand of RNA associated with polyribosomes in some viruses; envelope acquired by budding from plasma membrane. RNA-dependent RNA polymerase associated with virion.

> Parainfluenza virus: *Severe respiratory infections (croup, bronchiolitis, bronchitis, pneumonia) in children; common cold in adults*
> Mumps virus: *Mumps (epidemic parotitis)*
> Respiratory syncytial virus: *Severe respiratory infections (bronchiolitis and pneumonia) in children; common cold in adults*
> Measles virus: *Measles (rubeola)*

11. RHABDOVIRUS—linear, single-stranded RNA; probably replicate in cytoplasm. "Bullet-shaped" virion; acquire envelope by budding from plasma membrane.

> Rabiesvirus: *Rabies*

12. LEUKOVIRUS (ONCORNAVIRUS)—linear, single-stranded RNA; replicate in nucleus; acquire envelope by budding from plasma membrane. RNA-directed DNA polymerase and DNA-dependent DNA polymerase associated with the virion.

> Avian leukosis and sarcoma viruses: no disease in man?
> Murine leukosis and sarcoma viruses: no disease in man?
> Feline leukosis and sarcoma viruses: no disease in man?
> Mouse mammary tumor (Bittner) virus: no disease in man?
> Human leukosis, sarcoma and carcinoma viruses: leukemia, rhabdomyosarcoma, breast carcinoma?

13. ARENAVIRUS—strandedness and symmetry of RNA unknown (not helical); replicate in cytoplasm; pleomorphic; interior of particle appears unstructured and contains a variable number of electron-dense granules; acquire envelope by budding, chiefly from plasma membrane.

> Lymphocytic choriomeningitis (LCM) virus: *Aseptic meningitis*

Table 1—3 (continued)

Selected Viruses Associated with Major Virus Groups

14. CORONAVIRUS—strandedness of RNA unknown; probably helical symmetry;
     replicate in cytoplasm; surface carries characteristic pedunculated (petal)
     projections; maturation by budding into cytoplasmic vesicles.
          Human respiratory viruses: *Respiratory tract infections*

15. Unclassified Viruses
          Hepatitis viruses: *Infectious and serum hepatitis*

References

ANDREWS, C., and PEREIRA, H. G.: *Viruses of Vertebrates.* 3rd ed. Baltimore, Williams and Wilkins, 1972.

FENNER, F.: *The Biology of Animal Viruses.* Vol. I. New York, Academic Press, 1968.

LECHEVALIER, H. A., and SOLOTOROVSKY, M.: *Three Centuries of Microbiology.* New York, McGraw-Hill Book Company, 1965.

LURIA, S. E., and DARNELL, J. E., JR.: *General Virology.* 2nd ed. New York, John Wiley and Sons, 1967.

MELNICK, J. L.: Classification and nomenclature of animal viruses. Progr. Med. Virol. *15:*380, 1973.

MYRVIK, Q. N., PEARSALL, N. N., and WEISER, R. S.: *Fundamentals of Bacteriology and Mycology.* Philadelphia, Lea & Febiger, 1974.

WILDY, P.: Classification and nomenclature of viruses. In *Monographs in Virology.* Vol. 5. New York, S. Karger, 1971.

Chapter 2
Propagation and Quantification of Viruses

A. Methodology for Virus Cultivation

Since viruses are obligate intracellular parasites, the techniques for their propagation are more complex than those employed to culture bacteria. The three most common procedures used to cultivate animal viruses are (1) animal inoculation, (2) embryonated egg inoculation, and (3) inoculation of cell cultures.

1. Animal Inoculation

In the earliest attempts to propagate viruses, the definitive animal host of the agent was utilized. Such efforts were hampered by the complexity of the intact animal and the wide animal-to-animal variation in susceptibility, even within a single species. With the development of refined techniques for *in vitro* cultivation of cells capable of supporting virus replication, animals were no longer required for the routine propagation of most viral agents. However, animal inoculation is still invaluable for studying viral oncogenesis, pathogenesis of viral diseases, the immune response to viruses, the effect of environmental factors on viral infections, and the primary isolation of some agents.

The method used to inoculate animals depends on the sensitivity of the host to the agent as well as on the nature of the test or experiment. The following routes of inoculation are frequently employed: (1) intravenous, (2) intracerebral, (3) intraperitoneal, (4) intranasal, (5) intratracheal, and (6) intradermal. After virus replication has occurred, tissues from appropriate areas of the body are removed, minced or homogenized, and stored (usually in the frozen state) for subsequent use as a source of virus.

2. Egg Inoculation

Embryonated eggs have been used to cultivate viruses for over 50 years. Viruses from many groups have been cultured in various cavities of the embryonated egg or in the developing embryo itself (Fig. 2–1). Although

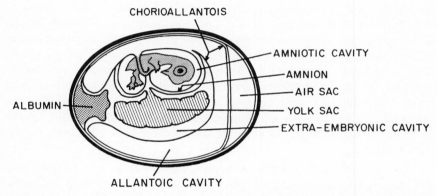

Figure 2–1. Embryonated chicken egg. A longitudinal section through an embryonated egg showing the arrangement of the embryo and embryonic membranes.

duck and turkey eggs, which have a longer incubation period than chicken eggs, have been used to cultivate some viruses, the chicken egg is usually employed.

The appropriate method of inoculation and the age of the embryo employed depend upon the agent being cultured. For example, primary isolation of influenza virus from throat washings is best accomplished by inoculation into the amniotic cavity of 7- to 8-day-old embryos; however, this virus replicates readily in the allantoic membrane of 12- to 13-day-old embryos after several passages ("adaptation") in the amnion. The most frequently employed sites of inoculation, other than the amniotic and allantoic cavities, include the chorioallantoic membrane and the yolk sac. Less commonly, virus may be injected directly into the developing embryo by either intravenous, intraperitoneal, or intracerebral inoculation. After virus replication has occurred in the cells of the membranes or embryo, virus may be released into the surrounding fluids which can be used as a source of virus. For example, influenza virus, which replicates in the respiratory system of the embryo and in the cells of the amniotic membrane, is released into the amniotic fluid which can be harvested with a syringe and needle. Other viruses, such as poxvirus and herpesvirus, which replicate in the chorioallantoic membrane, remain cell-associated in the lesions or "pocks" produced on the membrane. Grinding the infected membranes in an isotonic salt solution commonly serves to release such viruses.

3. Cell-culture Inoculation

The development of cell-culture techniques has reduced the cumbersome and expensive use of animals and embryonated eggs as means of propagating many viruses. Although there are inherent problems in the preparation and maintenance of tissue cultures suitable for virus propagation, their value is evidenced by the fact that more than 100 new viruses of human origin have been described since tissue-culture techniques have found routine application. The use of cell cultures not only has uncovered many new agents but also has greatly facilitated the study of long-recognized viruses such as poliovirus and has led to the development of vaccines for poliomyelitis and other viral diseases. Many details of host-cell virus relationships, mechanisms of pathogenesis, and an understanding of the molecular events involved in virus replication have been elucidated by the use of cell cultures.

There are three basic types of animal cell cultures: (1) primary and secondary cultures, (2) diploid cell strains, and (3) continuous cell lines. A *primary culture* is derived directly from the tissues of an animal or embryonated egg. The dissociated cells (usually obtained by treatment of tissue with trypsin) are suspended in a fluid growth medium and allowed to settle on solid surfaces such as those presented by a test tube, petri dish, or bottle. The cells attach to the container and divide mitotically to produce a monolayer of cells which constitutes the primary culture. A confluent primary culture of normal tissue may be subdivided to initiate a limited number of *secondary cultures*. Both primary and secondary cultures retain the normal diploid number of chromosomes characteristic of the parent tissue but usually undergo degeneration and cease to divide after prolonged maintenance in culture or following repeated subculture. However, some primary or secondary cultures undergo a change which permits prolonged serial culture for up to 50 times or more. They become altered morphologically even though they usually maintain the original number of chromosomes. Such altered cells are called *cell strains*.

During the course of culturing cell strains, *continuous cell lines* may emerge. Continuous cell lines represent cells which have assumed characteristics associated with malignant or premalignant cells. These cell lines grow faster than either primary cultures or cell strains and invariably are aneuploid; that is, have altered numbers of chromosomes. Continuous cell lines also can be obtained directly from primary cultures of malignant tissue or can be produced by infecting normal cells of primary cultures or cell strains with oncogenic viruses. Many continuous cell lines derived from normal, as well as from malignant, tissue produce tumors when transplanted into susceptible animals.

During serial culture of cell lines, variant cells often emerge which do not attach firmly to the culture vessels. These cells can be propagated in suspension cultures and are useful for obtaining high yields of some viruses and for experiments which require repeated sampling of a homogeneous cell population.

The type of culture used for propagating viruses is determined by the sensitivity of the cells to infection by the virus and by the nature of the experiments.

B.   Detection of Viral Replication in Cell Cultures

The effects of virus replication within a cell can range from complete destruction of the cell to no visible effect. The type of cytopathogenic effect (CPE) depends upon the virus and the cell system employed; however, morphologic changes that occur in a given system are usually constant and can be used as a basis for preliminary grouping.

The following are among the most frequently encountered morphologic changes which occur following viral infection: (1) Cell lysis or necrosis (Fig. 2–2). (2) Formation of multinucleate "giant cells" called *syncytia*.

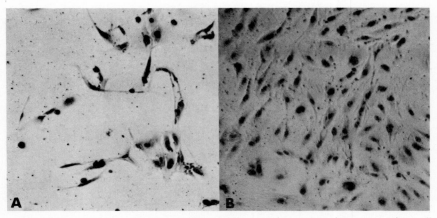

Figure 2–2. Viral cytopathic effect (CPE) showing enterovirus type with cell lysis. (A) Hamster cell culture infected with coxsackievirus for 24 hr. (B) Uninfected hamster cell culture. (Giemsa-stained preparations)

A syncytium is formed when viral-induced alterations in the cell membrane result in fusion of contiguous cells which initially are not destroyed but appear as a mass of cytoplasm containing a number of nuclei (Fig. 2–3). (3) Clusters or clumps of cells which occur when the membranes are altered and the cells adhere but do not fuse (Fig. 2–4). (4) *"Inclusion-body"* formation (Fig. 2–5). Intranuclear or intracytoplasmic structures may appear in virus-infected cells and can be of considerable diagnostic aid; for example, in rabies. In some cases, inclusion bodies may be the site of virus replication; in others, they may not be sites of replication but nevertheless contain masses of virus particles or viral components. In still

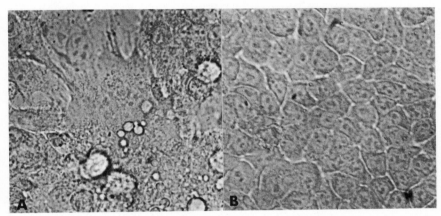

Figure 2–3. Viral cytopathic effect showing syncytium formation (giant cell). (A) HEp-2 cell culture infected with respiratory syncytial virus for 48 hr. (B). Uninfected HEp-2 cell culture. (Unstained preparations)

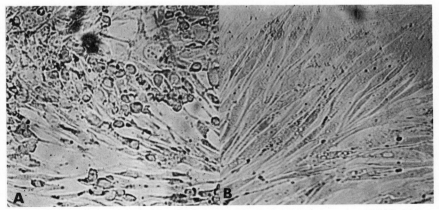

Figure 2–4. Viral cytopathic effect showing cell clumping. (A) Rabbit kidney cells infected with adenovirus type 3 for 3 days. (B) Uninfected rabbit kidney cell culture. (Unstained preparations)

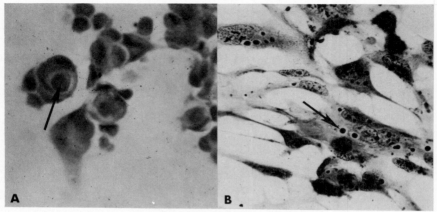

Figure 2—5. Inclusion-body formation. (A) Intranuclear inclusion bodies in cells infected with herpes simplex virus. (B) Intracytoplasmic inclusion bodies in cells infected with vaccinia virus. The arrows indicate the inclusion bodies. (Stained preparations)

other infections, the inclusion bodies appear to be remnants of virus multiplication since they develop after replication is completed.

In the absence of or prior to morphologic changes, the membranes of virus-infected cells may contain either virus components or partially extruded virus particles which have affinity for red blood cells. Such cells are said to be *hemadsorption positive* (Fig. 2–6). In some cases, hemadsorption tests are the sole means of detecting viral infection.

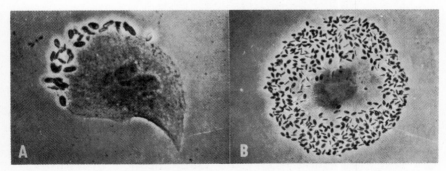

Figure 2—6. Hemadsorption of HeLa cells infected by Newcastle disease virus. HeLa cells exposed to x-irradiation continue to increase in size but fail to multiply. These "giant" HeLa cells were infected with Newcastle disease virus and incubated. The hemadsorption test was performed after 5 hr (A) and 6½ hr (B) using chicken erythrocytes. (A) The initial point of erythrocyte attachment represents the first area of the plasma membrane to be modified by the incorporation of viral hemagglutinin. (B) As incubation is continued, the entire circumference of the cell membrane is modified and finally the center of the cell surface. The area over the nucleus is the last region to become hemadsorption positive. (Reprinted with permission from Marcus, P. I.: Dynamics of surface modification in myxovirus-infected cells. Symp. Quant. Biol. *27*:351, 1962.)

Cellular metabolic alterations are a frequent consequence of viral infections and can result either in an increase or decrease in the pH of the culture fluid. In the case of some viruses, that produce cell degeneration, there is a decrease in the accumulation of acid end products as cell degeneration progresses; the pH is not lowered as it is in uninfected cell cultures. In contrast, other viruses, notably the adenoviruses, stimulate the production of acid end products, and the pH attained is lower than the pH of uninfected culture fluids.

Cells infected with some viruses, especially some of the oncogenic agents, show excessive division which results in the formation of foci composed of heaps of "transformed" cells (Fig. 2–7). Normal cells possess

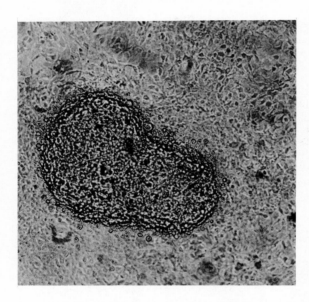

Figure 2–7. Focus of transformed cells. Culture of fathead minnow cells infected with Lucké renal tumor virus.

the property of contact inhibition which causes the cells to grow as monolayers; transformed cells have lost this function and pile up to form multicellular layers.

C.   Principles Employed in the Quantification of Viruses

Quantification of viruses can involve either a determination of the number of particles without regard to infectivity or an assay of the amount of infectious virus present.

1. Virus Particle Enumeration

a. **Electron Microscopy.** The electron microscope can be used to count the number of virus particles in a highly concentrated purified

VIRUS HEMAGGLUTINATION TITRATION

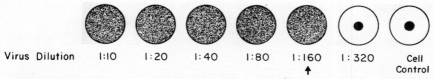

Figure 2—8. Diagram of virus hemagglutination titration. Red blood cells are added to serial dilutions of virus. Hemagglutination results when sufficient virus binds red blood cells to form a lattice. In the control tube, the red cells settle in a characteristic button.

suspension. One method involves adding a known number of latex particles, similar in size to the virus, to the preparation containing the virus to be counted. By determining the virus to latex particle ratio, the number of virus particles in the original suspension can be calculated with a reasonably high degree of accuracy.

b. Hemagglutination. Viruses which agglutinate red blood cells can be quantified by hemagglutination tests. Both infectious and inactivated virus can cause hemagglutination, thus this test can be used only to enumerate the physical particles and not their viability. Serial dilutions (usually twofold) of the virus are prepared, and red blood cells of the proper kind are added. If enough virus is present to bind red cells in the form of a lattice, the virus-cell complexes will settle in the tube in a characteristic pattern. After appropriate incubation, the tubes are examined from the bottom to determine the highest dilution of virus which causes hemagglutination (Fig. 2–8). This dilution is called the *hemagglutination titer* and is used to express the amount of virus in the original virus suspension.

2. Virus Infectivity Assays

a. Plaque or Focal Assays. The most precise measure of viral infectivity is achieved by procedures which determine the capacity of a suspension of virus to establish foci of infection on a monolayer of host cells. Suitable dilutions of virus are added to monolayers of susceptible cells. Following adsorption of the virus to the cells, an agar medium is added to the cultures, and incubation is carried out for several days to several weeks depending on the virus being assayed. If virus is transferred from cell to cell without being released into the medium, a fluid medium without agar can be used. As the virus in the initially infected cells replicates, its progeny infect neighboring cells and eventually produce a detectable focus of infection called a *plaque*. Each plaque usually results from the progeny of one infectious virus particle, which is commonly called a *plaque-forming unit* (PFU). Viruses that cause lysis or necrosis of cells produce clear plaques which can be counted after the addition of a stain to differentiate living from dead cells (Fig. 2–9). Viruses, such as the

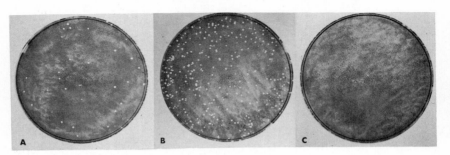

Figure 2–9. Plaque assay for viral infectivity. Sample A represents a tenfold dilution of sample B. Note small clear areas (plaques) in the monolayer where cells have been destroyed. (C) Uninfected cell control.

tumor viruses, which cause cell proliferation will produce foci of "transformed" cells. Noncytocidal and nononcogenic viruses may produce plaques which can be detected indirectly. For example, cells infected with viruses which insert hemagglutinin into the cell membrane bind red blood cells and can be detected by applying the hemadsorption test to the monolayer. After unattached red cells are washed from the cell monolayer, the foci with adsorbed red cells can be counted, and the number of infectious particles can be calculated.

b. Pock Assays. Some viruses form localized lesions on the chorioallantoic membrane of the embryonated egg. The titer of infectious virus is determined by counting the lesions, called "pocks," which develop after the addition of known dilutions of virus. The pock assay was commonly used before the development of the tissue culture plaque assay but is seldom used now since it is less convenient and accurate than the plaque assay.

c. Quantal Assays. Quantal assays (dilution to extinction) depend on an "all-or-none" response in which viruses are allowed to multiply for a period of time sufficient to permit detection of the effect of a single infectious virus particle by the amplification effect of its replication. Serial dilutions of virus are prepared, and susceptible cells are incubated with a measured volume of each of several dilutions of virus. After appropriate incubation, each culture, egg, or animal is examined to determine whether it exhibits an effect attributable to virus replication. The criteria most frequently employed for determining the end point in quantal titrations are (1) development of CPE in cell cultures, (2) death or characteristic disease in animals, (3) appearance of lesions on embryonated egg membranes or the embryo, and (4) development of effects detected by *in vitro* procedures, such as hemagglutination or hemadsorption tests. The highest dilution of virus which causes a visible effect must contain at least one infectious virus particle. The titer is often expressed as the 50% infectious dose (ID_{50}), which is the reciprocal of the highest dilution of virus that produces an effect in 50% of the cell cultures, eggs, or animals inoculated. Although the precision of quantal assays can be improved by using large numbers of test subjects, a reasonably accurate estimate of the concentration of infectious virus can be obtained by statistical analysis of the data obtained from a relatively small number of subjects.

References

FENNER, F. J., and WHITE, D. O.: Cultivation and assay of viruses. In *Medical Virology*. New York, Academic Press, 1970.

GOODHEART, C. R.: Assay of virus suspensions. In *An Introduction to Virology*. Philadelphia, W. B. Saunders Company, 1969.

HABEL, K., and SALZMAN, N. P.: *Fundamental Techniques in Virology*. New York, Academic Press, 1969.

SCHMIDT, N. J.: Tissue culture methods and procedures for diagnostic virology. In *Diagnostic Procedures for Viral and Rickettsial Infections*. 4th ed. E. H. Lennette and N. J. Schmidt, eds. New York, Amer. Public Health Assoc., 1969.

Chapter 3

Viral Replicative Cycles

The viral replicative cycle can be studied most conveniently by employing cell cultures; however, the events observed *in vitro* may differ from those which occur in intact animals because in the latter homeostatic control mechanisms, as well as the genetic makeup and immune status, can influence the outcome of a viral infection.

A normal viral replicative cycle can be divided into five merging phases: (1) adsorption, (2) penetration, (3) uncoating, (4) biosynthesis, and (5) maturation and release. The events which occur during each phase and the duration of the cycle vary depending on the type of nucleic acid in the viral genome, the group of virus being studied, the temperature of incubation, and the host cell type. A defect in any step can result in an abortive or defective replicative cycle.

It is important that students of medicine understand the molecular aspects of viral replication in order to understand the pathogenesis of viral diseases and the principles that relate to the action of chemotherapeutic agents. In this regard, it is notable that even at this early date understanding of the virus-specific events, which occur in infected cells, has led to the development of some chemotherapeutic agents for viral infections.

A. Adsorption

Initiation of infection demands that the virus make contact with and attach to susceptible cells. Initial contact between virus particles and cells results from random or brownian movement. The forces responsible for binding virus particles to the cell membrane are thought to be electrostatic; for example, strongly acidic phosphate groups on the cell surface have been shown to interact with amino groups on the virus. Sulfhydryl groups in the capsid protein of some enteroviruses also have been implicated in attachment since SH-blocking agents abolish the infectivity of these viruses.

Collision of virus particles with a cell does not always result in attachment. In some virus-cell systems, there are *receptor sites* on the cell surface for which the viruses have an affinity; the complementary portions of the virions are known as *virus-attachment* or *reacting sites*. Cell receptor sites have been demonstrated for members of the picornavirus, orthomyxovirus, and leukovirus groups and probably exist for agents in other groups.

The receptor sites for poliovirus can be isolated from susceptible cells by fractionation procedures. The receptor sites appear to have a role other than just serving as sites of attachment. If isolated plasma membrane fragments carrying receptor sites are incubated with poliovirus *in vitro* at 37° C, the virus is irreversibly altered. Although no morphologic changes are visible in electron micrographs, virus particles eluted from plasma membrane fragments are no longer infectious and do not attach to cells that normally support viral replication. Evidently interaction with cell receptor sites does not disrupt the viral protein coat, for RNA is not released and the particles are resistant to treatment with ribonuclease (RNase). Poliovirus capsids normally are resistant to the proteolytic enzyme trypsin. However, the capsids of eluted poliovirus are sufficiently altered so that trypsin treatment results in nucleic acid release. Furthermore, eluted particles no longer combine with specific Ab. Collectively, these observations suggest that the interaction of virus with the cell membrane results in a reorientation of structural units of the capsid and may initiate the first step in uncoating by rendering the virus particle susceptible to cellular proteolytic enzymes.

The envelopes of orthomyxoviruses and some of the paramyxoviruses contain a hemagglutinin as well as a neuraminidase capable of destroying cell receptor sites. It was first hypothesized that cell attachment was an enzyme substrate-mediated event; however, subsequent studies showed that viruses can infect cells containing receptors treated with periodate which renders the receptors insusceptible to neuraminidase. Furthermore, results of experiments with antiserum specific for the hemagglutinin and neuraminidase indicate that infectivity is neutralized only by the antihemagglutinin. Thus, it can be concluded that the hemagglutinins are essential for attachment and that neuraminidase is required neither for attachment nor entry.

B.   Penetration

There are at least four mechanisms by which viruses can penetrate cells: (1) On the basis of electron microscopic studies, it has been observed that some viruses are engulfed by a process of phagocytosis called "viropexis" (Fig. 3–1). (2) Penetration of viruses can involve the fusion or inter-

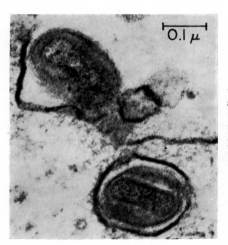

Figure 3–1. Phagocytosis of vaccinia virus. A particle contacting the surface and another in a vesicle are evident (× 120,000). (Reproduced with permission from Dales, S.: The uptake and development of vaccinia virus in strain L cells followed with labeled viral deoxyribonucleic acid. J. Cell Biol. *18*:51, 1963.)

action of the viral lipoprotein envelope with the cell membrane (Fig. 3–2). This fusion results in alteration of both viral envelope and the cell membrane at the point of contact and permits passage of the naked nucleocapsid

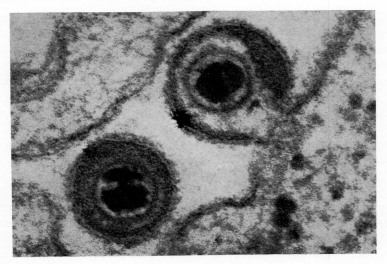

Figure 3—2. Fusioñ of virus envelope with cell membrane ($\times$ 180,000). (Reproduced with permission from Morgan, C., Rose, H. M., and Mednis, B.: Electron microscopy of herpes simplex virus. I. Entry. J. Virol. 2:507, 1968.)

directly into the cytoplasm. (3) Penetration also can involve the interaction of the virion with receptor sites on the cell membrane. It has been postulated that uncoating is initiated at the cell surface by host cell enzymes, and as a consequence the RNA is released directly into the cell. The residual capsid material which remains attached to the surface of cells infected with high multiplicities of virus may inhibit the attachment of additional virions. (4) Some viruses can enter cells by direct penetration of the intact virion through the cell membrane into the cytoplasm.

C. Uncoating

Before viral nucleic acid can be replicated and before viral coded proteins can be synthesized, the envelope and all or parts of the capsid material surrounding the genome must be removed. The initial steps leading to capsid disruption can begin during adsorption and penetration and may result in release of RNA into the cytoplasm (e.g., poliovirus). In the case of certain enveloped viruses, the envelope is removed at the cell surface, and the intact nucleocapsid penetrates the cell.

Those viruses which gain entrance to the cell by viropexis are exposed to the lysosomal enzymes that are transferred to the virus-containing vacuole. The uncoating of some viruses (e.g., adenovirus) does not require protein synthesis; therefore, the capsids must be disrupted either by pre-existing cellular enzymes or by physical forces. In contrast, the uncoating of vaccinia virus, which gains entrance by viropexis, is a two-stage process. The first stage, during which the outer membrane and some protein are removed, occurs within the phagocytic vacuole and does not require *de novo* protein synthesis. As this first stage of uncoating occurs, the phagocytic vacuole breaks down and virus cores, which are still resistant to DNase, are released into the cytoplasm. In order that uncoating be completed, new mRNA and protein must be made. It has been established that poxvirus cores can initiate mRNA synthesis as a result of the activity of a DNA-dependent RNA polymerase associated with the partially uncoated virion. Evidently mRNA released from the cores is translated into the enzyme(s) required for the final stage of poxvirus uncoating.

In the case of reovirus, the genome is never uncoated completely. The outer capsid is removed, and transcription takes place within the core particles which appear to remain intact throughout the replicative cycle. At no time is free double-stranded parental RNA found in the cytoplasm.

Infectious nucleic acid can be extracted from some viruses by a process of "artificial uncoating" employing treatment with phenol or other deproteinizing agents. The host cell range for infectious nucleic acid is usually much wider than for complete virus because nucleic acid penetration does not require specific receptor sites. However, infectious nucleic acid has a lower efficiency of infection than the corresponding virions because they lack the protection provided by the capsid. The role of infectious nucleic acid in the spread and transmission of viral diseases is unknown.

D. Biosynthesis

The site of viral synthesis varies depending upon the nucleic acid composition of the virus and the group to which the virus belongs; however, the following generalizations can be made: (1) most of the deoxyriboviruses synthesize their DNA in the nucleus of the host cell and their protein components in the cytoplasm; an exception is the poxviruses which synthesize all of their components in the cytoplasm; (2) most of the riboviruses synthesize all viral components in the cytoplasm; exceptions are the orthomyxoviruses and some of the paramyxoviruses and leukoviruses in which part of the replicative cycle takes place in the nucleus.

1. Protein Synthesis

Viral replication involves not only the synthesis of virion nucleic acid and capsid proteins but also the enzymes needed to catalyze the synthesis of viral components and maturation protein(s) required for virus assembly. In addition, some virus-induced regulator proteins are needed, either to inhibit certain cellular processes or to accomplish the sequential synthesis of viral-specific products. In some systems, mRNA must be synthesized before viral-specific protein can be made; in others, parental RNA can act directly as mRNA.

The new proteins observed following viral infection may be virus coded or they may be host coded but virus induced. Since the genomes of many viruses do not contain enough genetic information to code for all of the newly synthesized proteins present in infected cells, it must be assumed that the mRNA for some virus-induced proteins is transcribed from the host cell genome.

The translation of information encoded in the mRNA present in a normal cell requires over a hundred molecular components. Among these are more than 50 species of transfer RNA (tRNA), the enzymes necessary for attaching the amino acid residues to the tRNAs, the ribosomal proteins, and ribosomal RNA, as well as the factors involved in the initiation, elongation, and termination of the polypeptide chain. For many years, it was assumed that translation of virus proteins was accomplished by utilizing the unaltered transcription and translation mechanisms of the cell. Within the last decade it has been demonstrated that virus-specific polypeptides are not always synthesized solely by utilizing the pre-existing host-specified population of aminoacyl-tRNAs, aminoacyl-tRNA synthetases, and tRNA methylases. However, synthesis of viral proteins occurs by the same basic mechanism as normal cellular protein synthesis.

2. Nucleic Acid Transcription and Replication

Viruses can be divided into six classes on the basis of (1) nucleic acid type and (2) mechanism of gene transcription.

a. Class I Viruses. *Class I viruses have a double-stranded DNA genome. The DNA of these viruses is transcribed asymmetrically to give rise to mRNA.* Double-stranded virus DNA is probably duplicated by semiconservative replication described for other species of DNA (Fig. 3–3). New mRNA and, in some cases, tRNA must be synthesized prior to DNA replication.

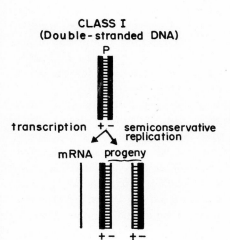

CLASS I
(Double-stranded DNA)

P

transcription +－ semiconservative replication

mRNA progeny

+－ +－

Figure 3–3. Replication of Class I, double-stranded DNA viruses. Parental nucleic acid is represented by the heavy lines; newly synthesized nucleic acid is represented by the light vertical lines. The horizontal lines indicate hydrogen bonding of double-stranded nucleic acid.

In the case of vaccinia virus, newly synthesized RNA can be extracted from infected cells within an hour after infection. The DNA-dependent RNA polymerase which transcribes the virus DNA is associated with the core of the infecting virion. Evidently, virus-specific RNA synthesis is initiated in vaccinia-infected cells before the inner protein coat is removed. This is indicated by the observation that the new single-stranded RNA from vaccinia-infected cells can be hybridized with viral DNA.

In addition to virus-specific single-stranded RNA, double-stranded RNA also can be isolated from vaccinia-infected cells. Although small amounts of double-stranded RNA can be isolated from normal cells, virus-infected cells contain ten times as much double-stranded RNA. Since the newly synthesized double-stranded RNA from infected cells can be melted and annealed to similarly treated virion DNA, it must be virus specific. The biological function of the virus-specific double-stranded RNA in vaccinia-infected cells remains to be established.

Although DNA-dependent DNA polymerase also can be found associated with highly purified vaccinia virions, its significance in viral replication has not been established. Since this polymerase is not associated with the core, it is possible that the enzyme found associated with virus particles represents polymerase which was adsorbed or accidentally incorporated into the virion and plays no essential role in the initiation of viral replication. Accordingly, it appears likely that the polymerase synthesized following viral infection, rather than that which is associated with the virion, is involved in the synthesis of progeny double-stranded DNA.

In summary, it can be concluded that double-stranded viral DNA serves as a template, not only for the synthesis of new viral DNA, but also for transcribing into mRNA the genetic information controlling the synthesis of capsid proteins and probably some of the enzymes involved in the replicative cycle.

b. Class II Viruses. *Class II viruses have a single-stranded DNA genome. Messenger RNA is transcribed from a newly synthesized double-stranded DNA intermediate.* The parvovirus group is comprised of the single-stranded DNA viruses that infect mammalian cells. The replicative cycle of these agents probably is similar to that described for the much studied single-stranded DNA bacteriophage (Fig. 3–4).

The results of studies with bacteriophage established that parental DNA serves as template for the formation of a complementary strand which is bound to the parental form by hydrogen bonding. This double-stranded intermediate is called the "replicative form" (RF). By semiconservative replication of the RF, additional molecules of double-stranded DNA are produced. These newly formed DNA molecules which do not contain the parental DNA are in some way different from the original replicative form in that they do not replicate to yield additional double-stranded

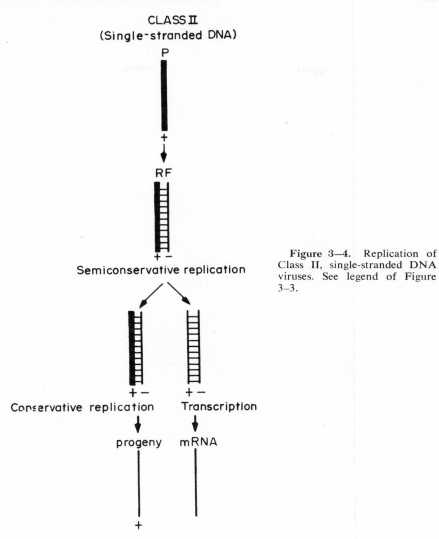

CLASS II
(Single-stranded DNA)

P

+

RF

+ −
Semiconservative replication

Conservative replication   Transcription

progeny   mRNA

+

Figure 3—4. Replication of Class II, single-stranded DNA viruses. See legend of Figure 3–3.

molecules. Evidently their function is to serve as templates for the transcription of mRNA, which is translated into virus-specific proteins. Single-stranded progeny nucleic acid is produced by conservative replication using as template the negative strand of the double-stranded DNA intermediate which contains the parental genome.

In summary, based on the data obtained with bacteriophage, both conservative and semiconservative nucleic acid replication are required for the production of progeny Class II viruses. Whereas DNA-dependent DNA polymerase activity has been shown to be associated with the Kilham rat virus, a parvovirus, no RNA polymerase activity has been detected. Additional information is needed before the mechanism by which the single-stranded animal DNA viruses replicate can be be elucidated.

    c. Class III Viruses. *Class III viruses have a double-stranded RNA genome. Messenger RNA is produced by asymmetric transcription of the genome.* Double-stranded RNA virus replication requires the synthesis of single-stranded mRNA and double-stranded virion nucleic acid (Fig. 3–5). The reoviruses were the first of the double-stranded RNA

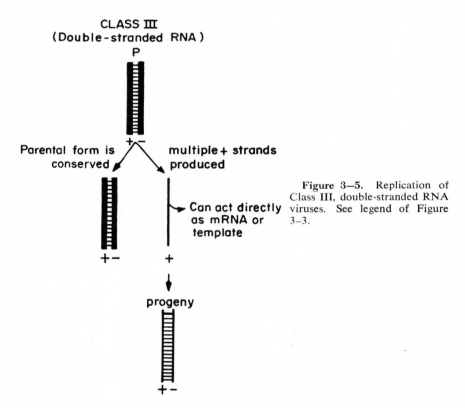

Figure 3—5. Replication of Class III, double-stranded RNA viruses. See legend of Figure 3–3.

viruses to be isolated and have been studied more extensively than other diplornaviruses. The reovirus genome is composed of 10 weakly linked, double-stranded RNA segments which are enclosed within a double-layered capsid. The RNA segments extracted from reovirions can be grouped into three classes (L, M, and S) on the basis of size. During uncoating, the outer capsomeric layer of the virion is removed by pre-existing cellular enzymes. The resulting subviral particle (SVP) is comprised of the inner capsomeric layer, double-stranded RNA, and an RNA-dependent RNA polymerase. The intimate association of the reovirus double-stranded genome with the polymerase within the subviral particle permits the transcription of single-stranded RNA without the participation of newly synthesized or preformed host enzymes.

Transcription of single-stranded viral RNA from the parental double-stranded RNA template begins in the cytoplasm of infected cells within an hour after infection. The transcription products are all single-stranded and do not self-anneal because only one strand of the parental genome is copied. On the basis of size, the transcripts fall into three classes (l, m, and s) which correspond to the three classes of double-stranded RNA (L, M, and S) isolated from mature virus particles. This observation indicates that the mRNA is transcribed from each of the 10 genome RNA segments. In the synthesis of reovirus RNA, the parental double-stranded genome is fully conserved and does not contribute directly to the single-stranded RNA pool.

A large fraction of the newly synthesized single-stranded viral RNA acts as mRNA, whereas the remaining RNA serves as template for progeny RNA synthesis. Some of the "early" RNA presumably functions as a messenger for the production of new polymerase molecules which could explain the increased rate of RNA synthesis observed later in the infection.

In summary, only one strand of the parental genome is transcribed. Some of the newly synthesized strands of RNA function as mRNA; the remaining strands function as a template for the synthesis of a complementary strand resulting in the production of new double-stranded viral genomes.

d. **Class IV Viruses.** *Class IV viruses are single-stranded RNA viruses whose mRNA is identical in base sequence to virion RNA. Parental RNA can act directly as mRNA.* Viruses belonging to this group are exemplified by poliovirus. The single-stranded parental RNA (positive strand) serves both as mRNA and as template for the synthesis of a complementary (negative strand) which in turn is copied to produce progeny RNA (Fig. 3–6). In this group of viruses, the RNA-dependent RNA polymerase is synthesized prior to viral RNA replication and is not associated with the virion.

The search for a poliovirus double-stranded replicative form similar to that found in bacteriophage led to the isolation of fully double-stranded RNA molecules which were called the *replicative form* (RF). Since maximal amounts of RF are detected after the peak of RNA replication, at least some RF appears to be an end product, rather than an intermediary in virus replication. However, some of the RF population must be a result of the first step in replication.

Evidently some of the negative strands of the RNA synthesized lead to the formation of intermediates which possess properties of both single-

CLASS Ⅳ
(Single-stranded RNA-poliovirus)

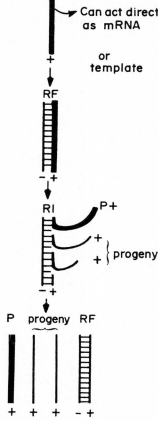

Figure 3—6. Replication of poliovirus, a Class IV, single-stranded RNA
virus. See legend of Figure 3–3.

and double-stranded RNA. Such forms, called *replicative intermediates*
(RI), are produced by the simultaneous production of multiple positive
strands of RNA from the negative strand of the RF. The multibranched
structure of poliovirus RI is apparent in electron micrographs of purified
material (Fig. 3–7). The single-stranded tails visualized in electron micrographs are presumed to be nascent single strands of viral RNA in the
process of dissociating from the RI and represent the ribonuclease-sensitive
portions of the RI. The precise mechanism by which the RI functions
has yet to be determined but the end result is the production of single-
stranded progeny RNA identical in base sequence to the parental RNA.
Progeny RNA can function as mRNA for production of more virus pro-

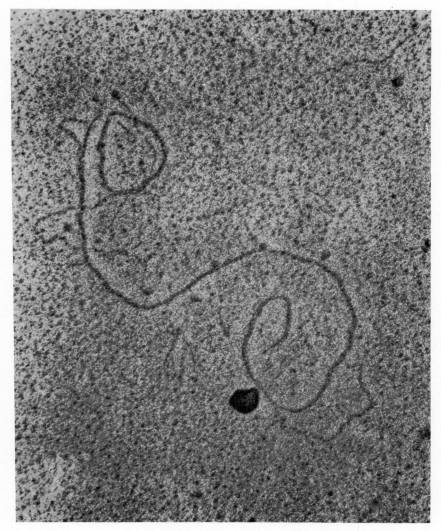

Figure 3–7. Poliovirus replicative intermediate. The illustration contains a single molecule of RI with possibly four branches. (Reproduced with permission from Bishop, J. M., and Levinton, L.: Replicative forms of viral RNA structure and function. Progr. Med. Virol. *13*:1, Karger, Basel 1971.)

tein, as template for the production of additional RF or become encapsidated to produce progeny virions.

The functional virus-specific proteins are formed by cleavage of precursor proteins, which in turn are derived from single large polypeptides translated from the polycistronic mRNA. One of the gene products is

RNA-dependent RNA polymerase(s) which catalyzes the synthesis of the negative strand required for progeny production.

In summary, the single-stranded viral genome can function as mRNA or as template for the synthesis of negative strands. The negative strands of replicative intermediates are the templates for the production of new viral genomes (positive strands).

e. **Class V Viruses.** *Class V viruses have a single-stranded RNA genome. Most, if not all, of the virion RNA is complementary in base sequence to the mRNA.* Single-stranded RNA viruses in this class differ from Class IV viruses in that RNA complementary to virion RNA functions as mRNA (Fig. 3–8). Virion-associated, RNA-dependent RNA polymerases which catalyze the production of mRNA have been found

CLASS V
(Single-stranded RNA-Influenza)

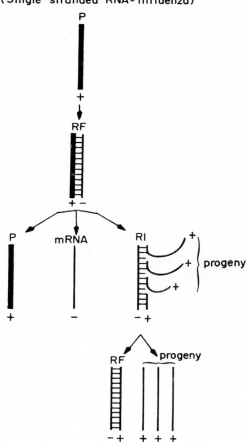

Figure 3—8. Replication of influenza virus, a Class V, single-stranded RNA virus. See legend of Figure 3–3.

in members of the paramyxovirus, rhabdovirus, diplornavirus, and ortho-myxovirus groups. Such enzymes probably are the rule rather than the exception when infectious nucleic acid cannot be isolated from virus particles and when the first function performed after infection is the transcription of the parental genome.

There are important differences between the virus groups within Class V with respect to virion compositions and genome replication. The sole criterion for grouping these agents into a single class is that the mRNA is complementary to virion RNA. The replication of influenza (an ortho-myxovirus) and Sendai (a paramyxovirus) will be discussed as repre-sentatives of Class V viruses.

The RNA extracted from influenza virions can be resolved into at least five distinct RNA segments. The segments probably are linked within the virions by way of a structural protein backbone.

All of the RNA in isolated influenza virus virions is positive stranded since no self-annealing can be detected. However, intracellular single-stranded RNA may be composed of as much as 10% negative strands. Negative strands can be detected within minutes after infection, apparently before positive strands appear. Although the virion-associated polymerase probably initiates RNA synthesis, a viral-induced RNA-dependent RNA polymerase is also synthesized in infected cells. The newly formed poly-merase activity can be detected approximately one hour after infection and increases in parallel with viral RNA synthesis. The virion-associated polymerase and the induced polymerase may be identical.

Influenza virus RNA synthesis and virus multiplication are inhibited by the addition of actinomycin D at the time of infection. This observation suggests that virus replication requires the synthesis of cellular mRNA and, presumably, cell-coded protein(s). The role of the cell-coded pro-tein(s) is unknown.

One model for the replication of influenza virus RNA assumes that negative-stranded RNA is synthesized while the positive strand is still attached to the protein backbone and that the newly formed negative strand displaces the parental RNA from the backbone The negative strand would subsequently serve as template for the production of progeny positive strands. When RNA is extracted from infected cells, molecules analogous to the RI and RF found in poliovirus-infected cells are ob-tained. Although the RI may be associated with protein in influenza virus-infected cells, the basic mechanism of genome replication is probably similar to that described for the Class IV, single-stranded RNA viruses.

The RNA extracted from Sendai virions, in contrast to that from influenza virus, is not segmented, and each nucleocapsid contains either positive or negative strands of RNA. Mature virions, however, may con-tain more than one nucleocapsid; thus, positive and negative strands of

RNA could exist in separate helices within a single virus particle. Lack of infectivity of paramyxovirion RNA and the fact that 80 to 90% of the RNA produced following infection is complementary to genome RNA indicate that the majority of RNA in the virions cannot function as mRNA.

A virion-associated polymerase catalyzes the synthesis of several species of complementary RNA which are smaller than genome RNA. The transcription of genomic RNA occurs in partially double-stranded structures called "transcriptive intermediates." At least some of the complementary RNA is associated with polyribosomes and functions as mRNA. Replicative intermediates also can be isolated from Sendai virus-infected cells. The observation that genome replication does not occur in the absence of protein synthesis suggests that the enzymes involved in the synthesis of progeny RNA and mRNA are different, since mRNA can be synthesized in the absence of protein synthesis. The RNA destined to become virion RNA rapidly becomes associated with protein to form nucleocapsid. This explains why free genome RNA does not accumulate in the cytoplasm.

In summary, the replicative cycle of Class V viruses involves the synthesis of negative strands of RNA complementary to the virus genome. The negative strands can function as mRNA or can serve as template for the production of positive progeny strands.

f. Class VI Viruses. *Class VI viruses have a single-stranded RNA genome but have RNA:DNA hybrids and double-stranded DNA forms as intermediates in the replicative cycle. The mRNA has not been well characterized but appears to be identical to genome RNA.* The single-stranded RNA viruses in this group possess several unique properties: (1) during replication an RNA:DNA hybrid intermediate is formed which serves as template for the production of double-stranded DNA (Fig. 3–9); (2) the DNA intermediate is integrated into the host cell genome; (3) many of these viruses can cause transformation of cells both *in vitro* and *in vivo.*

The genome is a single-stranded RNA molecule (70S) composed of linked segments of 35 and 20S subunits of RNA. Replication requires an RNA-directed DNA polymerase (reverse transcriptase) which is involved in the synthesis of the RNA:DNA hybrid template and a DNA-dependent DNA polymerase which is required for the synthesis of double-stranded DNA (provirus). These and other enzymes are contained in the virions. In Rous sarcoma virus, the DNA intermediate is made during the first 8 to 12 hours after infection and becomes covalently linked to host cell DNA, probably by way of endonuclease and ligase activities possessed by infectious virions. Synthesis of DNA is required only during the first 12 hours after viral infection. However, DNA transcription into RNA is required throughout the replicative cycle. The relationship of virion RNA to mRNA is not known, but available evidence suggests that both transcription and replication involve DNA-directed RNA synthesis. Negative

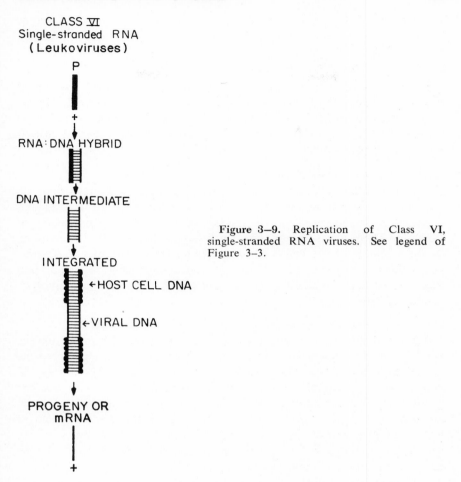

CLASS VI
Single-stranded RNA
(Leukoviruses)

P

+

RNA:DNA HYBRID

DNA INTERMEDIATE

INTEGRATED

←HOST CELL DNA

←VIRAL DNA

PROGENY OR
mRNA

+

Figure 3—9. Replication of Class VI, single-stranded RNA viruses. See legend of Figure 3–3.

strands of RNA have not been found in infected cells or in purified virions which suggests that the parental or progeny RNA can function as mRNA.

The discovery that the RNA of the oncogenic viruses can direct the synthesis of DNA has implications far beyond the immediate province of molecular biology. For example, DNA produced by mammalian oncogenic virus RNA may be transmitted indefinitely without evidence of cell alteration or malignancy; alternatively the regions of the cell genome carrying virus-coded information could become activated many years later and cause "spontaneous" cancer in man.

In summary, these RNA viruses replicate by way of an RNA:DNA hybrid and a double-stranded DNA intermediate which is integrated into the host cell genome. Progeny RNA is transcribed from the integrated viral DNA. The specialized event which permits integration of viral DNA into the host cell genome provides a mechanism by which viral genetic information can be transmitted genetically without phenotypic expression.

E. Maturation and Release

The process of virion maturation is determined in part by the site of virus replication and whether or not the nucleocapsid is surrounded by an envelope. The maturation (assembly) of representative naked and enveloped DNA and RNA viruses will be described. A prototype virus is indicated for each category.

1. Naked DNA Virus (Adenovirus)

The polypeptide precursors of adenovirus proteins are synthesized on cytoplasmic polyribosomes and are transported rapidly to the nucleus where they are incorporated into the capsid and internal components of the virus. The production of arginine-rich maturation factor(s) is required for the assembly of the structural proteins and DNA into infectious virus. The virions accumulate in the nucleus and remain cell-associated until they are released gradually as a consequence of cell death and autolysis of infected cells.

2. Enveloped DNA Virus (Herpesvirus)

Proteins synthesized in the cytoplasm are transferred to the nucleus where the nucleocapsids are assembled. The nucleocapsids migrate to the nuclear membrane which has incorporated virus-specific Ags during the course of the infection. By a budding process, the particles become enclosed in an envelope composed of the inner nuclear membrane which contains viral Ags. The enveloped virions leave the nucleus enclosed within cytoplasmic vesicles or vacuoles which appear to open at the cytoplasmic membrane and permit virus release from the cell. If the nucleocapsid leaves the nucleus through a break in the nuclear membrane. it may become enveloped at cytoplasmic or plasma membrane sites. An alternate mechanism for virus release is by way of the perinuclear cisternae, which are continuous with the endoplasmic reticulum and allow the gradual release of virions from the intact cell.

3. Complex DNA Virus (Vaccinia Virus)

Both viral DNA and protein components are synthesized in the cytoplasm and appear as dense granules and fibrils in foci called *factories* or *viroplasm*. At maturation, randomly arranged filaments become surrounded by a newly synthesized multilayered membrane to produce spherical "immature particles." The particles undergo internal differentiation to form the inner membrane, the lateral bodies, and the nucleoid or core which contains the DNA. The external membrane of the virion develops its characteristic mature appearance, and the particles accumulate in the cytoplasm. Some virions may be released slowly from microvilli on the cell surface, but most of the virus particles remain within the cell. The virus can spread directly from cell to cell through intercytoplasmic bridges even in the presence of specific neutralizing Ab.

4. Naked RNA Virus (Poliovirus)

Poliovirus RNA and protein precursors are synthesized in membrane-bound cytoplasmic structures, the virus-synthesizing bodies (VSB), in which virion maturation occurs. The capsomeres are formed by self-assembly from monomers of precursor proteins (structural units) which are present in pools within the VSB. As viral RNA is synthesized, it is rapidly enclosed in capsids which are formed by the assembly of capsomeres. Mature virus particles accumulate in the cytoplasmic matrix or within cytoplasmic vacuoles and may resemble intracellular crystals. Lysis of the cell results in the simultaneous and rapid release of large amounts of infectious virus.

5. Enveloped RNA Virus (Parainfluenza Virus)

These viruses are assembled from RNA and proteins produced in the cytoplasm. Their organization into helical nucleocapsids occurs rapidly in the cytoplasmic matrix, presumably by self-assembly. Some virus Ags are incorporated into the cell plasma membrane to form "spikes." The nucleocapsids become aligned in close proximity to the altered cell membrane. Virus maturation is completed when one or more of the nucleocapsids becomes encompassed by a portion of the "spike-containing cell membrane" (Fig. 3–10). Infectious virus is released gradually by a process of exocytosis (budding).

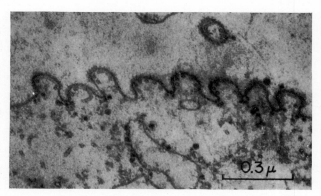

Figure 3–10. A row of eight budding particles showing many cross-sections of nucleocapsid aligned under the cell membrane (× 63,000). (Reproduced with permission from Compans, R. W., Holmes, K. V., Dales, S., and Choppin, P. W.: An electron microscopic study of the moderate and virulent virus-cell interactions of the parainfluenza virus SV5. Virology *30*:411, 1964.)

F. Abnormal Replicative Cycles

1. Abortive Infections

The infection of cells with virus does not always result in the production of infectious progeny. In nonpermissive cells, some or all of the viral components may be produced, but virus assembly or maturation either does not take place or yields only noninfectious virus particles. This type of virus-host cell interaction is referred to as an *abortive infection.* A virus which undergoes an abortive replicative cycle in one cell type may replicate normally in another. Thus the defect which prevents infectious virus production in these systems is usually a property of the cell and not the virus.

2. Defective Viruses

In other systems, the virus is genetically defective and is unable to cause the synthesis of some product essential for the production of infectious progeny. These viruses can replicate normally if the cells are infected with a "helper virus" which can code for the missing product. The Bryan high titer strain of Rous sarcoma virus (RSV) is an example of a virus defective in its capacity to synthesize essential envelope components. Infectious RSV particles are produced only in cells coinfected with Rous associated virus (an avian leukosis helper virus) or in cells which contain "chick helper factor." The helper factor is endogenous leukosis virus genetic material that is integrated into the cell genome and is transcribed and translated into the necessary envelope components (Chapter 24). Rous virus can be surrounded by envelopes containing Ags determined by any avian leukosis virus (Phenotypic Mixing, Chapter 4). Thus, immunologically distinct pseudotypes of RSV containing identical genomes can be produced depending upon which helper virus is involved.

The oncogenic DNA viruses exemplify the extreme state of defectiveness. In transformed cells, the virus genome may be integrated into the host cell genome and replicated with it during mitosis. Although viral-specific mRNA and Ags are present in transformed cells, no infectious virus is produced. In some cases the integrated virus can be "rescued" by culturing the nonproducing cells with cells that support the normal replication of the virus.

3. Viral Interference

Cells infected by more than one virion may support the normal replication of both viruses or one virus may inhibit or enhance the multiplication of the other. Virus-induced inhibition of viral replication is called the *interference phenomenon.* Viral enhancement will be discussed in Chapter 4.

There are three major categories of interference depending upon the relatedness of the viruses involved. *Autointerference* may be observed when a cell is infected with one type of virus at high multiplicities. *Homologous interference* occurs between viruses in the same taxonomic group. Homologous interference can be heterotypic or homotypic. Heterotypic interference occurs between two different types of virus belonging to the same group, for example influenza type A and type B. Homotypic interference occurs between different strains of a single type of virus; for example, between influenza types A_1 and A_2. *Heterologous interference* occurs between a wide range of unrelated viruses.

Viral interference can be effected at the level of adsorption or, more commonly, at some later intracellular step in the replicative cycle. The most important mediator of interference in natural viral infections probably is interferon (Chapter 7). Interferon is a virus-induced, cell-coded protein which mediates inhibition of virus replication at the intracellular level and may be involved in any or all of the types of interference named above. It undoubtedly is responsible for most heterologous interference. However, since some viral interference occurs when interferon production is absent or suppressed, factors other than interferons must be involved in the phenomenon of interference.

Interference which blocks virus adsorption or penetration results from competition for or destruction of receptor sites and thus can occur only between viruses which have common receptor sites. This type of interference, called *viral attachment interference,* is involved in some kinds of autointerference as well as some types of homologous interference.

Homologous interference sometimes occurs only if the interfering virus is allowed to replicate for a short time before the challenge virus is added. The most likely explanation for this observation is that there is competition for substrates or viral replicating sites which are required by both viruses for multiplication.

A special type of autointerference occurs when concentrated preparations of influenza virus are passaged serially. Increasing amounts of noninfectious (defective) virus are produced with each passage. The defective particles are deficient in one particular segment of RNA. The "incomplete" influenza virus interferes with the production of infectious virus; therefore, each passage contains decreasing amounts of infectious virus.

The interference phenomenon undoubtedly has practical significance in natural viral infections. On the one hand, it may be important in containing viral infections and mediating recovery from clinical illness before protective levels of Ab are produced. In contrast, its effect may be detrimental when polyvalent vaccines are administered. For example, heterotypic interference may develop if equal amounts of all three types of attenuated poliovirus are administered simultaneously. This problem has been overcome by applying knowledge of the dynamics of viral interference. The composition of the vaccine is adjusted so that the interfering type is present in lower concentration than the other types. Another problem which may be encountered in administering active vaccines is that viruses present in the host may interfere with the replication and effectiveness of the vaccine.

Much effort has been expended in attempts to utilize interferon prophylactically or therapeutically for human viral infections. This aspect of viral interference will be discussed at greater depth in Chapter 7.

References

ARLINGHAUS, R. B., WANG, C. S., and NASO, R.: *In vitro* polypeptide synthesis programmed with Rauscher leukemia virus RNA. In *Molecular Studies in Viral Neoplasia.* 25th Annual Symposium on Fundamental Cancer Research (March 8-10, 1972). Univ. of Texas at Houston, M. D. Anderson Hospital and Tumor Institute, Houston, Texas. To be published.

BALTIMORE, D.: RNA-dependent DNA polymerase in virions of RNA tumor viruses. Nature *226*:1209, 1970.

BALTIMORE, D.: Expression of animal virus genomes. Bacteriol. Rev. *35*:235, 1971.

BALUDA, M. A.: The DNA intermediate in the replication of avian RNA tumor virus. In *Molecular Studies in Viral Neoplasia.* 25th Annual Symposium on Fundamental Cancer Research (March 8-10, 1972). Univ. of Texas at Houston, M. D. Anderson Hospital and Tumor Institute, Houston, Texas. To be published.

BANERJEE, A. K., and SHATKIN, A. J.: Transcription *in vitro* by reovirus-associated ribonucleic acid-dependent polymerase. J. Virol. *6*:1, 1970.

BISHOP, D. H. L., OBIJESKI, J. F., and SIMPSON, R. W.: Transcription of the influenza ribonucleic acid genome by a virion polymerase. II. Nature of the *in vitro* polymerase product. J. Virol. *8*:74, 1971.

BISHOP, J. M., and LEVINTOW, L.: Replicative forms of viral RNA. Structure and function. Progr. Med. Virol. *13*:1, 1971.

BLAIR, C. D., and DUESBERG, P. H.: Myxovirus ribonucleic acids. Ann. Rev. Microbiol. *24*:539, 1970.

CHAN, V. F., and BLACK, F. L.: Uncoating of poliovirus by isolated plasma membranes. J. Virol. *5*:309, 1970.

CHOW, N., and SIMPSON, R. W.: RNA-dependent RNA polymerase activity associated with virions and subviral components of myxovirus. Proc. Nat. Acad. Sci. USA *68*:752, 1971.

COLBY, C., and DUESBERG, P. H.: Double-stranded RNA in vaccinia infected cells. Nature *222*:940, 1969.

COMPANS, R. W., HOLMES, K. V., DALES, S., and CHOPPIN, P. W.: An electron microscopic study of moderate and virulent virus-cell interactions of the parainfluenza virus SV5. Virology *30*:411, 1966.

DALES, S.: The uptake and development of vaccinia virus in strain L cells followed with labeled deoxyribonucleic acid. J. Cell Biol. *18*:51, 1963.

DARLINGTON, R. W., and MOSS, L. H., III: The envelope of herpesvirus. Progr. Med. Virol. *11*:16, 1969.

DUESBERG, P. H.: The RNAs of influenza virus. Proc. Nat. Acad. Sci. USA *59*:930, 1968.

DUESBERG, P. H., and COLBY, C.: On the biosynthesis and structure of double-stranded RNA in vaccinia virus-infected cells. Proc. Nat. Acad. Sci. USA *64*:396, 1969.

ETCHISON, J., DOYLE, M., PENHOET, E., and HOLLAND, J.: Synthesis and cleavage of influenza virus proteins. J. Virol. *7*:155, 1971.

FAZEKAS DE ST. GROTH, S.: Viropexis, the mechanism of influenza virus infection. Nature *162*:294, 1948.

FENNER, F.: *The Biology of Animal Viruses.* Vol. I. New York, Academic Press, 1968.

GREEN, M.: Oncogenic viruses. Ann. Rev. Biochem. *39*:701, 1970.

HANAFUSA, T., HANAFUSA, H., MIYAMOTO, T. and FLEISSNER, E.: Existence and expression of tumor virus genes in chick embryo cells. Virology *47*:475, 1972.

JOKLIK, W. K.: The intracellular uncoating of poxvirus DNA. I. The fate of radioactively-labeled rabbitpox virus. J. Mol. Biol. *8*:263, 1964.

JOKLIK, W. K.: The intracellular uncoating of poxvirus DNA. II. The molecular basis of the uncoating process. J. Mol. Biol. *8*:277, 1964.

KATES, J. R., and McAUSLAN, B. R.: Messenger RNA synthesis by a "coated" viral genome. Proc. Nat. Acad. Sci. USA *57*:314, 1967.

KATES, J. R., and McAUSLAN, B. R.: Poxvirus DNA-dependent RNA polymerase. Proc. Nat. Acad. Sci. USA *58*:134, 1967.

MORGAN, C., and ROSE, H. M.: Structure and development of viruses as observed in the electron microscope. VIII. Entry of influenza virus. J. Virol. *2*:925, 1968.

MORGAN, C., and HOWE, C.: Structure and development of viruses as observed in the electron microscope. IX. Entry of parainfluenza I (Sendai) virus. J. Virol. *2*:1122, 1968.

MORGAN, C., ROSENKRANZ H. S., and MEDNIS, B.: Structure and development of viruses as observed in the electron microscope. X. Entry and uncoating of adenovirus. J. Virol. *4*:777, 1969.

MORGAN, C., ROSE, H. M., and MEDNIS, B.: Electron microscopy of herpes simplex virus. I. Entry. J. Virol. *2*:507, 1968.

PONS, M. W.: Isolation of influenza virus ribonucleoprotein from infected cells: demonstration of the presence of negative-stranded RNA in viral RNP. Virology *46*:149, 1971.

ROBINSON, W. S.: Ribonucleic acid polymerase activity in Sendai virions and nucleocapsid. J. Virol. *8*:81, 1971.

ROBINSON, W. S.: Sendai virus RNA synthesis and nucleocapsid formation in the presence of cycloheximide. Virology *44*:494, 1971.

ROBINSON, W. S.: Intracellular structures involved in Sendai virus replication. Virology *43*:90, 1971.

SALZMAN, L. A.: DNA polymerase activity associated with purified Kilham rat virus. Nature New Biol. *231*:174, 1971.

SALZMAN, N. P., SHATKIN, A. J., and SEBRING, E. D.: The synthesis of a DNA-like RNA in the cytoplasm of HeLa cells infected with vaccinia virus. J. Mol. Biol. *8*:405, 1964.

SCHARFF, M. D., SHATKIN, A. J., and LEVINTOW, L.: Association of newly formed viral protein with specific polyribosomes. Proc. Nat. Acad. Sci. USA *50*:686, 1963.

SHATKIN, A. J.: Viruses with segmented ribonucleic acid genomes: multiplication of influenza versus reovirus. Bacteriol. Rev. *35*:250, 1971.

SINSHEIMER, R. L., STARMAN, B., NAGLER, C., and GUTHRIE, S.: The process of infection with bacteriophage ØX 174. I. Evidence for a "replicative form." J. Mol. Biol. *4*:142, 1962.

SPIEGELMAN, S., BURNY, A., DAS, M. R., KEYDAR, J., SCHLOM, J., TRAVNICEK, M., and WATSON, K.: Characterization of the products of RNA-directed DNA polymerases in oncogenic RNA viruses. Nature *227*:563, 1970.

SPIEGELMAN, S., BURNY, A., DAS, M. R., KEYDAR, J., SCHLOM, J., TRAVNICEK, M., and WATSON, K.: DNA-directed DNA polymerase activity in oncogenic RNA viruses. Nature *227*:1029, 1970.

STONE, H. O., PORTNER, A., and KINGSBURY, D. W.: Ribonucleic acid transcriptases in Sendai virions and infected cells. J. Virol. *8*:174, 1971.

TAN, K. B., and McAUSLAN, B. R.: Binding of deoxyribonucleic acid-dependent deoxyribonucleic acid polymerase to poxvirus. J. Virol. *9*:70, 1972.

TEMIN, H. M.: Mechanism of cell transformation by RNA tumor viruses. Ann. Rev. Microbiol. *25*:609, 1971.

TEMIN, H. M.: RNA-directed DNA synthesis. Sci. Amer. *226*:25, 1972.

TEMIN, H. M.: The RNA tumor viruses—background and foreground. Proc. Nat. Acad. Sci. USA *69*:1016, 1972.

TEMIN, H. M., and MIZUTANI, S.: RNA-dependent DNA polymerase in virions of Rous sarcoma virus. Nature *226*:124, 1970.

TOOLAN, H. W.: The Picodna viruses: H, RV, and AAV. Int. Rev. Exp. Path. *6*:135, 1968.

VELICER, L. F., and GINSBERG, H. S.: Synthesis, transport, and morphogenesis of type 5 adenovirus capsid proteins. J. Virol. *5*:338, 1970.

WARD, R., BANERJEE, A. K., LaFIANDRA, A., and SHATKIN, A. J.: Reovirus-specific ribonucleic acid from polysomes of infected L cells. J. Virol. *9*:61, 1972.

Chapter 4

Viral Genetics

The development of bacteriophage genetics established the basic principles which catalyzed the rapid progress in animal virus genetics. Meaningful genetic studies with animal viruses have been possible for a little over a decade, primarily because of two key technical developments. The first was the development of sensitive plaque assays for quantification of infectious virus. The second was the recognition and selection of stable genetic markers which are easy to detect and result from single mutations.

The two major mechanisms for genetic modification of viruses are *mutation* and *recombination*. The interaction of viruses or their products may also result in nonheritable phenotypic changes in the progeny. Some of the phenomena now known to be the consequence of gene product interactions were once thought to have a genetic basis. An understanding of the possible consequences of genetic interactions between viral nucleic acids, as well as the interaction of viral gene products, is important in interpreting the results obtained when cells are infected with more than one virus, an inevitable event in established infections.

In view of the potential for genetic change among viruses, the remarkable genetic stability of most viruses is singularly surprising and suggests that genetic change is usually met by rigorous selective pressures. For example, only one antigenic type of mumps virus is known to exist. A possible exception to this rule may be influenza virus with its numerous antigenic variants.

A.   Mutation

Mutations are defined as "heritable changes in the genome which do not result from the incorporation of genetic material from another organism." At the molecular level, a mutation is a chemical alteration in the base sequence of the nucleic acid of the genome. Mutations can arise from changes affecting a single nucleotide (a point mutation) or from larger alterations such as deletions or inversions which may involve hundreds or thousands of nucleotides. Spontaneous mutations occur in animal viruses at approximately the same rate as in other organisms (e.g., mutation rates per gene range from 10^{-5} to 10^{-8} each time a nucleic acid molecule is replicated).

A common cause of point mutations is incorrect base-pairing during either replication or repair of nucleic acid. Spontaneous mispairing can occur when the bases shift from their common tautomeric form to a more rare form. Mutation rates can be increased by treating viruses or their nucleic acid with various physical or chemical agents called *mutagens*. Mutagens mediate mutagenesis either by directly altering a base so that mispairing occurs or by indirectly provoking the repair of nucleic acid which has been damaged by the mutagen. Some analogues to the bases which normally are found in nucleic acid can pair with the normal nucleotides well enough to be substituted for the natural base but poor enough to cause incorrect base-pairing at a later time. Mutations can be recognized only if they result in detectable changes in the phenotype of the organism. Changes in the nucleic acid which do not cause phenotypic effects are referred to as "silent mutations."

A mutation is important medically when its expression gives a virus an advantage which results in increased virulence. Of equal importance are mutations which result in a decrease in virulence (attenuation). Attenuated viruses which retain the Ags that induce the production of protective Abs are essential for the production of living vaccines.

The mutations which have been detected in animal viruses affect a wide array of virus properties, including plaque-and-pock-type, antigenic composition, enzymatic activities, host range, and virulence. Conditional lethal mutants constitute a separate class from the mutants described above. These are viruses that have mutations which are lethal under certain conditions but which can replicate and yield mutant progeny under other conditions. For example, temperature-sensitive conditional lethal mutants have been isolated from a number of animal viruses. These mutants will grow normally at a low temperature but not at a high one, while the parental wild type grows at both temperatures. Many of the conditional lethal mutants obtained from animal viruses are unsuitable for genetic characterization, usually for one of two reasons. Either they revert to wild-type virus with high frequency (10^{-4}) or they are "leaky," i.e., some virus is produced even under the restrictive conditions.

Recently, much effort has been directed towards the selection of mutants with reduced virulence for use in living vaccines. Attenuated virus vaccines, such as the Semple rabies vaccine, which was empirically developed by Pasteur in 1885, were used long before the molecular mechanisms involved in mutation were understood. With our present knowledge of genetics and the ability to culture viruses *in vitro,* it is possible to select mutants on the basis of altered cultural characteristics, such as temperature or pH sensitivity. Mutants selected for phenotypic alterations detectable *in vitro* frequently are found to have an associated reduction in virulence. Thus potential vaccine strains can be selected *in vitro* from viruses with multiple phenotypic changes (co-variation). Final selection of suitable vaccine strains requires extensive animal testing and characterization of the virus.

B.   Genetic Interactions Involving Recombination

Recombination is the exchange of genetic material between two viruses which have infected the same cell. The result of recombination is the production of genetically stable progeny (*recombinants*), which possess characters not found together in either parent. The mechanism for recombination between viruses with nonsegmented genomes involves the breakage and reunion (crossing over) of the nucleic acid molecules from the two viruses (Fig. 4–1). In the case of viruses which have segmented genomes, recombination can result from the encapsidation of progeny nucleic acid segments produced by different parents.

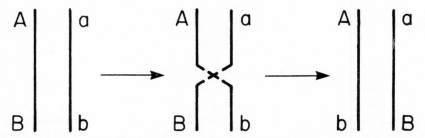

Figure 4–1. Recombination between viruses results from the breakage and reunion (crossing over) of homologous regions in the nucleic acid molecules from two viruses.

Recombination can occur when (1) both viruses are active (i.e., infectious), (2) one virus is active and one inactive, or (3) both viruses are inactive. The viruses which are involved in recombination may be mutants of the same virus, different strains of the same virus or, more rarely, unrelated viruses. A special type of recombination can occur between the nucleic acid of some viruses and the host cell genome (Chapters 3 and 24).

1. Recombination between Active Viruses

Two mutants of the same virus may recombine to produce wild-type progeny. For example, two temperature-sensitive mutants of poliovirus type 1 may recombine during replication at a permissive temperature to yield progeny which replicate at the restrictive temperature. This type of genetic interaction is of importance primarily to investigators interested in constructing genetic "maps" of viruses and in studying the functions of viral genes and gene products.

Recombination also can occur between immunologically distinct strains of the same virus or, less frequently, between unrelated viruses. For example, "hybrids" produced by the genetic interaction of two strains of influenza virus (A_0 and A_1) may possess the hemagglutinin of one parent and the neuraminidase of the other. Influenza virus provides an example of the occurrence of recombination in nature. Avian influenza viruses have been found which contain a neuraminidase indistinguishable from that of a human strain. This observation suggests, but by no means proves, that recombination may play a role in the production of the new strains of influenza A virus which cause the cyclic epidemics of influenza in man.

2. Recombination Involving Inactive Viruses

a. **Multiplicity Reactivation.** The production of infectious virus by a cell "coinfected" with two or more inactive viruses of the same strain is multiplicity reactivation. The reactivated virus is produced as a result of recombination between the damaged nucleic acids of viruses which have suffered lethal mutations in different genes; e.g., following exposure to UV-irradiation. As the damage to the nucleic acids of the inactivated virus population is increased, a larger number of particles are required per cell to produce a genome capable of producing infectious progeny.

Since the administration of vaccines produced by UV-irradiation of virulent viruses could result in the production of infectious virus by way of multiplicity reactivation, this method of inactivation is not used for the production of vaccines.

b. **Cross-reactivation or Marker Rescue.** Cross-reactivation is a consequence of genetic recombination between an active and a different, but related, inactive virus. This phenomenon results in the production of active progeny possessing one or more genetic traits from the inactive parent. Cross-reactivation can be used to obtain influenza virus strains which possess characteristics suitable for vaccine production. For example, one strain of influenza A virus which replicates well in embryonated chicken eggs was inactivated by UV-irradiation. The inactivated virus was mixed with an active strain of influenza virus which replicated poorly in eggs but which contained the desired hemagglutinin (immunogenic Ag). Since the more rapidly growing parent was inactivated, it failed to replicate but contributed the trait of rapid growth to the strain possessing the desired immunogenic Ag.

C. Gene Product Interactions

In addition to interactions involving genetic recombination, there can be interactions between viral-induced gene products (proteins) produced in cells infected with more than one virus.

1. Phenotypic Mixing

Phenotypic mixing is the incorporation of the genome of one virus into a capsid or envelope which contains components produced by another virus. The altered phenotype is not a stable change because, upon subsequent passage, the phenotypically mixed virus will produce progeny enclosed in capsids or envelopes coded by the parental genome (Fig. 4–2).

Phenotypic mixing is detected by infecting cells with high dilutions of the test virus to prevent mixed infections. If the test virus capsid contains capsomeres produced by two viruses (for example, poliovirus 1 and 2), the virus will be neutralized by antiserum to either virus. In contrast, the progeny will have capsids determined by the genotype of the phenotypically mixed parent and will be neutralized by only one type of antiserum.

a. Transcapsidation. The mismatching of entire capsids between two viruses replicating in the same cell is transcapsidation. This phenomenon is commonly observed when cells are mixedly infected with enteroviruses. Progeny virus released from cells infected with poliovirus and coxsackievirus or echo- and coxsackieviruses often have the genome of one virus enclosed within the capsid of the other. In some instances, genomes also may be enclosed in "mixed" capsids composed of capsomeres produced by both viruses. This latter type of interaction has been observed following infection of cells with different serotypes of poliovirus or different adenoviruses (Fig. 4–2).

b. Mosaic Envelopes. Mosaic envelopes contain a mixture of peplomeres (viral Ags) produced by at least two viruses. This type of phenotypic mixing occurs in cells mixedly infected with viruses which acquire their envelopes by budding through the cell membrane. For example, cells infected with influenza A and influenza B viruses will incorporate into the plasma membrane peplomers ("spikes") produced by both viruses.

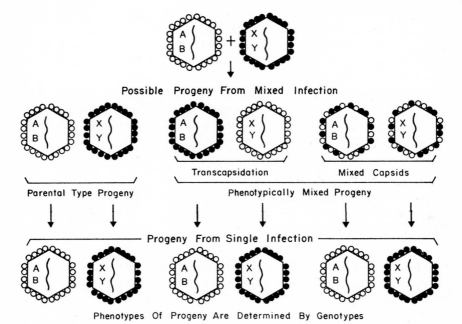

Figure 4–2. Phenotypic mixing. When cells are simultaneously infected with more than one virus, the progeny from the mixed infection may include (1) viruses identical to the parental type, (2) viruses which contain the genome of one virus and the capsid of another (transcapsidation), and (3) viruses with capsid components of both viruses (mixed capsids). When cells are infected with high dilutions of the progeny from mixed infections, the phenotypes of the viruses produced in the singly infected cells are determined by the genotypes of the infecting virus.

Some of the progeny particles will possess envelopes which contain viral Ags which are characteristic of both parental viruses.

Phenotypic mixing of viral capsids and envelopes in nature could have important consequences since it could alter the host range of virus and greatly complicate the serological diagnosis of some diseases.

2. Polyploidy and Genotypic Mixing (Heteropolyploidy)

Polyploidy and genotypic mixing result from the incorporation of more than one complete genome into the same virus particle. There is no recombination between the two genomes and progeny of both types are produced upon subsequent passage (Fig. 4–3).

In cells infected with genetically different forms of a virus, "heteropolyploid" particles may be produced by the accidental incorporation of two different nucleocapsids into the same envelope at maturation. Cells singly infected with the genotypically mixed viruses will yield progeny identical to both original parents as well as more genotypically mixed

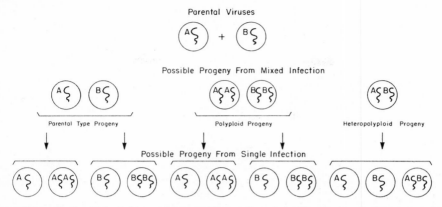

Figure 4–3. Polyploidy and genotypic mixing. In cells simultaneously infected with variants of a virus, the progeny from the mixed infection may include (1) viruses identical to the parental types, (2) polyploid particles produced by the incorporation of two nucleocapsids of the same virus into one envelope at maturation, and (3) heteroploid particles produced by the incorporation of two different nucleocapsids into one envelope. Cells singly infected with the progeny from a mixed infection may produce more parental type viruses, polyploid particles, or heteropolyploid particles, depending upon the genotype of the infecting virus particle.

viruses. The production of polyploid particles is a common occurrence in cells singly infected with some viruses, for example the paramyxoviruses. Enveloped virions which contain multiple nucelocapsids are readily detected with the electron microscope.

3. Complementation

Complementation refers to the interaction of two viruses which results in the production of infectious progeny of one or both types under conditions in which normal replication ordinarily would not occur. Complementation can involve (1) an active and a defective virus, (2) an active and an inactive virus, (3) two defective viruses or two conditional lethal mutants (Fig. 4–4). The viruses may be related or unrelated. There is no exchange of nucleic acid between the viruses; therefore, the genotypes are not altered.

In all cases of complementation, one virus induces the production of some essential gene product which the other requires and is unable to synthesize. The nature of the essential protein varies; in one system, it may be a capsid or envelope component and in another an enzyme. The mechanisms of complementation in many virus systems are not known.

Since the genotype of the viruses is not altered, the progeny of defective viruses will also be defective and will have the same gene product requirements as the parental virus. For example, Rous sarcoma virus is defective

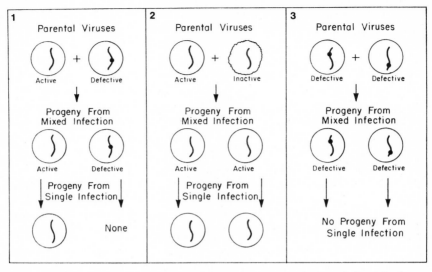

Figure 4—4. Complementation patterns. Mutations which result in defectiveness are indicated by ⊙ . A defective capsid is indicated by ⊙ . (1) In cells infected with an active and a defective virus, the gene product produced by the active virus can be utilized by the defective virus so that progeny defective viruses are produced as well as active viruses. However, in cells singly "infected" with the defective progeny no virus is produced because no wild-type allele of the active virus was present to complement the mutant cistron in the defective virus. (2) Cells infected with active virus and virus inactivated by methods which damage the capsid but not the nucleic acid yield active virus progeny of both types which will replicate normally in singly infected cells. (3) Two viruses defective in different cistrons may complement each other in mixed infections so that defective progeny of both types are produced. In single infections, neither defective virus will replicate because each still requires the gene product produced by the other virus.

in certain cell types because it is unable to code for the synthesis of envelope protein(s) necessary for infectivity. The avian leukosis viruses, which act as helper viruses, provide the missing protein, and complete Rous sarcoma virus is produced by unilateral phenotypic mixing. However, the progeny are incapable of independent replication upon subsequent passage unless a helper virus is present.

In contrast, when viruses are inactivated by methods which do not damage the nucleic acid, the progeny produced by complementation will be active viruses. The "activation" of an inactivated poxvirus by a related active poxvirus is an example of this type of complementation. When rabbits are injected with a mixture of heat-inactivated virulent myxoma virus and active avirulent fibroma virus, the animals die from progressive disease caused by the activated virulent virus. This phenomenon initially appeared to be an example of genetic cross-reactivation but is now known to be due to complementation. Poxviruses contain a DNA-dependent RNA polymerase which is heat labile. The active fibroma virus contains functional polymerase and produces mRNA which is translated into the enzymes required to uncoat the poxviruses. After uncoating, the undamaged nucleic acid from inactive virus can function and infectious progeny are produced.

The complementation reactions which occur between the adenoviruses and active SV_{40} or defective hybrid SV_{40}-adenovirus particles are of particular interest because of the oncogenic potential of these viruses. Human adenoviruses are defective in monkey cells but can be rescued by SV_{40}, which replicates in but does not destroy the simian cells. The adenovirus also can be rescued by defective SV_{40}-adenovirus hybrids which are formed during serial passage of adenovirus in monkey cells which harbor SV_{40}. Complementation of the adenovirus involves a step prior to DNA replication. The defective hybrids can themselves be complemented by the rescued human adenovirus which provides capsid proteins that the hybrid is unable to produce.

Tests for complementation between mutants, which may exhibit similar phenotypes, can be used to study the functional organization of the viral genome. Complementation between mutants has proved most useful as a preliminary step in genetic mapping. The use of temperature-sensitive mutants for both genetic and functional studies of the animal viruses has increased during the last decade. The results obtained from investigations of the mechanisms by which host-defective viruses are rescued by other viruses have already provided some insight into the possible mechanisms of cellular transformation and viral oncogenesis.

4. Enhancement

Enhancement is the increased production of one virus as a result of coinfection with a second noncytocidal virus. The phenomenon is limited to certain combinations of viruses. For example, infection of cells with parainfluenza-1 virus prior to inoculation of vesicular stomatitis virus (VSV) results in increased yields of VSV. In contrast, prior infection with other parainfluenza viruses or orthomyxoviruses has no enhancing effect on VSV.

The precise mechanisms by which enhancement is mediated are not known in all cases and may vary from system to system. One "enhancing" virus, parainfluenza-1 virus, inhibits the production and action of interferon. A cellular protein, called "enhancer," is produced in embryonated eggs infected with parainfluenza-1 virus and is released into the allantoic fluid. The enhancer, rather than the direct action of the virus, appears to have an anti-interferon effect.

Although both enhancement and complementation result in increased virus yields, they appear to be different phenomena. In complementation an essential protein is produced by one virus and used by another; in enhancement the action or production of an inhibitory protein (interferon) appears to be blocked by the enhancing virus.

References

COOPER, P. D.: Genetic analysis of animal viruses: new approaches and new vistas. Brit. Med. Bull. *23*:155, 1967.

FENNER, F.: *The Biology of Animal Viruses.* Vol. I. New York, Academic Press, 1968.

FENNER, F.: The genetics of animal viruses. Ann. Rev. Microbiol. *24*:297, 1970.

FENNER, F., and SAMBROOK, J. F.: The genetics of animal viruses. Ann. Rev. Microbiol. *18*:47, 1964.

FENNER, F., and WHITE, D. O.: *Viral genetics. In Medical Virology.* New York, Academic Press, 1970.

RAPP, F., and MELNICK, J. L.: Papovavirus SV40, adenoviruses and their "hybrids": transformation, complementation, and transcapsidation. Progr. Med. Virol. *8*: 349, 1966.

Principles of Immunity to Viruses

Host resistance to viral infections is complex and encompasses all the nonspecific mechanisms of resistance which are expressed upon initial encounter with a virus as well as the specific mechanisms which come into play during the course of the infection and upon subsequent exposure to the same virus.

The importance of the specific immune response in protection against reinfection with viruses was clearly demonstrated by Jenner, who introduced vaccination for the prevention of smallpox in 1798. Until recently, the eradication of virus during primary infection and protection against reinfection were believed to depend primarily on specific Ab. This assumption was based on the fact that serum Ab is first detected on about the 5th day during virus infections and reaches a maximum titer by the 14th day; clinical recovery, following virus eradication, commonly occurs during this period.

The observation that hypogammaglobulinemics recover normally from many virus infections and the fact that a number of clinical conditions are associated with enhanced susceptibility to viruses led to a renewed interest in the role of specific cell-mediated immunity in virus infections. In addition, the discovery of interferon suggested that this nonspecific antiviral substance also is an important determinant of host resistance. Collectively, these findings prompted a reevaluation of the concepts of viral immunity. It is apparent that the total immune response to viruses represents an interplay of both baseline innate and acquired immune systems (Fig. 5–1).

A. Mechanisms of Nonspecific Resistance

1. Innate Immunity to Viruses

Innate immunity is defined as "that immunity which is constitutive for the species and is expressed toward a primary infection before acquired immunity develops." Some of the factors of the host which contribute to innate immunity are discussed below.

a. **Anatomical and Chemical Barriers.** The intact skin and mucous membranes of the host provide the first line of defense against virus infection. In addition to these passive mechanical barriers, "chemical barriers" such as lactic acid in sweat and fatty acids in sebaceous secretions probably play a significant role in preventing virus from making contact with susceptible cells.

In the respiratory tract, the mucociliary escalator, which prevents particles of 5 to 10 μm or more from penetrating the lower lung, may participate in the mechanical removal of viruses that impinge on the mucous blanket. Any virus which escapes these barriers and reaches the lower lung will encounter alveolar macrophages and may be destroyed.

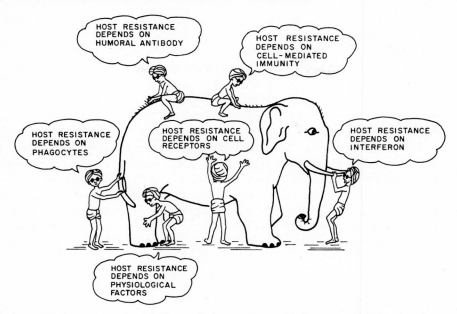

Figure 5–1. Host resistance to virus infections. The complexity of the immune response is schematically illustrated in terms of the fable about six blind men attempting to define the nature of an elephant. The intent of the illustration is to emphasize that the total immune response to viruses involves the interplay of specific and nonspecific immune mechanisms. (Adapted with permission from Glasgow, L. A.: Interrelationships of interferon and immunity during viral immunity. J. Gen. Physiol. *56:*212 Suppl., 1970.)

However, some viruses replicate in macrophages which can then act as vehicles for virus dissemination.

   b. Age and Physiological Condition of the Host.   Age and physiological condition are also important determinants of resistance to viruses. Many virus infections are more severe in neonates, infants, and the elderly than in young adults. It is difficult to assess the relative importance of nonspecific and specific immune factors with respect to age-dependent changes in resistance since both are undoubtedly involved. Malnutrition can interfere with the efficiency of both nonspecific and specific immunity. Even the mechanical barriers provided by the skin and mucous membranes are impaired in many types of nutritional deficiency states.

   Hormonal changes can affect the pathogenesis and severity of certain viral diseases. For example, pregnant women are prone to develop paralytic poliomyelitis rather than the less severe forms of the disease. Also, patients receiving corticosteroid therapy are subject to more frequent and severe viral diseases than normal individuals, probably because steroids inhibit the nonspecific inflammatory response as well as the specific immune response to viruses.

c. Genetic Composition. Genetic composition is of primary importance in determining resistance to certain viral agents. For example, some racial groups differ markedly in their susceptibility to diseases such as yellow fever and measles. However, since accurate human genetic data are difficult to obtain, the best examples illustrating the role of genetics in determining resistance are provided by inbred animal models.

The observation that the susceptibility of mice to Gross leukemia virus is linked with certain histocompatibility genes prompted a major search for a similar association between the HL-A system and disease in man. An association between HL-A 4c and Hodgkin's disease, which probably has a viral etiology, has been recently reported. Subsequent studies have suggested a positive correlation between HL-A2 and acute leukemia, which also appears to have a viral etiology. An evaluation of the significance of these findings must await the accumulation of more data from carefully controlled studies.

2. Determinants of Cell Resistance to Viruses

a. Receptor Site Requirements. Some viruses require specific cell receptor sites for virus attachment. Accordingly, cells which do not possess the receptors are resistant to these viruses. For example, primates are susceptible to poliovirus, whereas nonprimates are resistant because their cells lack the surface receptors for this virus.

b. Nonpermissive Host Cells. Since viruses utilize the substrates, energy supply, and organelles of host cells to synthesize virus macromolecules, cells which lack the necessary components for synthesis are nonpermissive (i.e., will not support virus multiplication even though virus attachment and penetration may occur; for example, small lymphocytes are usually nonpermissive). In contrast, the large lymphocyte, an activated cell, is permissive for a variety of viruses. Agents such as phytohemagglutinin and antilymphocyte serum, which transform small lymphocytes to large blast-like cells, enhance the susceptibility of these cells to some viruses.

The permissiveness of macrophages is of major importance in determining the outcome of certain virus infections. For example, in mice, susceptibility to some encephaloviruses and hepatitis virus is apparently determined by the capacity of macrophages to support virus replication. The susceptibility of the macrophage to virus is genetically determined. In the case of some Group B togaviruses, susceptibility of the macrophage to virus infection has been demonstrated to be under the control of a single gene with resistance being dominant. Susceptibility to a mouse hepatitis virus also is under single gene control but dominance in this case relates to susceptibility.

The presence in a host of special cells which are permissive for a given virus may explain, in part, the phenomenon of tissue tropism; nonpermissive cells could account for the pattern of resistance of various tissues observed in systemic virus infections.

3. Inflammation

Viruses which succeed in establishing an infection will invariably elicit some component of the inflammatory response. The particular events in inflammation which contribute to defense include (1) the early accumulation of neutrophils, which leads to a local increase in oxygen utilization and acid production, (2) the formation of a fibrin network in tissues, (3) the accelerated escape of fluid from vessels, and (4) the eventual extravascular accumulation of macrophages and lymphocytes. Collectively these responses may limit the spread of virus, dilute toxic factors, and provide antiviral substances, which can act either extracellularly or intracellularly. Factors such as acid metabolites, elevated temperature (fever), and lowered pH and oxidation-reduction potential in tissue provide unfavorable environmental conditions for the replication of many viruses. Thus the inflammatory response usually benefits the host by limiting the infection. On the other hand, an exaggerated inflammatory response may contribute to the pathogenesis of the disease (Chapter 6).

4. Interferon

Available evidence supports the concept that the interferon system is one of the most important elements of the host's nonspecific defense against viral infections. The term "interferon system" is used because this system can be divided into several components. Interferon is a protein(s) produced and released by cells following viral infection and in response to certain nonviral stimuli. Interferon is not itself directly antiviral, but instead reacts with uninfected cells to induce the formation of an "antiviral protein," which mediates antiviral activity. Recent evidence suggests that antiviral protein blocks either virus-specific transcription or virus-specific translation (Chapter 7).

Interferon has a broad antiviral spectrum and is effective, in varying degrees, against viruses in most of the major groups. Thus infection of cells with avirulent viruses can protect against unrelated virulent viruses. The prospects for using interferon therapeutically or prophylactically for human virus diseases are discussed in Chapter 7.

a. **Role of Interferon During the Establishment of Viral Infection.** Interferon is the first host defense mechanism that can be detected following primary infection of cells at the implantation site. Replication of virus in the initially infected cells is probably not inhibited but, as interferon is produced and released, it diffuses to surrounding cells and incites them to produce antiviral protein. Hence the cells in closest proximity to the interferon-producing cells become the most resistant to virus. If interferon succeeds in preventing or limiting viral infection at the implantation site, dissemination to distant sites will not occur or may be suppressed. Thus the early action of interferon can be critical in determining the outcome of a virus infection.

    b. Role of Interferon in Virus Dissemination. In systemic virus infections, virus can spread from the primary site of infection by way of the blood or lymph or by means of infected cells. Interferon is present in the serum within a few hours after the onset of viremia and rapidly circulates to target organs where it can protect cells against seeding of virus from the blood. Cells of the lymphoreticular system, including lymphocytes and macrophages, are excellent sources of interferon and would be expected to play an important role in controlling systemic spread of virus. The lymphoid series of cells are not only capable of producing interferon but also participate in the specific immune response. These cells, therefore, provide a bridge between the specific cellular and humoral immune systems and the nonspecific interferon system.

    c. Role of Interferon in Recovery from Established Virus Infection. Interferon produced locally in the target organs of established virus infections undoubtedly makes a major contribution to recovery. However, specific immunity acquired during the infection is probably the major factor involved in virus clearance even in a previously nonimmune host. A comparison of the interferon and Ab responses clearly reveals how the action of each would complement the other (Fig. 5–2). Interferon is

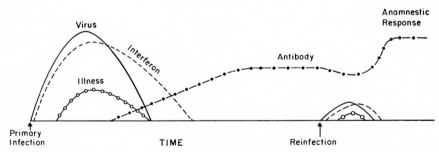

Figure 5–2. Host reaction to viral infection. Schematic representation of the relative occurrences of virus multiplication, illness, interferon, and Ab during a primary infection and reinfection. (Adapted with permission from Baron, S.: The defensive role of the interferon system. J. Gen. Physiol. *56:*196 Suppl., 1970.)

produced within hours after infection and acts intracellularly to block virus replication and cell-to-cell spread but exerts no direct effect on free virus. In contrast, Ab is produced later at sites distant from the target organ and can neutralize the infectivity of extracellular virus. Since a single Ab molecule probably can neutralize a virus particle, even small amounts of circulating Ab can promote clearance during viremia.

B. Mechanisms of Specific Immunity

The mechanisms of specific immunity are divided into those mediated by humoral Ab and those mediated by immune cells. Both depend upon the activity of small lymphocytes derived from stem cell precursors in the bone marrow (Fig. 5–3). It has been suggested that stem cell precursors

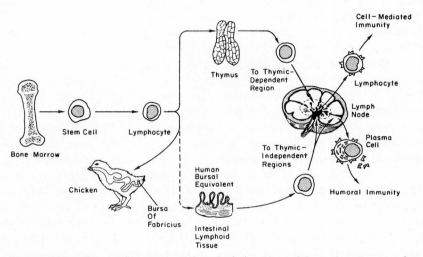

Figure 5–3. Schematic representation depicting the origin and pathways of the cells involved in humoral and cell-mediated immunity. (Adapted with permission from Bellanti, J. A.: Immunology. Philadelphia, W. B. Saunders Co., 1971.)

differentiate to form at least two distinct lymphocyte populations: the thymus-dependent lymphocytes (T-cells), which require an intact and functional thymus, and bone marrow-derived lymphocytes (B-cells), which develop independent of the thymus but in some instances require the help of T-cells. Since B-lymphocytes and their descendants (plasma cells) synthesize humoral Ab, any defect in the B-cell system will lead to a deficiency in humoral Ab synthesis. The T-cell system has a dual function; first it is required for the development of cell-mediated immunity, and second, thymus-dependent lymphocytes provide a necessary stimulus to B-lymphocytes to produce Abs in response to certain "thymus-dependent" Ags. Thus a defective T-lymphocyte system will lead to deficiencies in both cell-mediated immunity and in humoral immunity against the so-called "thymus-dependent" Ags.

1. Humoral Immunity

Specific Abs are produced in the host during and after viral infections. Convincing evidence for the importance of humoral Abs is the fact that immune gamma globulin administered passively will protect against infection or reduce the severity of an existing infection.

Doubts as to the importance of humoral Ab in preventing reinfection emerged when it was recognized that patients with hypogammaglobulinemia recover normally from many primary virus infections and become immune to reinfection. However, if sensitive serologic techniques are used, it can be demonstrated that these patients develop small amounts of Ab in response to virus Ags. These low levels of Ab probably are sufficient to convey immunity to reinfection by viruses which involve a viremic phase.

a. Role of Immunoglobulin Classes. *The class IgM* contains the largest of the immunoglobulin molecules and is the first Ab to be produced following primary antigenic challenge. Levels of IgM Ab upon secondary antigenic challenge are seldom any higher than those which develop after primary challenge. In contrast, in the case of IgG Abs, a secondary challenge results in a rapid and enhanced response due to immunologic memory (anamnestic response). Although IgM Abs are generally less efficient in neutralizing virus than IgG Abs, they are more efficient in fixing complement (C). For this reason, IgM Abs are especially important in complement-dependent destruction of virus-infected cells and possibly certain of the enveloped viruses. Although Abs of the IgM class cannot cross the placenta, the fetus is capable of producing Abs of this class of immunoglobulin during the second trimester of gestation. This is obviously important in the case of virus infections of the fetus. Elevated levels of IgM globulins occur within the fetus infected with such agents as rubella virus and may be an aid in the diagnosis of intrauterine infections.

Antibodies of *the class IgG* account for most of the antiviral activity in serum and the effectiveness of killed vaccines administered parenterally depends to a large extent on the development of IgG Ab. An important biological property of IgG is its ability to cross the placenta. Consequently, newborn infants are endowed with preformed maternal Ab at birth and are protected from many virus infections during the critical neonatal period when the infant's Ab-producing mechanisms are comparatively inefficient. Since passively acquired Ab can specifically inhibit active immunization of the infant with virus vaccines, vaccination schedules should be planned accordingly.

Most IgG Abs have the ability to fix C, which is believed to be essential for neutralization of certain viruses and for Ab-mediated cytolysis of virus-infected cells. However, on a molar basis IgG Abs are less efficient in fixing C than are IgM Abs.

Although small amounts of IgG and IgM are synthesized locally at secretory surfaces and released into external secretions, most of the IgG which can be detected in nasal secretions during viral respiratory tract infections is derived primarily from serum as a result of inflammation of the nasal mucosa.

Antibodies of *the class IgA* are present in mucosal and other external secretions as well as serum. The first evidence that nasal secretions possessed antiviral activity was reported over 50 years ago. Several workers in the late 1920s and 1930s measured Ab in various body fluids and Francis, in 1940, suggested that the antiviral properties of nasal secretions might be important in resistance to influenza. The first clear indication of the importance of locally produced Ab in virus infections was made by Fazekas de St. Groth and Donnelley in 1950. They showed that mice vaccinated by the intranasal route were more resistant to infection with influenza virus than those vaccinated by other routes.

The contemporary era of investigation in this field began with the discovery that a secretory form of IgA is present in relatively large quantities in many secretions including those of the bronchial mucosa, urinary tract, and the salivary, lacrimal, and mammary glands. Secretory IgA has structural and functional properties different from those of serum IgA (*Fundamentals of Immunology*).

In recent years secretory Abs have been shown to play an important role in the protection of the host against viruses, particularly those in which the infection is localized. For example, the presence of IgA in the nasopharynx correlates better with immunity to respiratory virus infections than does serum Ab. During immunization with the Sabin attenuated poliovirus vaccine, a state of local resistance develops in the alimentary tract along with the appearance of serum IgG Abs. This "gut immunity" is characterized by marked and sometimes effective resistance to virus implantation; but if infection occurs, the period of virus excretion is shortened. On the other hand, following parenteral immunization with the Salk inactivated poliovirus vaccine, the alimentary tract remains susceptible to reinfection although circulating IgG Abs develop to high titer. It has been proposed that secretory IgA Abs protect by preventing reinfection of the alimentary tract, whereas circulating IgG Abs act during the viremic stage to prevent, in the case of poliovirus, invasion of the central nervous system.

The fact that secretory IgA is produced locally indicates that the Ab-producing cells are stimulated by Ag locally. As would be expected, inactivated vaccines administered parenterally are effective for inducing serum Ab production but are relatively ineffective in inducing the synthesis of secretory IgA. However, secretory IgA is produced following parenteral administration of vaccines containing live attenuated viruses, such as the measles virus or poliovirus which infect, multiply, and spread widely throughout the body. The requirement for local stimulation of plasma cells prompted investigations on new approaches for inducing secretory IgA Ab in immunoprophylaxis. For example, the local application of influenza vaccine directly into the respiratory tract has been found to enhance secretory IgA Ab production and increase protection.

The IgD class of immunoglobulin was discovered in a patient with multiple myeloma and, subsequently, low levels of IgD were found in the serum of normal individuals. The biological function of this immunoglobulin is unknown.

Antibodies of *the class IgE* are present in the β-globulin fraction of serum and are responsible for allergic disorders such as hay fever; these Abs can be demonstrated in man by the Prausnitz-Küstner reaction. Like IgA, IgE is produced in the respiratory and intestinal tracts and is found in external secretions. The role which Abs of the class IgE may play in viral infections remains to be established with certainty. Indirect evidence for the participation of IgE Abs in viral infections is provided by observations on children with ataxia telangiectasia, one of the immune deficiency diseases. These patients have decreased levels of serum and secretory IgA and lack IgE. They are more susceptible to recurrent viral and bacterial sinopulmonary infections than are patients who are deficient only in IgA. The lack of IgE has been suggested as a possible cause for this increased susceptibility. However, these patients also have impaired cellular immunity which could account for their increased susceptibility to certain virus infections.

b. Mechanisms of Virus Neutralization. Virus neutralization is defined as the decrease in virus infectivity which follows the interaction of virus with specific Ab. The association of virus with Ab does not irreversibly alter either reactant since intact virus and Ab can be dissociated from viral Ag-Ab complexes by appropriate dilution or by physical or chemical treatment. The mechanism by which Ab neutralizes virus infectivity and ultimately effects its destruction depends upon the virus, the class of Ab, the ratio of Ab to virus, and how a particular host cell handles the Ag-Ab complex.

Inhibition of virus adsorption to cells is one important mechanism by which "neutralizing Ab" effects neutralization. The surface of the virion is composed of many repeating subunits which would suggest that Ab would have to coat the virus to prevent adsorption. However, some viruses can be neutralized by a single Ab molecule. Each IgG Ab molecule has two Ag binding sites permitting the establishment of two specific bonds with two determinant groups on a single virion. The stabilization of a virus-Ab complex has a high temperature coefficient and probably results in slight conformational changes in both molecules. These changes may be sufficient to inhibit the attachment of virus to cells by altering the configuration of the virus sites that combine with cell receptors.

Enhanced virus degradation is another important effect of neutralizing Ab, especially in those instances in which the interaction of virus with Ab does not prevent attachment. For example, vaccinia virions which have been completely coated with Ab can somehow adsorb to and penetrate susceptible cells even though the virion surface projections are obscured by Ab. Whereas Ab treatment of the virus decreases its adsorption to cells and prolongs its retention at the cell surface, the Ab-coated virus is eventually phagocytized (Fig. 5–4). In this case, Ab exerts its neutralizing effect intracellularly by interfering with post-engulfment stages in the normal vaccinia virus replicative cycle. Even virus which is adsorbed to cells prior to the addition of antiserum can be neutralized as long as it remains in the extracellular position. Antibody appears to neutralize vaccinia virus infectivity by preventing the normal release of functional virus cores from the phagocytic vacuole into the cytoplasm. Instead the virus-Ab complexes are degraded as a unit within the phagosome by lysosomal enzymes. During this abnormal "uncoating," the genome is gradually rendered acid soluble and the nucleic acid is not replicated.

In the case of poliovirus, Ab actually enhances the *in vitro* attachment of virus to cells. However, the RNA of neutralized virus is completely degraded before it is replicated. It has been suggested that Ab-coated virus attaches to the cells nonspecifically and is phagocytized and rapidly destroyed by lysosomal enzymes within the phagosome. In contrast, the RNA from nonneutralized virus is released directly into the cytoplasm following interaction of the capsids with specific cell receptors on the cytoplasmic membrane and does not encounter lysosomal enzymes.

Complement-mediated enhancement of virus neutralization is an important defense mechanism in the case of certain viruses, such as herpes simplex virus. The first IgM or IgG Ab produced ("early" IgM and IgG) possesses low neutralizing activity for herpesvirus *in vitro* in the absence of C. When C is added, both IgM and IgG Abs exhibit enhanced neutralizing activity. Late IgM Ab can neutralize herpesvirus in the absence of C, but its activity is enhanced by the addition of C. The quantitative effectiveness of late IgG Ab in neutralizing virus does not appear to be influenced by C; however, the rate at which virus is neutralized by late IgG is enhanced in the presence of C.

Complement-dependent enhancement of virus neutralization, which occurs with viruses such as rubella and influenza, may be due to complement-mediated lesions in the envelope of the virus which resemble the comple-

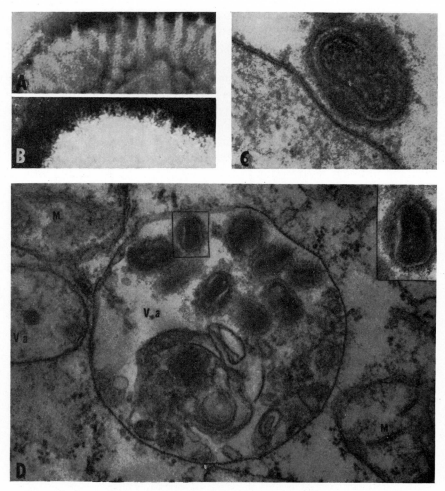

Figure 5–4. A, Portion of an unneutralized particle of vaccinia virus showing the surface ridges on tubules. Magnification: × 224,000. B, A vaccinia virus particle which has been exposed to specific antiserum. The surface projections have become obscured by a dense coat of fine fibrils. The print was purposely underdeveloped to emphasize the fine filamentous nature of the coat. Magnification: × 224,000. C, A vaccinia virus particle which has been exposed to specific antiserum is seen adsorbed to a partially invaginated outer cell membrane. Magnification: × 120,000. D, A group of vaccinia virus particles clumped by specific antiserum are seen within a phagocytic vacuole in a cell 3 hours after inoculation. (Va, vacuole; M, mitochondria). Each particle possesses the characteristic fuzzy coat, shown at a higher magnification in the insert. Magnification: × 48,000; insert × 96,000. (Reprinted with permission from Dales, S., and Kajioka, R.: The cycle of multiplication of vaccinia virus in Earle's stain L-cells. 1. Uptake and penetration. Virology 24:278, 1964.)

ment-induced lesions on erythrocytes. In the case of rubella virus, the envelope is completely removed in the presence of unheated antiserum (Fig. 5–5). These observations support the concept that Ab and C can lyse the envelopes of some viruses, which results in loss of infectivity. However, in herpesvirus, the maximal complement-induced enhancement of neutralization occurs at an early stage in the C activation sequence and adds antiviral activity to the list of biological functions associated with early C components (*Fundamentals of Immunology*). Since C is invariably present in the plasma, this system could be important in increasing the effectiveness of early Ab against some viruses and preventing virus dissemination.

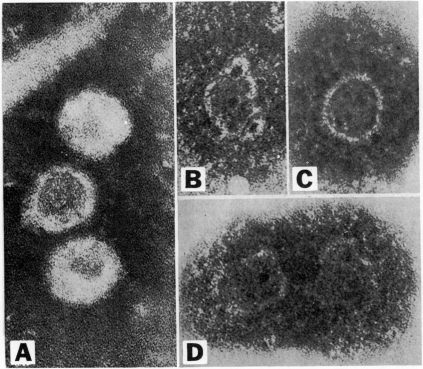

Figure 5–5.   A, Three rubella virions linked by Ab from heat-inactivated antiserum. Virus particles show typical light amorphous outer covering of intact virus. B, C, and D, Rubella virus particles after treatment with antiserum containing complement. Lesions typical of immune lysis can be seen in outer coverings of particles. In C, complement hole can be seen at periphery of internal component, although no envelope remains. Negatively stained preparations, × 300,000. (Reprinted with permission from Almeida, J. D., and Lawrence, G. D.: Heated and unheated antiserum on rubella virus. Amer. J. Dis. Child. *118:*101, 1969. Copyright 1969, American Medical Association.)

   c. Cytolysis of Virus-infected Cells.   Antibody-mediated destruction
of virus-infected cells is a complement-dependent reaction which can
either aid in recovery from infection or contribute to its pathogenesis
(Chapter 6). Cells which are infected with viruses that alter the antigenic
composition of the plasma membrane are susceptible to both Ab-mediated
and immune cell-mediated destruction.
   Cytolysis can occur when either specific antiviral IgG or IgM and C
are added to virus-infected cells possessing antigenically altered membranes.
However, IgM is more effective than IgG in initiating cell lysis because a
single IgM molecule bound to a cell surface determinant group is sufficient
to cause a complement-dependent target lesion, whereas 2 IgG molecules bound in close proximity are required.
   d. Nonneutralizing Antibodies.   Natural viral infections and immunization with attenuated vaccines lead to the induction of Abs against
both internal and surface components of the virion. Internal virus Ags
and even some surface Ags are nonimmunogenic; i.e., Abs produced
against them do not neutralize the virus. It has been suggested, however,
that some nonneutralizing antiviral Abs directed at surface components
may act as opsonins to enhance phagocytosis and degradation of the virus.
Some of the Abs detected in serologic tests used in the diagnosis of viral
infections are against nonimmunogenic internal or "hidden" Ags.
   Individuals infected or immunized with influenza virus develop Abs
against at least two envelope Ags, neuraminidase and hemagglutinin, both
of which are external antigenic components of the envelope. The Ab
against hemagglutinin is primarily responsible for virus neutralization.
In contrast, antineuraminidase Ab does not neutralize virus infectivity but
can inhibit the release of virus from infected cells thus reducing the virus
yield. Although antineuraminidase Abs do not prevent the initial steps in
infection, it is apparent that they could participate in later events related
to the release and spread of virus from the primary focus of infection.
   Virus complexed with Ab can exhibit different levels of infectivity in
different host cells. When the same virus-Ab mixture is assayed on two
different types of cells, the infectivity is not always the same. This fact indicates that neutralization of a virus may depend on how a particular host
cell handles the complex. In rare cases, the attachment of Ab to virus actually enhances the infectivity of the virus for some cells. The mechanism by
which Ab enhances infectivity is not known but could result from an
increase in virus uptake coupled with a depression of the normal degradation process of the virus-Ab complex.
   There is mounting evidence which indicates that Ab may contribute
to the clinical manifestations of some virus infections. Infants infected
with respiratory syncytial (RS) virus develop serious respiratory diseases,
such as bronchiolitis or pneumonia, during the first few months of life,

but less severe infections occur with increasing age. These infants become infected with RS virus even in the presence of maternally acquired anti-RS Ab. It has been suggested that the maternal IgG present reacts with the excess viral Ag in the lung. It is possible that these Ag-Ab complexes produce immunologic injury and contribute to disease manifestations characteristic of RS illness in early infancy. Similarly, some individuals immunized with inactivated measles vaccine, which results in the selective stimulation of IgG without concomitant stimulation of secretory IgA Ab, develop more severe infections when naturally infected with measles virus than do nonimmunized subjects (Chapter 6).

2. Cell-mediated Immunity

Cell-mediated immunity is effected by cells rather than humoral Ab. The possible importance of cell-mediated immunity in virus infections was recognized over 50 years ago. Evidence supporting the significance of this system is amply provided by observations on patients with either inherited or acquired defects in cellular immunity. These individuals show a striking inability to control many of the noncytolytic viruses, particularly those in which the virus nucleic acid becomes integrated into the host cell genome or which are transferred from cell to cell and thus do not encounter humoral Ab.

The cellular immune system represents a major mechanism for surveillance and rejection of foreign or antigenically altered host cells as well as the elimination of intracellular parasites. The precise mechanism by which cell-mediated immunity operates in viral immunity is not clear. However, in many noncytolytic virus infections, viral Ags may be present in cell membranes either as a result of incorporation of Ags into the membrane or as a consequence of gradual release of virus particles through the membrane. It would appear that cell-mediated events are particularly well suited for destroying these altered host "target cells" and aborting virus replication.

The cell-mediated immune system depends on specifically sensitized lymphocytes (T-cells) and activated macrophages. Evidently the first step in the effector activities of the immune T-lymphocyte involves the recognition of foreign Ag on the target cell surface by Ab-like receptors on the specifically committed lymphocyte. The lymphocyte interacts with Ags on the target cell which leads to its ultimate destruction. In the course of their activities, reacting T-cells undergo blast transformation and liberate lymphokines which chemotactically attract additional lymphocytes as well as macrophages. Specifically immune T-lymphocytes and B-lymphocytes also can produce interferon and Ab, respectively, following reaction with Ag. An increased mobilization of cells provides an amplification mechanism for the local production of interferon and perhaps specific Ab.

Interferon, in conjunction with circulating or cytophilic Ab produced locally at the site of infection, could protect macrophages and other cells and thus help localize the infection (Fig. 5–6). Alternatively, it is possible

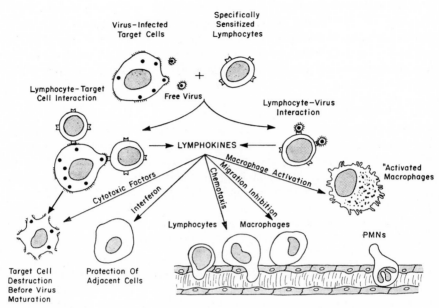

Figure 5—6. Schematic representation depicting the possible events involved in cell-mediated immunity.

that cytophilic Ab produced locally could attach to the surface of macrophages and enhance their capacity to destroy infected cells as well as virions.

Lymphokines which mobilize macrophages chemotactically may also be involved in their "activation." Activated macrophages have enhanced phagocytic and digestive capabilities and could converge and possibly destroy infected target cells before virus maturation and release occur.

The relative importance of Ab, cell-mediated immunity, and interferon is determined in part by the nature of the virus-host cell interaction and in part by the mechanisms concerned in the pathogenesis of the disease. In cytolytic infections accompanied by viremia and in infections of epithelial surfaces, Ab and interferon probably are more important than cell-mediated immunity. In contrast, cellular immune responses appear to play the dominant role in noncytolytic infections, where the cell membrane is antigenically altered and cell-to-cell transfer of viruses is the major mode of spread.

C. Alterations in the Immune Response as a Consequence of Disease or Therapy

1. The Immune Deficiency Diseases

The immunologic deficiency syndromes can be divided into those which involve (a) humoral Ab production (the B-cell system), (b) cellular immunity (the T-cell system), and (c) both humoral and cellular immunity (stem cell functions) (*Fundamentals of Immunology*).

a. **Defective Humoral Antibody Production.** The immune deficiency diseases which involve defects only in humoral Ab production can result in *agammaglobulinemia, hypogammaglobulinemia,* or *dysgammaglobulinemia.* Patients with agammaglobulinemia or hypogammaglobulinemia have reduced levels of all immunoglobulins. In contrast, those with dysgammaglobulinemia have deficiencies in one or more but not all of the immunoglobulin classes.

The term *agammaglobulinemia* is a misnomer, since these patients possess some gamma globulin in their serum. However, the term is retained for historical reasons in current classifications of immune deficiency disorders and refers to conditions in which there are fewer than 100 mg of IgG per 100 ml of plasma. Hypogammaglobulinemics are patients who have in their circulation between 100 and 500 mg of IgG per 100 ml of plasma. In view of the arbitrary nature of these definitions, the term *hypogammaglobulinemia* will be used in this text to refer to those conditions where all of the immunoglobulins are below normal.

Most patients with hypogammaglobulinemia suffer from frequent severe and recurrent bacterial infections but usually recover normally from virus infections and even develop immunity to reinfection.

Dysgammaglobulinemias are disorders which may be caused either by a decreased production or lack of one or more class of immunoglobulin or by the production of functionally abnormal immunoglobulin. Various types of dysgammaglobulinemias have been associated with an impaired capacity to control a number of virus infections and failure to develop a normal Ab response to virus vaccines (Table 5–1). It is not known why patients with selective immunoglobulin deficiencies are less able to resist viral infections than patients with hypogammaglobulinemia.

b. **Defective Cell-mediated Immunity.** There are two diseases which occur when the thymus gland fails to develop normally: (1) *congenital thymic aplasia* (DiGeorge syndrome) and (2) *thymic dysplasia* (Nezelof syndrome). Patients with these diseases show selective deficiencies of cell-mediated immunity but relatively intact humoral immunity.

Infants with congenital thymic aplasia are born without thymus and parathyroid glands (aplasia). This disease entity does not have a hereditary basis and probably represents a defect in early embryonic develop-

TABLE 5—1

Noninfectious Immune Deficiency Diseases Associated with Increased
Susceptibility to Virus Infections

A. *Impaired Humoral Ab Production with Normal Cell-mediated Immunity*
   1. Poliovirus, vaccine strain
   2. ECHO
   3. Serum hepatitis
   4. Cytomegalovirus
   5. Adenovirus
   6. Varicella
   7. Vaccinia

B. *Impaired Cell-mediated Immunity with Normal Humoral Immunity*
   1. Varicella
   2. Vaccinia
   3. Measles

C. *Impaired Humoral and Cell-mediated Immunity*
   1. Vaccinia
   2. Measles
   3. Varicella
   4. Cytomegalovirus
   5. Adenovirus
   6. Herpes simplex

Adapted from Glasgow, L. A.: Interrelationships of interferon and immunity during viral infections. J. Gen. Physiol. *56*:221 Suppl., 1970.

ment. In contrast, thymic dysplasia is an autosomal recessive disorder in which there is faulty development of the thymus gland. This defect presumably results from a failure in the migration of bone marrow stem cells to the thymus, a step prerequisite for the development of the thymus.

Unlike the infections observed in humoral Ab deficiencies, which are primarily bacterial in nature, children born with defects in the thymus gland manifest severe and persistent viral and fungal infections as well as bacterial infections.

c. **Defective Humoral and Cellular Immunity.** As would be expected, the prognosis for patients who possess profound deficiencies in both humoral and cellular immune responses is exceedingly poor.

Thymic dysplasia with hypogammaglobulinemia (Swiss type) is the most severe immunologic defect known. This is an hereditary disease which can be either an autosomal recessive or x-linked recessive disorder. Children born with this disease are characterized by the early onset of severe infections due to certain viral and fungal agents as well as pyogenic and enteric bacteria. Attempted immunization with any live attenuated virus or bacterial vaccine may be fatal.

The Wiskott-Aldrich syndrome is characterized by (1) recurrent infections with a wide variety of agents, including certain viruses, fungi, bacteria, and protozoa; (2) allergic reactions which include bronchial asthma and eczema; (3) reduced levels of circulating Ab, particularly IgM; and (4) thrombocytopenia. These patients may develop overwhelming viral infections involving viruses usually associated with benign clinical illnesses in normal patients. However, some of these patients can handle virus infection early in life without complication. These observations suggest that patients with Wiskott-Aldrich syndrome may develop late defects in cell-mediated immunity. Patients with this syndrome appear to have both a primary defect involving the afferent limb of the Ab response and a secondary and progressive immunologic defect involving the thymus-dependent lymphoid system.

Ataxia telangiectasia is a syndrome transmitted as an autosomal disorder. The victims of this disease appear to be clinically normal from birth until about 2 to 4 years of age. The immunologic disorder, which probably is not the central disturbance in the syndrome, is variable but usually is characterized by a deficiency in IgA, a lack of IgE, and impaired cell-mediated immunity. It is generally agreed that this immunologic deficiency disease is based on a defect in maturation of the thymus-dependent lymphoid tissues. Many of the patients studied had been immunized with the routine virus vaccines prior to the development of clinical illness and seemed not to have had undue complications. However, children with this disease usually experience a progressive bronchiectasis and eventually die of respiratory insufficiency and pneumonia. These chronic infections do not respond well to routine antibiotic therapy. It has been suggested that recurrent viral infections are due to decreased IgA and possibly IgE Ab production.

2. Effects of Viruses on the Immune Response

A number of viruses replicate in cells of the lymphoreticular system which are involved in both specific and nonspecific immunity. As would be expected, viruses which destroy or alter these cells alter the function of the immune system. There is mounting evidence that many leukemia and some nonleukemia viruses which infect lymphoid tissue in experimental animals can either suppress or enhance humoral or cell-mediated immunity. Similarly, viruses can either stimulate or depress interferon production and phagocytosis.

Patients with infectious mononucleosis, hepatitis, and congenital rubella may have enhanced levels of one or more immunoglobulin classes. In contrast, the frequency of hypogammaglobulinemia in congenital rubella suggests that this may be another congenital abnormality which can result from intrauterine infection with rubella virus. Many hypotheses have been proposed to explain how viruses alter humoral Ab production. The adjuvant effect of viruses may be a consequence of stimulation of the immune response afforded by viral nucleic acid. Depressed humoral Ab production obviously could result if either stem cells or B-cells were damaged or destroyed by virus infection.

One parameter of cell-mediated immunity is delayed hypersensitivity. Diminished reactivity to tuberculin has been reported in patients infected with influenza, measles, varicella, and polioviruses. Vaccination with attenuated measles or poliovirus vaccines also produces a temporary impaired response to tuberculin. Another alleged measure of the capacity to develop cellular immunity is the stimulation of lymphocyte blast transformation by phytohemagglutinin (PHA). It has been shown that lymphocytes from patients with infectious mononucleosis, infectious hepatitis, or congenital rubella are depressed in their ability to undergo blast transformation with PHA. Virus infection of the thymus gland or T-cell system could be an important cause of altered cell-mediated immunity

3. Effects of the Malignant State on Susceptibility to Viruses

Altered immune responses may accompany or even contribute to the neoplastic process. Their occurrence in cancer patients can also result from effects superimposed by chemotherapy or radiotherapy. Patients with lymphoid system malignancies are especially prone to infection. In fact, Hodgkin's disease was the first clinical condition in which immune deficiency was observed to be associated with an increased incidence of virus infection. An increase in the incidence and severity of varicella-zoster infections is particularly common in patients with Hodgkin's disease.

Zoster infections appear most frequently at a time when the cell-mediated immune response is maximally depressed as indicated by the presence of cutaneous anergy or abnormalities in lymphocyte transformation *in vitro*. However, viral dissemination reportedly occurs most frequently when two additional elements of the host's defense mechanism are impaired which result in: (1) failure to produce humoral varicella-specific complement-fixing Ab and (2) a reduced level of interferon in vesicle fluid.

An increase in the incidence and severity of varicella-zoster, herpes simplex, and cytomegalovirus infections has been observed in patients with other lymphomas. In chronic lymphocytic leukemia, varicella zoster and vaccinia infections may be severe. However, with a few notable exceptions, individuals with acute leukemia do not appear to have increased susceptibility to viruses. In fact, the beneficial effects of intermittent viral infections on the course of clinical leukemia have been reported for almost 70 years; recently, remissions were reported to follow naturally acquired or artificially transmitted infectious mononucleosis. Clinical improvement has also been reported to follow the inoculation of necrotizing viruses into a patient with acute myelocytic leukemia.

Almost all of the known antileukemia and anticancer agents have been shown to have strongly immunosuppressive side effects. Leukemic patients treated with steroids, drugs, or radiation may develop severe or fatal cytomegalovirus infections which can involve the lung, liver, gastrointestinal tract, and the heart. Varicella-zoster and vaccinia infections also cause severe disease in these patients. Measles infections in leukemic patients on steroid therapy may cause giant cell pneumonia which is frequently fatal. Even immunization of steroid-treated leukemic patients with attenuated virus vaccines can cause severe disease.

4. Immunosuppression Associated with Organ Transplantation

After organ transplantation between unrelated donors, the immune response is deliberately depressed to prevent rejection of the transplanted tissue. The ultimate goal of immunosuppression in these patients is the selective inhibition of cellular immunity with minimal disturbance of the humoral immune response. However, the regimens used, which include Imuran and steroids, affect the primary and secondary Ab responses as well as cellular immunity. Clinical trials with antilymphocyte serum (ALS) suggest that this material may be useful in preventing organ rejection and may be less toxic for the patients than immunosuppressive drugs. However, ALS may also suppress those immunologic mechanisms that are important in the recognition and destruction of potentially malignant cells, a natural mechanism of surveillance against tumors. For example, there are reports that patients given ALS have developed reticulum-cell sarcomas at the site of injection. Similar results have been obtained in experimental animals. Although a viral cause is strongly suggested in certain human lymphomas, no known cases of human reticulum-cell sarcoma have been proved to be of viral origin. Since this possibility cannot be excluded, the potential role of ALS in the induction of malignant lymphoid tumors and activation of potentially oncogenic latent viruses in man cannot be ignored.

Primary or reactivated herpesvirus infections present the most common viral complications in transplant patients not receiving ALS. Although individuals subject to recurrent herpes do not have an increase in herpes simplex reactivation following immunosuppression, herpes simplex pneumonia and disseminated fatal herpes simplex infections have been reported following lung and kidney transplantation, respectively.

Cytomegalovirus (CMV) infection, which is usually inapparent, is the most common infection following kidney transplantation; within two months after transplantation, 91% of these patients have serologic or virologic evidence of infection which probably represents reactivation of a latent virus. This virus is the most common agent associated with pulmonary infections in these patients and also may cause a transient hepatitis or a mononucleosis-like syndrome. There is also evidence of increased infection by human papillomavirus (a papovavirus) in renal transplant patients.

5. Miscellaneous States Associated with Impaired Viral Immunity

Miscellaneous states which are associated with impaired immunity and increased susceptibility to virus infections are listed below.

Neonates who acquire virus infections may experience unusually severe disease. Since host defense mechanisms are not fully developed during neonatal life, the spectrum of maternally acquired Ab largely determines the pattern of resistance to virus infections. For example, newborns with no passive immunity to herpes simplex are prone to develop severe primary herpes infections, whereas newborns with antiherpes IgG are more likely to experience attenuated infections.

In extreme *old age,* cell-mediated immune responses and humoral Ab production are depressed. The incidence of varicella-zoster is 5-fold greater in individuals over 80 years of age than in adults between 20 and 40. The elderly are also more prone to develop severe influenza, often with fatal complications.

Severe malnutrition depresses delayed-type hypersensitivity reactions and has been associated with fatal cases of measles and herpes simplex.

Burn patients sometimes develop fatal disseminated herpetic infections. Data from studies on the immune response following thermal injury in experimental animals have shown that a delay in Ab production occurs as well as diminution in delayed hypersensitivity reactions.

Patients with *eczema* and *atopic dermatitis* have impaired immunologic mechanisms which are believed to play a part in the enhanced dissemination of herpes simplex, vaccinia, and varicella viruses observed in these individuals.

Patients with *Down's syndrome* (mongolism) and *lepromatous leprosy* show an unusually high incidence of Australia Ag which is associated with serum hepatitis. It is possible that suppressed cellular immunity may contribute to the observed increase in chronic anicteric hepatitis observed in these patients.

Psychogenic factors such as stress and depression probably contribute to the exacerbation of herpes simplex infections.

D. Persistent Virus Infections and Latency

Under certain conditions, virus can persist in the body in spite of an apparently normal immune response. Following a primary virus infection, some viruses, such as herpes simplex and varicella-zoster, become latent (hidden) in certain tissues and may later be reactivated to cause clinical illness. In other systems, virus may persist in the absence of subsequent overt disease. It is not known whether the virus persists in an infectious form as a result of limited replication due to the presence of neutralizing Ab and interferon, or if it persists as an noninfectious entity transmitted vertically at cell division. For example, adenoviruses are latent in tonsils and adenoids of healthy individuals but can be "activated" by incubating the tonsil or adenoid tissue *in vitro.*

Not all persistent viruses are latent, and infectious virus can often be demonstrated in chronic infections. Cytomegalovirus is shed in the urine of chronically infected, asymptomatic individuals, and serum hepatitis virus persists for long periods after recovery from hepatitis. Congenital rubella patients with high levels of circulating Ab also shed infectious virus for months after birth.

The persistence of some latent viruses may result from the integration of virus-coded nucleic acid into the host cell genome. The nucleic acid apparently is replicated along with the cell genome prior to cell division and escapes the host's immune and interferon responses by remaining in cells without producing infectious virus (Chapters 3 and 24).

Another mechanism proposed to explain virus persistence in the presence of specific Ab involves a "steady-state" type of infection in which the host cells are not killed by the virus. Examples are the noncytolytic viruses which are transmitted from cell to cell and thus escape the neutralizing activity of humoral Ab. It is not clear why cellular immune mechanisms do not always destroy cells infected with such viruses, especially in those instances in which the antigenic composition of the plasma membrane is altered. A possible explanation is provided by observations that infectious virus in the circulation of mice infected with lactic dehydrogenase (LDH) virus cannot be neutralized by anti-LDH Ab alone but can be neutralized by anti-mouse globulin. Presumably cells carrying virus in their membranes are protected from attack by immune cells by a nonneutralizing Ab which the mouse produces. In an analogous situation, the presence of Ab (blocking Ab) against tumor cell Ags can prevent their destruction by cell-mediated immune mechanisms. Nonneutralizing Ab of this type has been shown to prevent the *in vitro* cytotoxic effect of immune lymphocytes on monolayers of cells carrying a persistent noncytocidal orthomyxovirus infection.

It has been suggested that some chronic virus infections are perpetuated by a continuing balance between viral multiplication and antiviral immunity. Virus multiplication in a chronically infected host would stimulate interferon and Ab production, which in turn would reduce viral replication. As virus multiplication is decreased, these immunologic responses would tend to lessen and thus preserve the balance. Any shift in this delicate balance could result in either the appearance of clinical illness or eradication of the infection.

E. The Interplay of Immune Mechanisms

Recent advances in immunology and virology permit the construction of a unified concept pertaining to the nature of host resistance to viruses based on the combined action of specific and nonspecific factors of immunity. Upon primary encounter with a virus, preexisting nonspecific defense mechanisms may prevent infection. If the virus surmounts these barriers, an infection may be established which induces nonspecific and specific immunologic systems of defense to respond.

Prevention of local dissemination of virus or viremia may be accomplished nonspecifically by the interferon system and various elements of the inflammatory response. Detectable specific immunologic events, consisting of the appearance of humoral Ab and cell-mediated immunity, occur 2 to 5 days after infection. The relative importance of each mechanism of defense will depend upon the virus involved, the portal of entry, mode of dissemination, and the host.

References

ALMEIDA, J. D., and LAWRENCE, G. D.: Heated and unheated antiserum on rubella virus. Amer. J. Dis. Child. *118*:101, 1969.

AVILA, F. R., SCHULTZ, R. M., and TOMPKINS, W. A. F.: Specific macrophage immunity to vaccinia virus: macrophage-virus interaction. Infect. Immun. *6*:9, 1972.

BARON, S.: Host defenses during virus infection. In *Modern Trends in Medical Virology*. R. B. Heath and A. P. Waterson, eds. New York, Appleton-Century-Crofts, 1967.

BARON, S.: The defensive role of the interferon system. J. Gen. Physiol. *56*:193 Suppl., 1970.

BELLANTI, J. A.: Immune deficiency disorders. In *Immunology*. Philadelphia, W. B. Saunders Co., 1971.

BELLANTI, J. A.: Immune mechanisms in viral diseases. In *Immunology*. Philadelphia, W. B. Saunders Co., 1971.

BLANDFORD, G., and HEATH, R. B.: Immunoglobulins in virus disease. In *Modern Trends in Medical Virology*. R. B. Heath and A. P. Waterson, eds. New York, Appleton-Century-Crofts, 1970.

BLUMBERG, B. S., and MELARTIN, L.: Australia antigen and hepatitis—studies in asymptomatic people and lepromatous leprosy patient. Arch. Intern. Med. (Chicago), *125*:287, 1970.

COOPER, M. D., CHASE, H. P., LOWMAN, J. T., KRIVIT, W., and GOOD, R. A.: Immunologic defects in patients with Wiskott-Aldrich syndrome. In *Immunologic Deficiency Diseases in Man*. D. Bergsma, ed. Birth Defects Original Article Series, IV. New York, The National Foundation, 1968.

DALES, S., and KAJIOKA, R.: The cycle of multiplication of vaccinia virus in Earle's strain L-cells. 1. Uptake and penetration. Virology *24*:278, 1964.

DANIELS, C. A., BORSOS, T., RAPP, H. J., SNYDERMAN, R., and NOTKINS, A. L.: Neutralization of sensitized virus by purified components of complement. Proc. Nat. Acad. Sci. USA *65*:528, 1970.

DEODHAR, S. D., KUKLINCA, A. G., VIDT, D. G., ROBERTSON, A. L., and HAZARD, J. B.: Development of reticulum-cell sarcoma at the site of antilymphocyte globulin injection in a patient with renal transplant. New Eng. J. Med. *280*: 1104, 1969.

DOWNIE, J. C.: Neuraminidase- and hemagglutinin-inhibiting antibodies in serum and nasal secretions of volunteers immunized with attenuated and inactivated influenza B/Eng./13/65 virus vaccines. J. Immunol. *105*:620, 1970.

FAZEKAS DE ST. GROTH, S., and DONNELLEY, M.: Studies in experimental immunology of influenza. III. The antibody response. Aust. J. Exp. Biol. Med. *28*:45, 1950.

FENNER, F.: *The Biology of Animal Viruses*. New York, Academic Press, 1968.

FRANCIS, T., JR.: The inactivation of epidemic influenza virus by nasal secretions of human individuals. Science *91*:198, 1940.

FUDENBERG, H., GOOD, R .A., GOODMAN, H. C., HITZIG, W., KUNKEL, H. G., RIOTT, I. M., ROSEN, R. S., ROWE, D. S., SELIGMANN, M., and SOOTHILL, J. R.: Primary immunodeficiencies. Report of a World Health Organization committee. Pediatrics. *47*:927, 1971.

GLASGOW, L. A.: Interrelationships of interferon and immunity during viral infections. J. Gen. Physiol. *56*:212 Suppl., 1970.

GLASGOW, L. A.: Immunosuppression, interferon, and viral infections. Fed Proc. *30*:1846, 1971.

GOOD, R. A.: Disorders of the immune system. In *Immunobiology*. R. A. Good, ed. Stamford, Conn., Sinauer Associates, 1971.

HAMPAR, B., NOTKINS, A. L., MAGE, M., and KEEHN, M. A.: Heterogeneity in the properties of 7S and 19S rabbit-neutralizing antibodies to herpes simplex virus. J. Immunol. *100*:586, 1968.

HEHLMANN, R., KUFE, D., and SPIEGELMAN, S.: Viral-related RNA in Hodgkin's disease and other human lymphomas. Proc. Nat. Acad. Sci. USA *69*:1727, 1972.

HELLSTRÖM, K. E., and HELLSTRÖM, I.: Immunologic defenses against cancer. In *Immunobiology*. R. A. Good, ed. Stamford, Conn., Sinauer Associates, 1971.

JOHNSON, R. T.: *Inflammatory Response to Viral Infections*. Assoc. Res. Nerv. Ment. Dis. L. P. Rowland, ed. Vol. XLIX. Baltimore, Md., Williams & Wilkins Co., 1971.

KILBOURNE, E. D., LAVER, W. G., SCHULMAN, J. L., and WEBSTER, R. G.: Antiviral activity of antiserum specific for an influenza virus neuraminidase. J. Virol. *2*:281, 1968.

MARCUS, P. I., ENGELHARDT, D. L., HUNT, J. M., SEKELLICK, M. J.: Interferon action: inhibition of vesicular stomatitis virus RNA synthesis induced by virion-bound polymerase. Science *174*:593, 1971.

MERIGAN, T. C., and STEVENS, D. A.: Viral infections in man associated with acquired immunological deficiency states. Fed. Proc. *30*:1858, 1971.

MIMS, C. A.: Host defenses against viruses and the latter's ability to counteract them. In *Microbial Pathogenicity in Man and Animals*. H. Smith and J. H. Pearce, eds. New York, Cambridge Univ. Press, 1972.

NOTKINS, A. L., MERGENHAGEN, S. E., and HOWARD, R. J.: Effect of virus infections on the function of the immune system. Ann. Rev. Microbiol. *24*:525, 1970.

PETERSON, R. D. A., and GOOD, R. A.: Ataxia telangiectasia. In *Immunologic Deficiency Diseases in Man*. D. Bergsma, ed. Birth Defects Original Article Series, IV. New York, The National Foundation, 1968.

PORTER, D. D.: Destruction of virus-infected cells by immunological mechanisms. Ann. Rev. Microbiol. *25*:283, 1971.

ROSSEN, R. D., KASEL, J. A., and COUCH, R. B.: The secretory immune systems: its relation to respiratory viral infection. Prog. Med. Virol. *13*:194, 1971.

STEVENS, D. A., LEVINE, P. H., LEE, S. K., SONLEY, M. J., and WAGGONER, D. E.: Concurrent infectious mononucleosis and acute leukemia. Amer. J. Med. *50*: 208, 1971.

TOMASI, T. B., JR.: The concept of local immunity and the secretory system. In *The Secretory Immunologic System*. D. H. Dayton, P. A. Small, Jr., R. M. Chanock, H. E. Kaufman, and T. B. Tomasi, Jr., eds. Proceedings of a conference on the secretory immunologic system held December 10-13, 1969, at Vero Beach, Florida.

WALFORD, R. L., FINKELSTEIN, S., NEERHOUT, R., KONRAD, P., and SHANBROM, E.: Acute childhood leukemia in relation to the HL-A human transplantation genes. Nature *225*:461, 1970.

WEISER, R. S., MYRVIK, Q. N., and PEARSALL, N. N.: *Fundamentals of Immunology.* Philadelphia, Lea & Febiger, 1969.

WILLIAMS, R. C., KENYON, A. J., and HUNTLEY, C. C.: Immunoglobulins, viruses and speculation on their interrelationship in certain human and animal disease states. Blood *31*:522, 1968.

Pathogenesis of Viral Infections

When a susceptible individual becomes infected with a virus, and a certain threshold of virus replication is reached, disease usually becomes apparent. In some cases pathologic changes may be induced by the virus in the absence of detectable virus multiplication. The summation of viral-induced events which result in the symptoms associated with a given stage of disease is determined by the biochemical, immunologic, physiologic, and cytologic changes induced by the infecting virus. The pathogenicity of the virus at the level of the multicellular host is determined by several factors: (1) susceptibility of cells, (2) availability of susceptible cells to the virus, (3) effects of toxic products produced by virus-cell interaction, and (4) the physiologic and immunologic responses of the host.

Viral infections can be subdivided into the following major types: inapparent (subclinical or latent) and apparent (acute or chronic). An *inapparent infection* is one which is not associated with clinical signs of disease. This term is used in contrast to *apparent infection* where there are obvious clinical signs of disease (e.g., cell destruction in poliomyelitis or cell proliferation in human wart virus infections). Apparent infections can be subdivided into *acute* and *chronic*. An *acute infection* usually lasts for a relatively short period of time (days to weeks) and is generally followed by disappearance of the virus from the tissues and organs of the host (e.g., influenza). In contrast, a *chronic viral infection* is characterized by slowly progressing infection which persists for months or years (e.g., infectious hepatitis).

A *latent infection* is a type of inapparent infection in which production of infectious virus is not detectable, and the host and virus appear to be in equilibrium with each other. However, if this equilibrium should be disturbed and multiplication of infectious virus occurs, then apparent disease can develop. There are two general patterns of latent infections recognized in man. One pattern is exemplified by herpes simplex virus type 1, the etiologic agent of coldsores, and the second pattern by varicella virus, the etiologic agent for chickenpox and shingles. Both viruses establish latency by infecting sensory ganglia. Herpes simplex virus type 1 is acquired early in life, establishes a latent infection in trigeminal ganglia, and under conditions of physical, physiologic, or environmental stress abandons its latent state and causes apparent *recurrent* infections (e.g., coldsores).

However, in the case of varicella virus, the first attack by the virus causes chickenpox. Following recovery from chickenpox and production of lifelong immunity to this form of the disease, the virus remains latent in the cells of the dorsal root ganglia, but subject to reactivation by trauma, stress, or malignancy. Reactivation of the latent varicella virus results in a second disease called shingles (herpes zoster). The interval between the two diseases may vary from a few months to as long as 40 years or more.

A.   Virus Entry, Dissemination, Excretion, and Transmission

Since viruses must become intracellular before they can produce disease, it is important that students of medicine know how viruses (1) enter tissues, (2) are disseminated in the host, (3) are excreted, and (4) are transmitted to other individuals.

Under natural conditions, infection of a susceptible host is usually initiated by a small number of virus particles. At the onset of infection, the number of primary foci of infected cells will be few in comparison with the number of cells which ultimately become infected during the height of the disease. Viruses enter the host by a variety of routes: (1) mucous membranes (respiratory tract, alimentary tract, conjunctivae), (2) skin, (3) genital tract, or (4) placenta (Table 6-1). Entry of a particular virus is governed by several factors such as source of infecting virus (direct contact, air or aerosols, water, fomites, insects), distribution of susceptible cells in the host, stability of virus to various conditions (surface integuments, body secretions, pH, temperature, humidity), and age, physiologic and immunologic status of the host.

TABLE 6—1

Entry of Viruses in Man

Route	Viruses
Mucous membranes	
Respiratory tract	Rhinoviruses
	Adenoviruses
	Herpesviruses
	Orthomyxoviruses
	Paramyxoviruses
	Coronaviruses
	Reoviruses[1] (Diplornaviruses)
	Enteroviruses[1]
	Variola
	Rubella
	Mumps
	Rabies[1]
Alimentary tract	Enteroviruses
	Reoviruses (Diplornaviruses)
	Infectious hepatitis virus[1]
	Serum hepatitis virus
	Adenoviruses
Conjunctivae	Rhinoviruses
	Herpesviruses
	Adenoviruses
Skin: as the result of:	
Abrasion	Human papillomavirus
	Molluscum contagiosum
	Orf
Arthropod bite	Togaviruses (Arboviruses)
Animal bite	Rabies, B virus (simian herpes)
Hypodermic needle	Serum hepatitis virus[1]
	Infectious hepatitis virus
Genital tract	Condyloma accuminatum (human papilloma)
	Herpes simplex type 2
Placenta	Rubella[1]
	Cytomegalovirus[1]

[1] Enter more commonly by another route.

1. Mucous Membranes

a. Respiratory Tract. The respiratory tract and alimentary tract are the principal sites of entry for the majority of viruses infecting man. Entry of viruses into the respiratory tract occurs via aerosols or droplets from the nasopharynx of infected individuals. This is an important route of entry for many common respiratory viruses of man; e.g., rhinoviruses, adenoviruses, orthomyxoviruses, paramyxoviruses, coronaviruses, and certain enteroviruses. Evidence suggests that rabies virus may also infect man by this route. The pathogenesis of orthomyxoviruses (influenza A virus) is a suitable model for respiratory viruses. Influenza A virus enters in the form of wet or dry aggregates (droplets) and localizes in the respiratory tract. The virus then attaches to the N-acetyl neuraminic acid receptor on the cell surface of epithelial cells of the upper and (to varying degrees) the lower respiratory tract. Upon entry of the virus core (nucleocapsid), new infectious virus is produced and spreads from cell to cell through intercellular and superficial fluid layers. Multiplication of the virus and its subsequent spread to other cells in the respiratory tract is restricted by (1) specific secretory IgA, (2) production of interferon (natural antiviral component) by infected cells, and (3) mucus which contains a natural glycoprotein that can neutralize the infectivity of extracellular influenza A virus. The consequences of virus multiplication, which is almost always limited to the respiratory tract, are cell necrosis and desquamation of the epithelium of the alveoli, bronchioles, and trachea. The disease is easily spread to other individuals because large amounts of virus are shed in droplets discharged by talking, sneezing, and coughing. Since the incubation period for influenza is short (2 to 3 days), the disease can easily become epidemic in a few weeks. Some viruses (mumps) enter the respiratory tract via droplets, produce a primary infection of the epithelial cells, and then spread via the blood to infect other organs.

b. Alimentary Tract. Enteroviruses are the major group of viruses which infect man by way of the alimentary tract. Because enveloped viruses (e.g., herpes simplex) are inactivated by acid conditions in the stomach, the only viruses which successfully infect the alimentary tract are the nonenveloped viruses (e.g., poliovirus, adenoviruses, reoviruses, and hepatitis viruses). Virus infection occurs by way of fomites or consumption of contaminated food or drink. In the case of poliovirus infection, the virus initially multiplies in the pharynx and lymphoid tissues (tonsils and Peyer's patches) and then in the epithelial cells lining the small intestine. Spread of virus to the draining lymph nodes leads to viremia and dissemination of virus throughout the body. During the viremic stage of the disease, the infection may spread to the anterior horn cells of the spinal cord and motor cortex of the brain. The probability of neural damage with paralysis is influenced by several factors including age, pregnancy, trauma, and inoculations. Excretion of virus occurs in the feces.

c. **Conjunctivae.** The conjunctivae may serve as a portal of entry for many of the viruses which cause upper respiratory tract infections including the rhinoviruses (common cold), herpesviruses, and certain adenoviruses. The source of infection can be nasopharyngeal secretions (e.g., rhinoviruses), latent infections of the trigeminal nerve root ganglia (e.g., herpesviruses), water from swimming pools or dust (e.g., adenoviruses). Also, the conjunctiva is a sensitive indicator of some systemic viral diseases such as measles and certain enteroviruses.

Herpes simplex virus type 1 is an etiologic agent of keratoconjunctivitis, causing serious eye infection which can lead to blindness. The basic lesion is a "dendritic ulcer," a creeping tree-like ulcer of the cornea. Spread of virus to the deeper layers of the cornea results in severe necrosis. Recurrent infections of the cornea are common in some patients because of reactivation of a latent herpes simplex virus in the trigeminal nerve root ganglia.

2. Skin

The normal skin acts as a natural barrier against most virus infections. Viruses may enter through the skin by way of (1) abrasions (e.g., molluscum contagiosum, orf, human papillomavirus), (2) bites of infected arthropods (e.g., togaviruses), (3) animal bites or licks on an abraded area (e.g., rabies), or (4) hypodermic needles (e.g., hepatitis viruses). Most viral skin diseases (e.g., measles, rubella, varicella, smallpox) occur following entry of virus by the respiratory route and subsequent systemic spread of the virus by way of macrophages, lymphocytes, or other leukocytes. Rabies virus spreads in man by way of dorsal root ganglion cells of peripheral nerves serving the inoculated area. The only localized viral infections of the skin in man are caused by the human papillomavirus and the proliferative inflammatory lesions of the skin produced by poxviruses (e.g., vaccinia, molluscum contagiosum, and orf). More commonly, the rashes seen in the exanthemata of childhood (e.g., varicella, measles, rubella) are considered to be allergic in nature resulting from a "IgE-like" Ab on mast cells reacting with viral Ag(s) in the skin or associated with the capillary endothelium. The viral Ag(s) originates from viruses which have attached to cells of the vascular walls and produced a focus of infection.

With respect to excretion and transmission of virus responsible for skin infections, it is notable that poxviruses (e.g., orf, variola) are sufficiently resistant to drying that they persist in an infectious state in scabs and exfoliating epidermis or bedding and clothing for extended periods. Varicella virus also is transmitted by materials from lesions, whereas measles virus is excreted and transmitted by secretions from the nose, throat, or the conjunctivae.

3. Genital Tract

Two human viruses, a papillomavirus which causes genital warts (condyloma acuminatum) and herpes simplex virus type 2, are spread by sexual intercourse. The virus of condyloma acuminatum causes a marked proliferation of cells of the epidermis with extensive hyperkeratosis. Virus is found mainly in the keratinized layers of the wart. Acidophilic inclusions may be found in cell nuclei and more rarely in the cytoplasm. This is the only type of human wart that becomes malignant. Herpes simplex virus type 2 is acquired early in adulthood and is usually retained in the body for life. Although rare, severe and often fatal disease can be acquired by the infant at the time of birth from virus present in the mother's vagina. The infant's skin becomes covered with vesicles which rupture to form ulcers. Systemic dissemination of the virus often occurs which can develop into hepatitis, meningitis, encephalitis, or meningoencephalitis.

4. Placenta

Entry of virus through the placenta represents a specialized route of infection. Rubella virus may cross the placenta and exert its teratogenic (production of abnormal development) action especially on the lens, heart, and brain of the fetus. Cytomegalovirus also crosses the placenta and infects the fetus which usually dies *in utero* or may be born with permanent neurologic sequelae attributable to microcephaly and microgyria (convolution of the brain). The virus can sometimes be isolated from the mother's urine. The fact that subsequent babies are not affected by cytomegalovirus infection indicates that active infection of the mother persists for only a few months. Several other viruses may infect the fetus and lead to abortion. For example, if a virus infection occurs late during pregnancy, the baby may be born with an acute viral disease caused by herpes simplex virus type 2; a similar circumstance can occur with varicella virus or poliovirus. There is speculation that leukoviruses also may be passed *in utero*. Evidence for this mode of transmission has been obtained with viruses causing leukemia (Chapter 24) in animals.

B. Factors Influencing the Incubation Period

The *incubation period* of a viral infection is the interval between infection and the first manifestation of symptoms. It will be short (1 to 3 days) in diseases in which the symptoms are due to viral growth at the site of entry, as in respiratory tract infections (Table 6-2). In contrast, a moderate to long incubation period (5 to 30 days) is associated with generalized infection (chickenpox, measles, rubella, mumps). In these diseases virus

TABLE 6–2

Periods of Incubation and Communicability of Some Common
Viral Diseases in Man

Disease	Mode of Transmission	Incubation Period[a] (Days)	Period of Communi-cability[b]	Incidence of Subclinical Infections[c]
Influenza	Respiratory	2–3	Short	Moderate
Common Cold	Respiratory	1–3	Short	Moderate
Bronchiolitis	Respiratory	3–5	Short	Moderate
Eastern equine encephalitis	Mosquito bite	3–5	Short	Low
Dengue	Mosquito bite	5–8	Short	Moderate
Herpes simplex infection	Contact	5–8	Long	Moderate
Enterovirus infection	Alimentary	6–12	Long	High
Poliomyelitis	Alimentary	5–20	Long	High
Measles	Respiratory	9–12	Moderate	Low
Smallpox	Respiratory	12–14	Moderate	Low
Chickenpox	Respiratory	13–17	Moderate	Moderate
Mumps	Respiratory	16–20	Moderate	Moderate
Rubella	Respiratory	17–20	Moderate	Moderate
Mononucleosis	Contact	30–50	? Long	High
Hepatitis (infectious)	Alimentary	15–40	Long	High
Hepatitis (serum)	Hypodermic needle	50–150	Very Long	High
Rabies	Animal bite, Respiratory	30–100	None	None
Warts	Contact	50–150	Long	Low

[a] Until first appearance of prodromal symptoms. Diagnostic signs (e.g., rash or paralysis) may not appear until 2 to 4 days later.
[b] Most viral diseases are highly transmissible for a few days before symptoms appear. Short = 1–4 days. Moderate = 5–9 days. Long = 10–30 days. Very long = months–years.
[c] High ≈ 90%; low ≈ 10%.
(Modified from Fenner, F., and White, D.: Medical Virology. New York, Academic Press, 1970.)

enters the respiratory tract and then spreads in a stepwise fashion in the host before producing disease in the target organ. The length of the incubation period can be influenced by other factors; for example, the direct intravenous injection of togaviruses by an infected arthropod would result in a short (1 to 4 days) incubation period. On the other hand, the long incubation period which characterizes human papillomavirus infection (warts) is due to the unusually slow growth rate for these viruses. A phenomenon of great importance, which at present is poorly understood, is the unusually long incubation period of the so-called neurologic virus diseases (Chapter 22) in which virus-cell interaction is initially non-cytocidal and symptoms of disease are not apparent for many months or even years after infection.

C. Pathogenetic Patterns

Viruses characteristically infect certain organs of the body and not others (i.e., display tropism) and may follow prescribed pathogenetic patterns. Poliomyelitis can serve as a useful example to illustrate the pathogenetic pattern of viral disease (Fig. 6–1). In this disease, virus enters by way of the alimentary tract and multiplies in the oropharyngeal mucosa, the tonsils, Peyer's patches, or lymph nodes which drain these tissues. Virus then begins to appear in the throat and feces and is spread

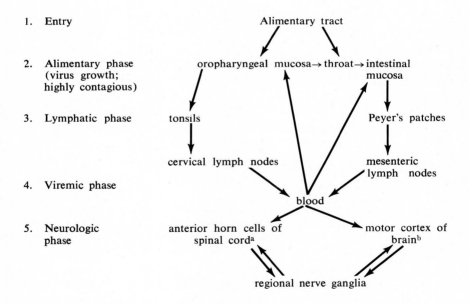

Figure 6–1. Pathogenetic pattern of poliovirus in a nonimmune individual.

[a] Infection of anterior horn cells of spinal cord or brain stem results in bulbar polio; usually fatal due to cardiac and respiratory failure.
[b] Infection of motor cortex results in encephalitic type; only 1 to 2% infections invade CNS and give rise to paralytic clinical syndrome.

via the blood to other susceptible tissues (distant lymph nodes and CNS). If virus multiplication reaches a high level in the CNS, the disease may become fatal or motor neurons are destroyed and paralysis follows. Involvement of the CNS may be prevented by poliovirus-neutralizing Abs induced by prior infection or by vaccination.

D. Concepts of Viral Pathogenesis

There are two primary types of pathogenesis which may follow virus-host interactions: (1) cell injury or destruction and (2) neoplastic transformation. In discussing mechanisms of pathogenesis of disease both viral aspects and host responses to the virus-host cell complex must be considered.

1. Virus-related Pathogenesis

a. **Cell Injury or Destruction.** The majority of human viral illnesses are acute rather than chronic in nature. Cellular injury or destruction during acute disease may be caused in several ways: (1) general toxic effect produced directly by virions (e.g., penton protein of adenoviruses) or by toxic products released from the infected cells which also may be responsible for symptoms of fever, headache, and malaise which accompany many viral diseases; (2) synthesis of a virus-coded protein(s) which specifically blocks cellular biosynthesis; (3) induction of chromosomal aberrations in host cells thereby inhibiting cell mitosis; or (4) production of viral inclusion bodies (i.e., intracellular masses of new viral material) which may disrupt the structure and function of host cells to cause their death.

In some cases of exanthematous disease caused by rubella, rubeola, variola, varicella, and certain togaviruses, a severe form of viral disease occurs which involves hemorrhagic eruptions and disseminated intravascular coagulation. The organs most frequently involved include the kidney, brain, pituitary, lungs, liver, adrenals, and intestinal mucosa. The generalized spread of exanthematous viruses is sometimes associated with a defective immune response or RES suppression by radiation, drugs, or corticosteroid therapy. Following viremia, the endothelial cells of the visceral blood vessels become infected. When infected endothelial cells are injured, platelets agglutinate and thrombi are formed at the site. The mechanisms of pathogenesis may include (1) direct agglutination of platelets by the virus, (2) cell injury which may predispose to platelet agglutination and thrombus formation, or (3) replication of the virus in endothelial cells which may form Ag-Ab complexes capable of initiating intravascular coagulation. The morbidity and mortality associated with the severe forms of exanthematous diseases can be reduced by anticoagulant therapy (e.g., heparin).

b. Neoplastic Transformation. The interaction between potential on-cogenic (cancer-producing) viruses and host cells can result in virus multiplication with or without transformation of the cell. For example, it is known that in animals infected with leukoviruses most organs are producing new infectious virus. However, the incidence of neoplastic transformation is low in terms of the total number of cells infected. Although cancer cells may produce infectious virus, multiplication of the virus is not required for neoplastic transformation. However, the presence of virus genetic information is required. Neoplastic transforma-tion, manifested by alterations in the cell plasma membrane, changes in cell morphology and orientation, presence of tumor-specific Ags, and the capacity to grow at an increased rate *in vivo,* is dependent upon integra-tion and expression of the virus genome. Neoplastic transformation of Ab-precursor cells by leukoviruses may reduce the total number of Ab-producing cells, the amount of Ab produced per cell, and the class of immunoglobulin produced. Presumably a combination of these effects accounts for the immunodepression associated with leukemia.

2. Host-related Pathogenesis

a. Inflammatory Reactions. During the course of a virus disease in-fected cells become altered, thereby eliciting an inflammatory response which is generally related to release of virus or diffusion of certain by-products from the injured or destroyed cells. The nature of the in-flammatory response may give a specific clinical character to the lesions produced by a given virus (e.g., localized lesions with herpes simplex and maculopapular lesions with measles). Infection of neuronal cells in man by poliovirus causes an inflammatory response characterized by an intense perivascular infiltration of inflammatory cells which may result in accumulation of macrophages and host cell death. In contrast to acute bacterial diseases, the inflammatory cells in viral infections are pre-dominately mononuclear cells consisting of macrophages, plasmacytes, and lymphocytes. A transitory polymorphonuclear cell infiltration of the infected site may occur on occasion. Leukopenia is a general characteristic of the acute phase of viral infections; the leukocyte count often decreases to 3000 per mm^3.

b. Humoral- and Cell-mediated Immunopathology. In some viral diseases immune mechanisms of the host are responsible for the patho-genesis of disease. This view has evolved from the consideration that maternal serum Ab (IgG) passively acquired by young infants does not provide protection against the most severe form of obstructive bronchiolitis associated with respiratory syncytial (RS) virus infections but instead may cause the condition. Children over two years of age seem to develop a less severe form of the disease because they lack specific maternal IgG Ab which is evidently responsible for injury in young infants. Injury results from complement lysis due to the reaction of maternal IgG with virus Ag(s) on the surface of infected cells or with extracellular soluble Ag(s) to form cytophilic immune complexes. Other respiratory viruses do not produce RS virus-like disease because of their failure to cause a high incidence of infection during the first year of life when specific maternal IgG is present in the infant's serum.

The pathogenesis of some viral diseases may be directly related to immunologic alterations induced by the infecting virus. For example, it is known that viruses can profoundly affect humoral immunity (e.g., rubella, leukoviruses), cellular immunity (measles, influenza, varicella, polio, hepatitis, and Epstein-Barr (EB) viruses) and phagocytosis by the RES (e.g., mumps, influenza, and coxsackievirus). Several hypotheses have been proposed to explain the mechanisms of immunodepression by viruses: (1) alteration in Ag uptake, (2) depression of Ab synthesis, (3) destruction of Ab-producing cells and their precursors, and (4) competition between the infecting virus and immunizing Ag for noncommitted Ab-producing cells. Lymphocytes from individuals infected with infectious hepatitis virus are defective in their ability to undergo blast transformation and neutrophils infected with mumps, influenza, or coxsackieviruses have a reduced capacity to phagocytize bacteria.

Virus-induced tissue damage can stimulate the production of tissue-specific immunoglobulins, particularly with enveloped viruses which form their outer coat from cell membranes. In this way the new virions from damaged cells carry cell Ags which stimulate the production of anti-cell immunoglobulins. Evidently virus-induced immunopathologic mechanisms play a role in the pathogenesis of (1) certain chronic virus infections (e.g., hepatitis), (2) disseminated intravascular coagulation in exanthematous diseases, (3) chronic viral glomerulonephritis, (4) "autoimmune" disease, and (5) malignancy.

There is strong evidence that delayed-type hypersensitivity to viral Ags may be important in the pathogenesis of some viral diseases. For example, in a small proportion of measles (rubeola) cases, postinfection encephalitis may occur 1 to 2 weeks following disappearance of the rash. Although measles virus cannot be isolated from the brain, lymphocytic infiltration and demyelination changes are apparent. Another example is vaccinia infection of the skin in which dermal swelling, edema, and vesicle formation in the epidermis are thought to represent a delayed-type hypersensitivity response. Arthus-type vascular lesions may also result from the complexing of circulating Ab with vaccinia virus Ags present in blood vessel walls.

E.   Pathogenesis of Congenital Viral Infections

Tremendous interest in the action of viruses on the fetus developed following the observations that cytomegalovirus, rubella, and possibly leukemia viruses (Chapter 24) are acquired from the mother *in utero*. Interaction between virus and fetus results in either (1) no effect on the fetus, (2) fetal death with abortion, or (3) fetal infection with resulting malformation. It has been firmly established that maternal infection with cytomegalovirus, rubella virus, or vaccinia virus can result in fetal damage. However, it should be pointed out that in most instances infection of the mother produces no detectable effect on the growth and development of the fetus.

Infection of the fetus may occur early or late in pregnancy; for example, infections with varicella, measles, or coxsackievirus have been reported to occur shortly before term.

Whereas many viruses fail to infect the fetus *in utero,* it is possible for the fetus to become severely infected during birth with herpes simplex virus type 2 from genital lesions in the mother's vagina.

Rubella and cytomegalovirus will be discussed in detail because the most comprehensive studies on congenital defects have been done with infants of mothers infected with these agents. Rubella or cytomegaloviruses enter the fetus from maternal blood by establishing foci of infection in the placenta. During early fetal development the viruses spread from cell to cell. During late fetal development the manner of spread is similar to that found after birth.

Rubella virus growing in fetal cells may cause cell necrosis and chromosome breaks with a concomitant loss of cell division or reduced mitotic rate. These effects are accompanied by drastic changes in the growth rate and development of fetal structures and are characterized clinically by hepatosplenomegaly, purpura, hemorrhage, jaundice, and other signs of disseminated infection involving the ears, eyes, bone structure, and heart. Severe cases are often fatal soon after birth. Unlike many nonviral teratogens, rubella virus may persist throughout early postnatal life and continue to damage tissues and influence development for several months. Persistence of infectious rubella virus in congenitally infected infants is probably due to chronic infection of thymus-derived lymphocytes since these infants are not able to mount a cell-mediated response against the virus. Although its inflammatory response is relatively weak, the fetus has some ability to repair viral damage by replacing necrotic cells. The outcome of infection depends on the effectiveness of reparative processes. The fetus is capable of producing IgM Abs to rubella virus, but the response is only primary and the amount of Ab made is minimal. However, the antiviral substance interferon is produced (Chapter 7). The synthesis of Ab and interferon depends on the stage of fetal development the greatest amounts being produced near term. After birth, rubella virus is slowly eliminated by immune mechanisms and by attrition of infected mitotically inhibited cell clones.

Cytomegalovirus infection in adults usually remains latent. However, during pregnancy latent infection occasionally becomes activated with resulting viremia and passage of virus across the placenta to the fetus. The important clinical features in neonates include hepatosplenomegaly, thrombocytopenic purpura, hepatitis with jaundice, microcephaly, and mental retardation. In contrast to rubella virus infections, most of the congenital abnormalities following cytomegalovirus infection are the result of destruction of formed organs rather than defects in organogenesis.

References

CHANOCK, R. M., KAPIKIAN, A. Z., and MILLS, J.: Influence of immunological factors in respiratory syncytial virus disease of the lower respiratory tract. Arch. Environ. Health. 21:347, 1970.

FENNER, F.: The Biology of Animal Viruses. Vol. II. The Pathogenesis and Ecology of Viral Infections. New York, Academic Press, 1968.

LEIDER, W., MAGOFFIN, R. L., LENNETTE, E. H., and LEONARDS, L. N. R.: Herpes simplex-virus encephalitis: its possible association with reactivated latent infection. New Eng. J. Med. 273:391, 1965.

McKAY, D., and MARGARETTEN, W.: Disseminated intravascular coagulation in virus diseases. Arch. Intern. Med. (Chicago) 120:129, 1967.

MIMS, C. A.: Aspects of the pathogenesis of virus diseases. Bacteriol. Rev. 28:30, 1964.

MIMS, C. A.: Pathogenesis of rashes in virus diseases. Bacteriol. Rev. 30:739, 1966.

MIMS, C. A.: Pathogenesis of viral infections of the fetus. Progr. Med. Virol. 10:194, 1968.

NOTKINS, A. L. MERGENHAGEN, S. E., and HOWARD, R. J.: Effect of virus infection on the function of the immune system. Ann. Rev. Microbiol. 24:525, 1970.

PORTER, D. D.: Destruction of virus infected cells by immunological mechanisms. Ann. Rev. Microbiol. 25:283, 1971.

SMITH, H.: Mechanism of virus pathogenicity. Bacteriol. Rev. 36:291, 1972.

SMITH, H., and PEARCE, J. H., eds.: Microbial Pathogenicity in Man and Animals. Symposium 22. New York, Cambridge University Press, 1972.

STEVENS, J. G., and COOK, M. L.: Restriction of herpes simplex virus by macrophages: an analysis of the cell-virus interaction. J. Exp. Med. 133:19, 1971.

Chapter 7

Control of Viral Infections

A. Approaches to the Control of Viral Infections

Considerable success has been achieved in the treatment of bacterial diseases by the use of chemotherapeutic agents. Consequently, an intensive search for chemical substances for use in the prevention or treatment of viral diseases has emerged. There are three practical approaches to the control of viral illnesses: immunologic, chemoprophylactic, and the use of interferon (Table 7–1). Immunologic procedures have afforded significant protection against many viral diseases (Table 7–2). Recent successes with drugs that modify the course of viral infections have been encouraging. The artificial induction of interferon, a natural antiviral agent, provides a new approach for enhancing resistance against viral diseases. In addition, general supportive therapy continues to be an essential part of the treatment of all viral diseases.

TABLE 7—1

Efficacy of Approaches Used for Controlling Viral Infections

Approach	Level of Effectiveness	Characteristic Antiviral Spectrum	Duration of Effect
Immunologic	Usually high	Very narrow	Relatively long
Chemoprophylactic	Moderate	Narrow	Very short
Interferon	Moderate to high	Very broad	Relatively short

B. Vaccines

1. Active Immunization

Active immunization with vaccines is a highly effective means for controlling a number of viral diseases. The concept of using viruses for human "vaccination" originated nearly two centuries ago when an English country doctor, Edward Jenner, scratched the arm of a Gloucestershire farm boy and deliberately contaminated the wound with pus from a milkmaid's cowpox sores in a trial to prevent smallpox. Since that time routine vaccination for smallpox has been a cornerstone of public-health practice. However, the American Academy of Pediatrics is currently supporting an earlier recommendation of the United States Public Health Service that routine vaccination of children for smallpox be discontinued. This change in policy is actually based on a review that six to eight deaths due to severe reactions to smallpox vaccination occur annually in the United States. This statistic weighed against the fact that the disease is currently endemic in only seven countries of the world (Ethiopia, Sudan, India, Nepal, Pakistan, Afghanistan, and Indonesia) prompted the new policy. Whereas routine vaccination for smallpox is being discontinued, the use of live-virus vaccines is being recommended for other diseases in need of control, especially in instances in which (1) the antigenic types of the etiologic agents are few, (2) there is systemic invasion of the host, and (3) highly effective immunity follows a natural infection; e.g., measles, mumps, rubella, poliomyelitis, and yellow fever. In contrast, a disease (1) which is caused by numerous antigenic types, (2) in which the infection is superficial, and (3) in which naturally acquired immunity is not long lasting generally can be successfully controlled by the use of killed-virus vaccines; e.g., influenza. Viruses of certain groups, such as the rhinoviruses and certain enteroviruses of many antigenic types, cannot be controlled in a practical way with either live- or killed-virus vaccines.

Vaccines consist of either live attenuated (reduced virulence) or inactivated (dead) viruses. The principles of animal virus genetics have been utilized for developing attenuated poliovirus vaccines. It is possible

TABLE 7—2

Present Status of Vaccines against Important Human Viral Infections

Virus	Vaccine status	
	Existing[a]	In Developmental Stage
Vaccinia	Live	Live, further attenuated; killed
Rabies	Killed; live	Killed, tissue-culture grown
Togaviruses		
Yellow fever	Live	None
WEE, EEE, VEE[b]	Killed (animal)	Live (animal); killed (man)
Japanese B encephalitis	Killed	Killed, tissue-culture grown; live, tissue-culture grown
RSSE[c]	Killed (Soviet)	Killed, tissue-culture grown
Rubella (German measles)	Live	None
Respiratory complex		
Influenza A and B	Killed; live (Soviet)	Live (hybrid virus) Killed; viral subunits
Adenovirus[d]	Live	Viral subunit
Parainfluenza 1, 2, and 3	None	Killed, purified and concentrated; live
Respiratory syncytial	None	Killed, purified and concentrated; live
Rhinovirus	None	Killed; live
Enteroviruses		
Polioviruses	Killed; live	None
ECHO and Coxsackie	None	None
Systemic paramyxoviruses		
Measles	Live; killed	Killed; viral subunits
Mumps	Killed; live	None
Herpesvirus group		
Herpes simplex	None	Killed
B virus (simian herpes)	None	Killed

[a] Now licensed in the U. S.
[b] Western, Eastern, and Venezuelan equine encephalomyelitis viruses
[c] Russian spring-summer encephalitis
[d] Removed from commercial distribution because of oncogenicity of most serotypes

(Modified from Hilleman, M. R.: Toward the control of viral infections of man. Science *164*:506, 1969.)

to obtain a wide variety of temperature-sensitive (ts) mutants (i.e., having inability to multiply at 40° C) from the wild-type polioviruses or select for genetic changes that affect the viral capsid. The ts mutants maintain immunogenicity but lose their neurovirulence properties. Although a single-step mutant has an appreciable leak or reversion rate back to the wild type, this problem is circumvented by selection of multiple-step mutants (e.g., mutants with altered capsids which are unable to grow at 40° C). Alternately, the procedure used for producing the attenuated viruses currently employed in many vaccines was deliberate and repeated serial passage of the original human wild-type virus in embryonated eggs or non-human tissue cultures. This procedure resulted in the chance selection of strains of viruses which have greatly reduced virulence for man (e.g., yellow fever, measles, mumps, and rubella vaccines). Once a suitable virus strain is developed and tested for safety, and its immunogenicity is established in animals and human volunteers, a large volume of a single seed stock of virus can be stored in an unaltered state for many years and used for production of large batches of vaccine from time to time.

Inactivated vaccines are preparations of "dead" virus in which virus infectivity has been destroyed, usually by treatment with formalin. The only inactivated-virus vaccine in widespread use today is influenza vaccine. A survey of the current status of vaccines available for use against important viral infections is presented in Table 7–2. The vaccines currently available for administration together with the schedules for immunization are listed in Table 7–3. Table 7–4 lists the advantages and disadvantages

TABLE 7–3
Immunization Schedules for Virus Vaccines

Vaccines	Recommendations for First Injection	Recommendations for Booster Injection(s)
Live Vaccines		
Smallpox	Before travel abroad[1]	? Presently not recommended[1]
Poliomyelitis	2 to 6 months of age	One year later and then every 5 years
Yellow fever	Before travel through endemic areas	Every 10 years
Measles[2]	1 year of age	? Presently not recommended
Rubella[2]	1 year of age	? Presently not recommended
Mumps[2]	1 year of age	? Presently not recommended
Inactivated Vaccines		
Influenza	Autumn before expected epidemic	2 months later and then annually if indicated
Rabies	Immediately after bite or lick by rabid animal	Daily for 14 days

[1] Vaccination required only when traveling to areas where smallpox is endemic or where smallpox cases have recently been reported.

[2] Measles, rubella, and mumps vaccines are now available in a trivalent virus vaccine.

TABLE 7—4

Advantages and Disadvantages of Live- vs. Inactivated-virus Vaccines

Advantages	Disadvantages
Live-virus Vaccines	
Administered in single dose[1]	Possibility of live virus reverting to virulence
Administered by natural or unnatural route	Possibility of natural spread[2]
Wide spectrum of immunoglobulins produced (IgG, IgM, IgA) and cell-mediated immunity	Cancer virus contaminants
Possibility of local suppression of wild-type virus infection	Viral interference by existing viral infection may prevent good immune response
	Lability of live virus
Inactivated-virus Vaccines	
Use of polyvalent vaccines	Booster doses needed
Stability	No development of secretory IgA
No natural spread	High concentration of virus-antigen needed

[1] Booster dose may be required.
[2] Particularly important with rubella if the vaccine strain were teratogenic.

of live-virus and inactivated-virus vaccines. There is a general consensus among clinical virologists that live-virus vaccines produce subclinical infections which probably lead to the same type of immune response as is seen following natural infection. Usually, a single dose of live-virus vaccine produces prolonged immunity; however, in the case of poliomyelitis and yellow fever, revaccination is recommended (Table 7–3). It is noteworthy that live-virus vaccines are not completely free of possible dangers or drawbacks such as contamination with live animal cancer viruses, interference by a preexisting virus (such as interference of poliovirus vaccine by enterovirus), and the lability of such vaccines. Inactivated-virus vaccines are free from most of the potential dangers associated with live-virus vaccines, but the disadvantages are that large amounts of virus Ag must be administered and several booster injections are required. Some of these difficulties may soon be overcome, particularly with influenza, through the use of disrupted virions as "subunit" vaccines. With the advent of many new vaccines and the expectation that others will be available in the near future (Table 7–2), efforts are being made to develop more simplified methods for vaccine administration through the use of combined polyvalent vaccines and intranasal administration of vaccines. Ex-

amples of combined vaccines include poliovirus-DPT (diphtheria, per-
tussis, tetanus) vaccine and a combination of measles, mumps, and rubella
in a trivalent vaccine. The intranasal administration of a live "hybrid"
influenza A virus vaccine is currently being tested for efficacy and safety
in human volunteers.

2. Passive Immunization

Protection against viral diseases can also be achieved by prophylactic
administration of immune serum. Inoculation of immune serum or immunoglobulin before infection or early in the incubation period may prevent or modify diseases with long incubation periods (greater than 12
days) such as measles, rabies, infectious hepatitis, poliomyelitis, and
mumps, as well as viral diseases which are associated with viremia (e.g.,
smallpox, encephalitis).

Human immunoglobulin has proved to be effective in the prophylaxis
of infectious and serum hepatitis. However, it should be emphasized that
passive immunization should only be regarded as an emergency procedure
for the immediate and short-term protection of unimmunized individuals
at special risk. Passive immunization is effective in measles if the immunoglobulin is administered within 5 or 6 days following exposure to the disease. Passive immunization is less effective against chickenpox and is of
questionable value in preventing congenital abnormalities in pregnant
women exposed to rubella. In suspected rabies, combined active and passive immunization should be considered. Because of the frequent complications associated with the use of rabies immunoglobulin of equine
origin, a human rabies immunoglobulin has been developed in volunteers
and is currently being tested for efficacy.

Because of the availability of viral vaccines, the use of immunoglobulin
is recommended only for the prophylaxis of infectious and serum hepatitis
and rabies virus infections.

3. Virus Neutralization by Specific Immunoglobulins

The mechanism of virus neutralization by specific Ab does not require
saturation of the virion with Ab molecules. In fact, a single Ab molecule
is usually sufficient to neutralize the infectivity of a virus particle. Neutralized virions may or may not adsorb and penetrate host cells, depending
on the number of neutralizing Abs attached to the virion. However, when
such virions become intracellular they are inactivated by cellular enzymes
and fail to initiate an infection.

Experiments with agammaglobulinemic patients indicate that they recover from viral infections in a normal fashion despite low levels of
immunoglobulin (Chapter 5). This observation has led to a reassessment
of the possible role of cell-mediated immunity and interferon activity in

recovery from viral diseases. Animal experiments involving lymphocyte transfer, neonatal thymectomy, and antilymphocyte serum support the view that cell-mediated immunity plays an important role in recovery from viral diseases. However, the precise mechanisms involved are not known.

C. Antiviral Prophylactic and Therapeutic Drugs

The discovery of antibiotics which are highly effective against bacterial diseases has stimulated an extensive search for drugs of comparable value for preventing or curing viral diseases. Modest success has been achieved, and the future looks promising.

The most encouraging results in chemoprophylaxis of viral infections have come from work with the following agents: (1) thiosemicarbazones (methyl-isatin-β-thiosemicarbazone, methisazone) given orally for protection against smallpox, (2) amantadine (Symmetrel) for prophylaxis against influenza, and (3) metabolic inhibitors (including iododeoxyuridine, trifluorothymidine) for treating corneal infections caused by herpes simplex virus type 1. The best hope for therapy of viral diseases depends on the development of drugs which can selectively block viral synthesis, reduce tissue damage, and enhance the resistance of the host. The search for useful antiviral drugs is made difficult by the very close relationship and dependence of viruses upon host cell biosynthetic processes, the fact that total virus multiplication in the host is nearly complete by the time

TABLE 7—5

Mechanism of Action of Prophylactic and Therapeutic Agents

Site and Action	Example
Neutralization of extracellular virus	Specific Ab*
Inhibition of virus penetration	Amantadine (Symmetrel)*
Inhibition of viral nucleic acid synthesis	Iododeoxyuridine (IUdR, Stoxil), trifluoromethyldeoxyuridine, cytosine arabinoside (ara-C)
Inhibition of viral transcription	Rifampin, actinomycin D
Inhibition of viral translation	Thiosemicarbazones, methisazone, puromycin, cycloheximide
Inhibition of virus release	Specific Ab against neuraminidase
Inhibition of cytopathic or histopathic effects	? Anti-inflammatory drugs
Suppression of symptoms in the host	? Anti-inflammatory drugs
Enhancement of host recovery	Agents that stimulate interferon* and/or immune responses

* Mainly effective only as prophylactic agents.

symptoms appear, and the emergence of drug-resistant mutants. Several compounds have been found which inhibit both cellular and viral biosynthetic events. For example, puromycin and cycloheximide block both cellular and viral protein synthesis, whereas actinomycin D inhibits transcription of DNA to mRNA. Although these drugs are not suitable for human use, they are valuable tools for use in elucidating the mechanisms involved in virus replication (Chapter 3).

It is now well accepted that there are several viral-specific sites concerned with virus replication which can be attacked by antiviral drugs (Table 7–5). The ideal antiviral drug is one which would inhibit intracellular viral multiplication without harming the host cells. An alternative approach to therapy is to seek means of counteracting the effects of viral pathogenesis rather than the virus itself. Since the pathogenesis of certain viral infections (e.g., viral exanthems) is concerned in part with specific hypersensitization and other immune phenomena (Chapter 6), anti-inflammatory drugs have been found to be beneficial.

1. Thiosemicarbazones

The thiosemicarbazones (Fig. 7–1) and Rifampin (discussed below) are of special interest because they provide a link between bacterial and

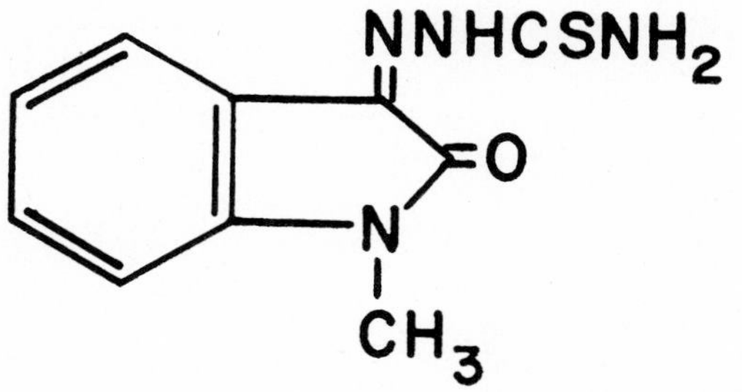

Figure 7–1. Structural formula of N-methyl-isatin-β-thiosemicarbazone (methisazone).

viral chemotherapeutic agents (Chapter 6, *Fundamentals of Bacteriology and Mycology*). Originally, the only known antimicrobial effects of the thiosemicarbazones was their tuberculostatic activity. It was later found that methyl-isatin-β-thiosemicarbazone (methisazone) was active against vaccinia or smallpox viruses when given orally or subcutaneously to infected mice. Further experimental studies in human smallpox contacts indicated that methisazone is effective in reducing the incidence of smallpox by 75 to 95% of household contacts. Vaccinia reactions in eczematous patients (eczema vaccinatum) and progressive generalized vaccinia (vaccinia gangrenosa) in patients with defective cellular immunity are unaffected by hyperimmune serum but have been treated successfully with methisazone. The drug acts by preventing the translation of viral-specific mRNA into capsid proteins and virus maturation is halted.

2. Rifampin

The antibiotic Rifampin (Chapter 6, *Fundamentals of Bacteriology and Mycology*) is highly effective for the treatment of tuberculosis. The observation that Rifampin specifically blocks initiation of bacterial transcription (DNA-dependent RNA polymerase activity) and the initiation of transcription required by certain bacteriophages prompted an investigation of the effect of this drug against mammalian viruses. The results showed that Rifampin selectively inhibits growth of poxviruses (vaccinia) and suppresses the transformation of cells by Rous sarcoma virus in tissue culture systems. The mechanism of action appears to involve the DNA-dependent. RNA polymerase activity associated with the capsid structure of sensitive viruses (Chapter 3). The concentration of Rifampin needed to inhibit activity of these viruses is enormously higher (100 μg/ml) than that needed to inhibit bacterial growth (0.025 μg/ml). This high concentration of Rifampin is not physiologically practical in man. Further work on finding more potent antiviral derivatives of Rifampin may uncover a drug which will be clinically useful.

3. Amantadine

This compound is a synthetic primary amine that has specific prophylactic activity against certain strains of influenza A$_2$ viruses. Amantadine (Symmetrel) (Fig. 7–2) appears to act by limiting virus penetration or

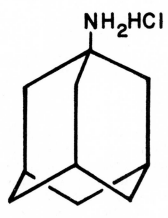

Figure 7–2. Structural formula of amantadine hydrochloride (Symmetrel).

by inhibiting uncoating of virus particles after their entrance into the host cell. It has been clearly demonstrated in several double-blind studies that Symmetrel given twice daily in 100-mg doses will decrease the clinical attack rate of natural or experimentally induced influenza in young adults by 50%. In addition, long-term studies have shown that treatment of older patients with similar doses of Symmetrel is associated with only minimal to moderate toxicity. Despite these favorable data, the drug is only prophylactic and, as a consequence, is not effective for treating clinical influenza. However, it is possible that treatment of debilitated persons with the recommended doses of Symmetrel may reduce the incidence of pneumonia and death. Studies to test this possibility are urgently needed.

4. Iododeoxyuridine

The demonstration that iododeoxyuridine (IUdR, Stoxil) inhibits vaccinia and herpesviruses in tissue culture, and the successful clinical application of this drug in the early treatment of vaccinial or herpetic eye infections in man, provided the first example of a rational approach to the development of an antiviral drug. IUdR is a halogenated pyrimidine (Fig. 7–3) which can become incorporated into newly synthesized viral

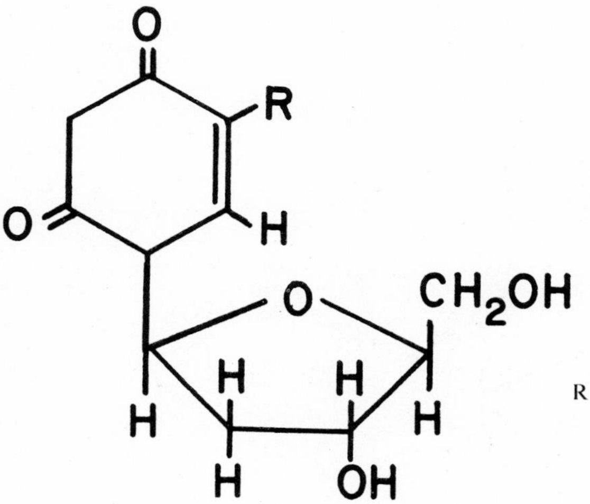

Figure 7–3.   Structural formula of iododeoxyuridine (IUdR, Stoxil) and other 5-substituted deoxyuridines.

R = CH₃: Thymidine
     I: 5-Iododeoxyuridine
     F: 5-Fluorodeoxyuridine
   Br: 5-Bromodeoxyuridine

DNA resulting in the production of abnormal or noninfectious DNA. Although the drug could have the same effect on cellular DNA synthesis, viral DNA synthesis in corneal cells proceeds at an accelerated rate and is more vulnerable to the action of IUdR than DNA synthesis by the slowly growing corneal cells. For this reason, IUdR should be applied only to corneal lesions caused by herpesviruses. Unsuccessful treatment with IUdR is usually due to emergence of drug-resistant viral mutants or progression of the lesion to the deep stromal layers of the cornea where infectious virus does not normally multiply. It should be pointed out that recovery from the disease depends on the natural defense mechanisms of the patient as well as on the drug. Since infection of the cornea with herpesviruses is a serious disease in man which often leads to blindness in untreated cases, IUdR is a potentially valuable drug for treating this disease. However, it is necessary to apply the drug repeatedly to the affected site and to use it only topically because systemic administration could result in neoplastic changes, infertility, or serious genetic mutation. The systemic use of IUdR should be restricted to patients with life-threatening viral infections caused by DNA viruses (e.g., herpes encephalitis, simian B virus infection, cytomegalic inclusion disease, varicella or herpes zoster complicating a malignant disease). Investigations in human volunteers employing another halogen-substituted drug, trifluoromethyldeoxyuridine, indicate that it may be a more effective chemotherapeutic agent than IUdR.

5. Cytosine Arabinoside

This drug is a pyrimidine nucleoside (Fig. 7–4) like IUdR but, in contrast to IUdR, cytosine arabinoside (ara-C) contains a metabolically normal base but an abnormal sugar (arabinose in place of ribose). Ara-C

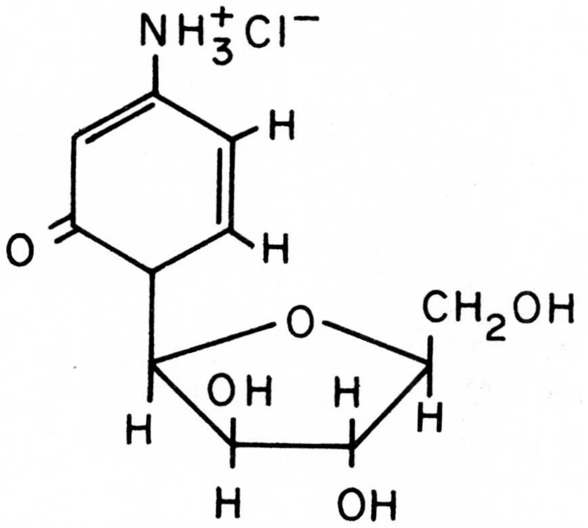

Figure 7–4. Structural formula of cytosine arabinoside (ara-C).

inhibits the multiplication of viruses (e.g., herpesviruses and vaccinia) by interfering with viral DNA synthesis. In general, the RNA viruses that have been tested are resistant to the inhibitory effect of ara-C, with the exception of Rous sarcoma virus, an RNA virus. Unlike many other RNA viruses, Rous sarcoma virus requires a DNA step during its replication cycle (Chapter 3). The mechanism of action of ara-C probably involves inhibition of the reduction of cytidine diphosphate to deoxycytidine diphosphate. Some reports indicate that ara-C is incorporated into both RNA and DNA of leukemic cells. The drug may inhibit cellular DNA synthesis; therefore, ara-C is useful primarily for superficial infections. Although ara-C is known to be rapidly deaminated in man to uracil arabinoside, which has little or no biological activity, cancer chemotherapists have demonstrated its beneficial effects in patients with acute lymphocytic leukemia.

The purine nucleoside adenine arabinoside (ara-A) is a new experimental antiviral drug with significant therapeutic activity against herpesvirus encephalitis and vaccinia virus encephalitis in animals. Following systemic administration, ara-A is rapidly deaminated to hypoxanthine arabinoside which retains significant biological activity, unlike uracil arabinoside, the by-product of ara-C metabolism. A comparison of the antiviral activity of IUdR, ara-C, and ara-A in experimental DNA virus infections in animals indicates that ara-A exhibits superior therapeutic activity. These results suggest that ara-A might be equally effective in man.

D. Interferon

By definition interferon is a low molecular weight protein (mol wt = 12,000 or 24,000) produced by living cells in response to a viral infection or other inducers such as fungal extracts containing the mycophage RNA (helenine and statalon). It is well recognized now that nonviral agents (e.g., *Hemophilus sp.,* endotoxin, rickettsiae) and synthetic copolymers of inosinic acid:cytidylic acid (poly I:C) are also capable of inducing interferon in cells. Interferon is a host cell-coded protein which protects other host cells by inhibiting the multiplication of both RNA and DNA viruses, irrespective of the nature of the inducing agent. There are three important aspects in discussing the antiviral activity of interferon: (1) production, (2) nature, and (3) mechanism of action (Fig. 7–5).

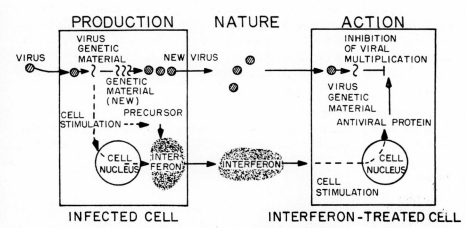

Figure 7–5. Production, nature, and mechanism of action of interferon against viruses. During infection of a cell, virus nucleic acid either derepresses a cellular gene(s) to produce interferon or induces the release of an interferon precursor molecule. Interferon is then released into the extracellular spaces and rapidly adsorbed by surrounding host cells where it derepresses a cellular gene(s) to produce a second component (AVP) which possesses antiviral activity. (Modified from Harris, M.: Interferon: clinical application of molecular biology. Science *170:*1068, 1970.)

1. Production

During a natural viral disease, the infecting virus nucleic acid stimulates the cell to synthesize interferon. It is believed that a family of interferon molecules can be synthesized by the cell. One class of interferon may exist in the precursor state and is released from cells following exposure to certain bacteria, endotoxin, or rickettsiae. The production of the other classes of interferon is initiated by infecting viruses, mycophage RNA, or poly-I:C. The genetic information for interferon synthesis resides in the host cell and not in the infecting virus. For example, in cells infected with an RNA virus like parainfluenza, actinomycin D (inhibitor of DNA-dependent RNA synthesis) blocks the production of interferon but does not prevent parainfluenza virus multiplication. Interferon does not directly inactivate viruses; therefore infected cells may continue to produce more virus and interferon simultaneously. However, the interferon they produce is released, is rapidly taken up by uninfected cells, induces resistance to virus replication, and thus promotes recovery from viral diseases (Fig. 7–5). In the absence of virus infection or a nonviral inducer, interferon production normally remains repressed in the cell. Experiments to measure the interferon yield in cell cultures derived from various organs and exposed to different strains of influenza virus showed that both virus and cells differ in their capacity to induce or produce interferon.

2. Nature

Some general properties of interferon are listed in Table 7–6. Different viruses apparently induce the same class of interferon in human cells. Interferon induced by one virus (e.g., influenza virus) will protect against many different DNA and RNA viruses (e.g., herpesviruses, polioviruses). In contrast to this lack of virus specificity, interferon is host-species specific; e.g., chick interferon will protect chickens but not humans from viral disease.

3. Mechanism of Action

It has been postulated that 4 cellular proteins are involved in interferon action: (1) a receptor site protein responsible for recognizing an interferon-

TABLE 7–6

Properties of Interferon

1. A protein with a molecular weight of 12,000 (monomer) or 24,000 (dimer).
2. Formed by living cells in response to an inducing substance.
3. Induces antiviral activity without being toxic for host cells.
4. The action of interferons against the growth of viruses in cells must operate through some intracellular mechanism involving both cellular mRNA and protein synthesis.

inducing molecule, (2) interferon itself, (3) a repressor of interferon synthesis, and (4) an antiviral protein postulated to be the mediator of interferon action. It is generally accepted that the mechanism of action of interferon requires the production of a second antiviral protein (AVP) since inhibitors of mRNA (actinomycin D) or protein (cycloheximide) synthesis completely block the action of interferon against viruses. Interferon by itself has absolutely no effect on viruses. Once interferon binds to cells, it is rapidly carried across the cell membrane to the cell nucleus. It has been postulated that interferon acts within the nucleus to activate the cell genome to synthesize mRNA which is then translated to AVP. The action of AVP is to inhibit virus-specific protein synthesis, but the exact mechanism is still open to question. Current published reports suggest that AVP generated in interferon-treated cells has a direct inhibitory effect on viral "transcriptase" activity.

E. Clinical Application of Interferon

Interferon is synthesized during most viral infections. It has been detected in the serum of patients with mumps, yellow fever, chickenpox, and influenza and in nonimmune individuals after vaccination with an attenuated strain of measles virus. Interferon has several advantages for clinical use: (1) it is weakly antigenic; (2) repeated doses can be administered; (3) it has little or no toxicity; (4) it is a highly active biological material. A major disadvantage is that animal interferons are inactive or at most only slightly active in humans; therefore, all interferons used in man must be made from human or possibly primate cells. The production of large quantities of interferon for human use has not yet been feasible.

References

CHANOCK, R. M.: Control of acute mycoplasmal and viral respiratory tract disease. Science. *169*:248, 1970.

COLBY, E., and MORGAN, M. J.: Interferon induction and action. Ann. Rev. Microbiol. *25*:333, 1971.

GELBAIN, H., and LEVY, H. B.: Polyinosinic-polycytidylic acid inhibits chemically induced tumorigenesis in mouse skin. Science. *167*:205, 1970.

HERRMANN, E. C., JR., and STINEBRING, W. R., eds.: Second conference on antiviral substances. Ann. N.Y. Acad. Sci. *173*:1, 1970.

HILLEMAN, M. R.: Toward the control of viral infections of man. Science. *164*:506, 1969.

KLEINSCHMIDT, W. J.: Biochemistry of interferon and its inducers. Ann. Rev. Biochem. *41*:517, 1972.

MYRVIK, Q. N., PEARSALL, N. N., and WEISER, R. S.: *Fundamentals of Bacteriology and Mycology*. Philadelphia, Lea & Febiger, 1974.

Chapter 8

Principles of Laboratory Diagnosis of Viral Infections

One obvious function of the diagnostic laboratory is to provide the physician with a definitive diagnosis when a virus is suspected as the etiologic agent of disease, especially if the disease is severe and the symptoms are vague. Of equal importance is the collection of data for studies that involve the detection and prediction of epidemics. Another essential function is to detect the emergence of antigenic variants of viruses, such as influenza virus, which might require alterations in the composition of vaccines. Finally, the diagnostic laboratory is always on the alert for isolates that may represent newly discovered viruses.

The effective use of the virus laboratory requires that the physician be well informed on several important points: (1) the appropriateness of the specimen(s) to be collected; (2) proper methods of collecting, preserving, and transporting specimens; (3) the need for supplying the laboratory with pertinent information about the patient's case history; (4) knowledge of the range and appropriateness of laboratory tests used in the diagnosis of virus diseases, and (5) proper interpretation of laboratory results. Despite the technological advances which have been made, most virus diagnostic procedures are still time-consuming and expensive. Since many virus diseases can be diagnosed on the basis of clinical symptoms alone, the services of the diagnostic laboratory are not routinely required. Accordingly, the physician should not request laboratory tests without reasonable justification.

There are essentially three lines of approach to laboratory diagnosis: (1) microscopic examination of specimens for possible pathologic alterations or the presence of virus; (2) isolation and identification of the definitive agent; and (3) demonstration of a rise in titer of specific Abs during the course of the illness. The approach followed in each case depends on the nature of the infection, the stage of the illness, and the value of the information which can be obtained in relation to the time and expense involved.

The results obtained from most conventional laboratory tests provide only a "retrospective" diagnosis because the illness has usually run its course before final laboratory results are available. The specific treatment of virus infections has been nonexistent until recently, but now that antiviral drugs are becoming a reality, there will be an increasing demand for the development of rapid diagnostic techniques.

A. Rapid Diagnostic Techniques in Clinical Virology

1. Conventional Microscopic Examination

Rapid procedures for diagnosing virus diseases are not new to the clinical laboratory; for example, histologic examination of brain tissue for Negri bodies (acidophilic cytoplasmic inclusion bodies) has been employed for the detection of rabies since their discovery by Negri in 1903. In general, histopathologic methods have a limited application in virology, since they can be used to establish an etiologic diagnosis of only a few diseases. However, conventional histologic procedures are still used to differentiate between chickenpox and smallpox by demonstrating the presence of nuclear or cytoplasmic inclusion bodies, respectively, in smears of vesicle fluid and skin scrapings. The cytologic examination of urine for the inclusion bodies found in cytomegalovirus infections also is still used to establish a rapid presumptive diagnosis of this disease.

Since errors in interpretation of stained smears can occur even in experienced hands, test results must always be evaluated in light of clinical and epidemiologic data. Confirmation of a presumptive diagnosis based on cytologic studies is desirable and is usually obtained either by virus isolation or by serologic procedures.

2. Fluorescent Antibody Techniques

Among the most promising procedures for the rapid and specific diagnosis of virus infections is the fluorescent Ab technique. Two variations of this procedure are currently used in the virus diagnostic laboratory. *Direct immunofluorescence* provides a means of "staining" specimens containing viral Ag with specific antiviral Ab "tagged" with a fluorescein derivative. When examined with a microscope equipped with an ultraviolet light source, the Ag-Ab complexes appear as bright fluorescent areas against a dark background.

The *indirect immunofluorescence* system or "sandwich" technique differs from the direct procedure in that the antiviral antibody is not tagged. Instead, after the specific Ab has combined with viral Ag, fluorescent-labeled antiglobulin is applied and combines with the antiviral immunoglobulin. The indirect method has the disadvantage of being a two-step procedure but is far more sensitive than the direct test (*Fundamentals of Immunology*). This variation has the further advantage of requiring only one tagged reagent that can be used against all specific antiviral sera when they have been prepared in the same animal. For example, antisera against many known viruses can be produced in rabbits; a single preparation of goat anti-rabbit globulin conjugated with fluorescein will react with virus particles coated specifically with Ab in these various antisera.

Immunofluorescence is now employed routinely in the diagnosis of rabies and, in the hands of experienced technicians, is equally as sensitive as the time-consuming mouse inoculation test. Fluorescent Ab procedures also have been used successfully in the rapid diagnosis of influenza and respiratory syncytial virus infections. Of special importance is the applicability of these procedures to the diagnosis of ocular herpetic infections and herpesvirus encephalitis since 5-iodo-2'-deoxyuridine therapy is reportedly effective if initiated soon after symptoms appear. Other applications of immunofluorescence for rapid diagnosis include suspected cases of smallpox and the suspected rubella patient who has been in contact with a susceptible pregnant woman. The use of fluorescent Ab techniques appears to provide one of the best means for coping with these "virus diagnostic emergencies."

3. Electron Microscopy

Although most of the viruses which infect man have been visualized with the electron microscope, the application of electron microscopy to the rapid diagnosis of virus infections is limited. At present, electron microscopy is mainly useful for assigning an unknown virus to its proper morphologic group. For example, the electron microscope has been used successfully to distinguish smallpox from other agents which may initially cause similar clinical symptoms. Examination of negatively stained vesicular fluid proved useful in diagnosing smallpox during the 1966 outbreak in Birmingham, England. The electron microscope, in conjunction with careful case histories, can be used to distinguish smallpox from nonvariolar conditions such as chickenpox, shingles, septic rashes, and vaccination reactions. The main advantage of this procedure is that specimens can be prepared and negatively stained within 5 minutes and, in most cases, only a few minutes of observation of the stained preparation are required to detect the presence of poxvirus.

The possibility of labeling specific Abs with ferritin provides the potential for the rapid specific diagnosis of many viral infections with the electron microscope. At the moment, however, the limited specificity of these procedures and the requirements for highly trained personnel and expensive equipment confine its use to major research centers.

4. Other Tests for Detecting Viral Antigens

Agar-gel precipitin and complement-fixation tests are standard techniques used for detecting viral Ag which appears rapidly in the blood and superficial lesions in smallpox. Precipitin bands are usually detectable within 24 to 48 hours.

It is possible that procedures which are used in clinical chemistry, such as radioimmunoassay, may ultimately provide a highly sensitive method for detecting trace amounts of viral Ag early in the disease. Although such procedures are expensive, they could circumvent much of the tedious work involved in the isolation and identification of viruses which presently can take many weeks to complete.

B.   Virus Isolation and Identification

1. Specimen Collection

Of all the procedures performed by the virus laboratory, virus isolation and identification are the most laborious and expensive. For these reasons every effort should be made to submit specimens that are most likely to contain the virus that is believed to be responsible for the disease.

The type of material to be collected depends on the nature of the illness. Thus, in upper respiratory diseases, throat washings or nasopharyngeal swabs are taken; in pulmonary infections, sputum or effusion fluids are collected; in paralytic diseases, cerebrospinal fluid (CSF) and feces are collected; in cases of encephalitis, blood and throat washings are taken; and when skin lesions are present, crusts and vesicular or pustular fluids are collected. These guidelines apply primarily to cases where the clinical picture or epidemiologic history provides a clue to the possible etiologic agent. The decision as to the type of specimen to collect in cases of generalized viral disease, which present no typical or characteristic symptoms, is more difficult. As a general rule, during the acute phase of a disease, virus usually can be isolated from throat washings, feces, or blood leukocytes.

Since specimens submitted for virus isolation will be inoculated into tissue cultures or animals, they should be collected aseptically to prevent contamination of material with extraneous bacteria. Obviously, in order to protect laboratory personnel, care should be taken to prevent contamination of the exterior of the container with the specimen.

The appropriate specimen should be obtained as soon as possible since, in general, virus is present in tissues and tissue fluids for only a few days before and after the onset of symptoms. For example, in Eastern equine encephalitis, virus is present in blood for only 24 to 48 hours during the acute stage of the disease and the chances of successful isolation are greatly reduced thereafter. In contrast, although the viremia in poliomyelitis is of short duration, virus may persist in stool specimens for as long as 40 days after the onset of symptoms. Specific information pertaining to specimen collection and laboratory diagnostic procedures will be presented in the chapters on the various viral diseases.

2. Storage and Shipment of Specimens

Many viruses are heat labile; therefore, *speed in delivering specimens to the laboratory is of utmost importance.* Ideally, the properly labeled specimens should be delivered to the laboratory immediately after collection. If this is not possible and there is a delay of a few hours, refrigeration at 4° C is recommended. If mail shipment is necessary, most specimens should be frozen as quickly as possible and shipped in an insulated container with dry ice. There are exceptions to this general rule; some viruses, such as respiratory syncytial virus, are inactivated by freezing and thawing. Thus, specimens obtained from children with severe respiratory tract infections should not be frozen since the etiologic agent would most likely belong to the paramyxovirus group. Another exception would apply to physicians who may not have ready access to a deep freeze and dry ice. Under these compromised conditions, specimens may be shipped by mail to a regional laboratory providing they arrive within 24 to 48 hours.

3. Laboratory Processing of Specimens

In the laboratory, the specimen must be inoculated into animals or cultures of susceptible host cells. The choice of the most appropriate cell system will depend to a large extent on the clinical information provided by the physician. The systems most frequently employed are tissue cultures, embryonated eggs, and newborn mice (Table 8–1).

Body fluids including cerebrospinal fluid, vesicular fluid, and serum may be inoculated directly into the selected culture system. Specimens such as throat washings, feces, and other materials which are contaminated with bacteria are centrifuged and treated with antibiotics before inoculation into the appropriate host cells. Tissue specimens are homogenized in a balanced salt solution and the supernatant fluid obtained after centrifugation constitutes the inoculum.

If the material being examined contains a virus, evidence of infection in an animal or tissue culture is recognized in one of several ways. The

TABLE 8—1

Protocol for Isolation of Common Viruses

I. Specimen collection
→
II. Specimen preparation
→
III. Inoculation into suitable host systems

MICE (1 to 3 days old)

Evidence of Infection (Paralysis, ruffled fur, death, etc.)

- Coxsackie A, B
- EEE, WEE, SLE
- Herpes simplex
- Colo. tick fever
- Yellow fever
- Rabies
- LCM
- EMC

TISSUE CULTURES (Primary, diploid, or continuous human cell lines; primary monkey kidney or chick embryo cells)

Cytopathic Changes		Hemadsorption	Hemagglutinins
Poliovirus	Adenovirus	Parainfluenza	Parainfluenza
Coxsackie B	Parainfluenza	Measles	Adenovirus (some types)
ECHO	Respiratory syncytial	Influenza B	Reovirus
EEE, WEE	Rhinovirus	Mumps	
Herpes simplex	Coronavirus		
Varicella zoster	Measles		
Vaccinia	Rubella (in rabbit cells)		
	Reovirus		

EMBRYONATED EGGS (Amniotic cavity or CAM)

Hemagglutinins	CAM Pocks	Death
Influenza A, B, C	Herpes simplex	EEE
Mumps	Vaccinia	WEE
	Variola	
	SLE	

IV. Preliminary identification by pathology and serology
→
V. Passage of harvested material to same or other host systems
→
VI. Specific identification by serologic procedures

ABBREVIATIONS:
CAM = chorioallantoic membrane
ECHO = Enteric cytopathogenic human orphan
EEE = Eastern equine encephalitis
EMC = Encephalomyocarditis
LCM = Lymphocytic choriomeningitis
SLE = St. Louis encephalitis
WEE = Western equine encephalitis

presence of a virus in cell cultures is most frequently indicated by the presence of viral hemagglutinins, cytolysis, cell aggregation, or syncytia. Mice may develop spastic or flaccid paralysis, humped backs, ruffled fur, or other evidence of infection or they may die depending on the pathogenic properties of the virus. In infected embryonated eggs, fluids may contain viral hemagglutinins, lesions may develop on the chorioallantoic membrane or the embryo may die (Chapter 2). The alterations induced in a test system, together with the patient's clinical condition, may permit the virologist to place the isolate within at least the correct major group and provide the physician with a presumptive diagnosis in most instances within 2 to 7 days. The final identification of an isolated virus is made by means of specific serologic tests with antisera prepared against known viruses. The tests used most frequently include those of complement-fixation, hemagglutination-inhibition, virus neutralization, fluorescent Ab, and less frequently, agglutination, precipitation, or flocculation.

4. Establishing the Significance of Virus Isolation

Before it can be established that a virus isolate is the cause of a patient's illness, a number of factors must be considered. Man, as well as laboratory animals and embryonated eggs, can undergo many inapparent, persistent, or latent virus infections. The patient may harbor an agent that is isolated and inadvertently incriminated as the cause of the current illness which in fact is due to another microbial agent. In addition, the inoculation of sterile specimens into an animal may upset the equilibrium between a latent virus and the animal's defense mechanisms and activate the virus which could be erroneously interpreted as the causative agent of the disease. Latent viruses in animal tissues used for preparing primary cell cultures also may be activated when the tissue is subjected to trypsinization and cultured *in vitro*.

To establish the causal significance of any virus isolate, the clinical symptoms exhibited must be compatible with the agent isolated and the patient should show an increase in Ab titer to the virus during the course of the illness. Hence specimens submitted for virus isolation should be accompanied by an acute phase serum sample followed by a convalescent phase serum sample so that serologic tests can be performed to determine whether or not a virus isolate is the cause of the patient's illness. Furthermore, if no virus is isolated, serum samples can be used to establish a retrospective diagnosis.

C. Serologic Diagnosis Employing Patients' Sera

The same serologic procedures that are used to identify viral isolates can be used "in reverse," namely by examining the patient's serum for Abs against known viruses or viral Ags. Serologic tests using patients' "paired sera" are the most used and have advantages over virus isolation methods because of their greater economy, dependability, and speed and especially because they can yield useful information even when virus isolation is not possible.

The serologic approach to virus diagnosis depends on the demonstration of a significant rise (fourfold or greater) in the titer of specific Ab in the patient's serum during the course of an infection. The first ("acute phase") specimen is obtained as early as possible in the illness; the "convalescent" phase specimen is obtained 1 to 3 weeks later. The "paired sera" usually are titrated simultaneously against known virus or viral Ag. The tests for Abs in patients' sera which are routinely employed include complement-fixation, hemagglutination-inhibition, virus neutralization, and immunofluorescence.

References

FENNER, F. J. and WHITE, D. O.: *Medical Virology.* New York, Academic Press, 1970.

GARDNER, P. S.: Rapid diagnostic techniques in clinical virology. In *Modern Trends in Medical Virology.* R. B. Heath and A. P. Waterson, eds. New York, Appleton-Century-Crofts, 1970.

HSIUNG, G. D., and HENDERSON, J. R.: *Diagnostic Virology.* New Haven, Conn., Yale University Press, 1964.

LENNETTE, E. H.: Laboratory diagnosis of viral infections. Amer. J. Clin. Path. *57:* 737, 1972.

LENNETTE, E. H., and SCHMIDT, N. J., eds.: *Diagnostic Procedures for Viral and Rickettsial Infections.* 4th ed. New York, American Public Health Assoc., 1969.

HORSTMANN, D. M., and HSIUNG, G. D.: Principles of diagnostic virology. In *Viral and Rickettsial Infections of Man.* F. L. Horsfall and J. Tamm, eds. 4th ed. Philadelphia, J. B. Lippincott Co., 1965.

SCHAEFFER, M.: Diagnosis of viral and rickettsial diseases. In *Applied Virology.* M. Sanders and E. H. Lennette, eds. Sheboygan, Wisc., Olympic Press, 1965.

SCHMIDT, N. J., and LENNETTE, E. H.: Advances in the serodiagnosis of viral infections. Progr. Med. Virol. *15:*244, 1973.

WEISER, R. S., MYRVIK, Q. N., and PEARSALL, N. N.: *Fundamentals of Immunology,* Philadelphia, Lea & Febiger, 1969.

Chapter 9

Properties of Viruses Associated with Respiratory Syndromes

Respiratory infections are the major cause of morbidity in man; more than 25% of all visits to or by physicians are motivated by symptoms of respiratory illness. It has been estimated that the common cold alone accounts for more than half of all absences from work and one quarter of the total time lost by industrial employees in the USA. Although they are seldom life-threatening, respiratory infections obviously are of great economic importance.

Of all the microbial agents, viruses are by far the most important cause of respiratory disease (only 5 to 10% of all respiratory infections are caused by bacteria). A number of different viruses can cause clinically indistinguishable respiratory illnesses; conversely, the same virus can provoke quite different syndromes. The age and immune status of the patient are important factors that can influence the severity of a virus infection. For example, croup (laryngotracheobronchitis) is a serious clinical manifestation of parainfluenza virus infection in children under 4 years of age.

Adults infected with this virus are usually asymptomatic because they possess specific neutralizing Abs. At most, infected adults exhibit symptoms of the common cold.

Patients with systemic virus infections, such as measles, smallpox, or poliomyelitis, may present the picture of the common cold during the prodromal period. Furthermore, some viruses can infect more than one organ system and cause clinically distinct diseases. These viruses will be characterized in the chapters concerning the syndrome with which they are most frequently associated.

Infections that are confined to the respiratory tract can be caused by viruses that are members of at least 6 of the major virus groups. The characteristics of the major groups were presented in Chapter 1; the individual viruses will be discussed below.

A.   Orthomyxovirus Group

1. Influenza Virus

Epidemics of respiratory disease similar to influenza have been recorded since 1173. The disastrous outcome of these epidemics probably led to the naming of the disease by the Italians in 1358. They called it an "influenza" meaning influence of the stars or heavenly bodies. In 1933, the virus that causes influenza was isolated in the ferret (the red-eyed skunk) and, in accordance with the name of the disease, was named influenza virus. The establishment of the infectious etiology of the disease led to the characterization of the virus.

Structure and Antigenic Properties.   Influenza virions are usually spherical and measure about 80 to 120 nm in diameter (Fig. 9–1). They consist of an outer lipoprotein envelope with evenly spaced surface projections (spikes) that contain the hemagglutinin and neuraminidase. The envelope surrounds an internal helical nucleocapsid composed of the protein structural units and 5 or more linked segments of single-stranded RNA (Chapter 3).

The influenza viruses are differentiated into 3 types (A, B, and C) on the basis of the specificity of a soluble Ag, the "S-antigen," associated with the internal ribonucleoprotein component of the virion. All type-A viruses contain the same S-antigen, which is antigenically distinct from the S-antigens in types B or C. Each type is subdivided into strains on the basis of minor differences in the surface viral Ag (V-antigens), which represent the hemagglutinin and neuraminidase. Major antigenic changes in V-antigens appear infrequently but are responsible for the pandemics of influenza that occur periodically. Although these variants retain the type-specific S-antigen, they are sufficiently different from their predecessors to be designated as new subtypes. For example, in 1947 subtype A_1

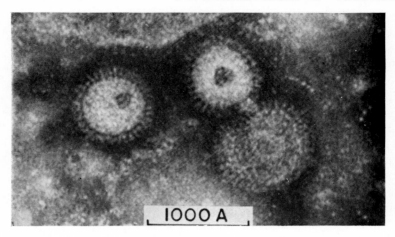

Figure 9—1. Electron micrograph of influenza virus. (Reproduced with permission from Horne, R. W.: The structure and composition of the myxoviruses. 1. Electron microscope studies of the structure of myxovirus particles by negative staining techniques. Virology *11:*79, 1960.)

emerged and replaced the original type A_0 isolated in 1933; in 1957, the A_2 (Asian) influenza virus became predominant. Influenza B viruses also exhibit antigenic variation but to a lesser degree than Influenza A. Influenza C viruses are relatively stable antigenically.

Recently it has been shown that the internal helix of influenza A virus is smaller in diameter than that of influenza C. In addition, the envelopes of influenza C seldom contain the spikes that are virtually always present on influenza A and B virions. On the basis of these differences, influenza C probably will be separated taxonomically from the other influenza viruses within the orthomyxovirus group. It has also been observed that influenza C infections in man are consistently less severe than those caused by the other orthomyxoviruses.

Host Range and Culture. Type A influenza viruses occur naturally in swine, horses, and birds, as well as in man. Types B and C appear to be parasites of man only. The influenza viruses can be propagated in embryonated eggs and ferrets and can be adapted to grow in the respiratory tracts of monkeys and many rodents. Influenza B virus also will replicate in primary monkey kidney or chick embryo cell cultures; influenza A can sometimes be adapted to grow in cell cultures, but the adaptation is often of short duration. The cytopathic effect of the influenza viruses is inconstant; virus replication is detected by the adsorption of guinea pig or group O human erythrocytes to infected cells.

B. Paramyxovirus Group

1. Parainfluenza Virus

The first human parainfluenza virus was isolated in 1955 from infants with croup. The virus, called croup-associated virus, was recognized by the characteristic syncytial cytopathic effect it produced in cell cultures. Subsequently, 3 additional antigenically distinct viruses were recovered from infants and children with respiratory disease. The viruses were recognized by the capacity of infected cells to adsorb guinea pig red blood cells. For this reason they were called "hemadsorption" viruses. Subsequently, the 4 viruses were grouped together and called parainfluenza virus types 1 to 4 because of their morphologic resemblance to influenza virus, with which they were first classified.

Structure and Antigenic Properties. The parainfluenza viruses are almost twice as large as influenza virus and are more pleomorphic. The spherical particles range from 100 to 300 nm in diameter, but filamentous and giant particles up to 800 nm have been observed. The helical nucleocapsid is surrounded by a loose, fragile envelope studded with short surface projections. Some virions may contain more than one nucleocapsid, i.e., are heteroploid. The RNA isolated from the paramyxoviruses is a single-stranded unsegmented molecule. A hemagglutinin and a neuraminidase are associated with the envelope; unlike influenza virus, most parainfluenza viruses are capable of hemolyzing erythrocytes from several animal species. The virion is relatively unstable at temperatures of 37°C and above and also is vulnerable to freezing and thawing, presumably because of the fragility of the envelope.

There is no single Ag common to the viruses in the paramyxovirus group. The 4 distinct serotypes of parainfluenza virus are differentiated on the basis of 2 type-specific Ags: a surface Ag (hemagglutinin) and an internal Ag (nucleocapsid). However, there is some immunologic cross-reactivity between the various types, since heterotypic Ab responses to infection with one type are observed in individuals previously infected with other types. There is also some immunologic relationship between the parainfluenza viruses and mumps virus but none with respiratory syncytial virus or the influenza viruses. In contrast to the antigenic variation observed in influenza A viruses, the parainfluenza viruses are antigenically stable.

Host Range and Culture. Viruses sharing the biologic and morphologic properties of the parainfluenza viruses isolated from man have been recovered from a number of animal species, including mice, swine, monkeys, and cows. Each of the viruses isolated from these animal species is antigenically related to one of the human parainfluenza virus types.

The parainfluenza viruses can be propagated most satisfactorily in primary cultures of human or monkey kidney cells; some types will replicate in continuous human cell lines or cell strains. Virus replication usually is detected by the hemadsorption technique, although syncytia may develop in infected cultures.

2. Respiratory Syncytial Virus

This virus was initially isolated in 1956 from a chimpanzee with an upper respiratory tract (URT) infection and subsequently from laboratory workers in contact with infected chimpanzees. Originally referred to as chimpanzee coryza agent, it is now called respiratory syncytial virus because of its pronounced tendency to form syncytia in tissue cultures. The virus is recognized as being one of the most important causes of severe lower respiratory tract infections in infants.

Structure and Antigenic Properties. Respiratory syncytial virus resembles the other paramyxoviruses morphologically. However, in contrast to the parainfluenza viruses, the respiratory syncytial virion does not possess hemolytic activity, a hemagglutinin, or neuraminidase despite the presence of surface projections on the envelope. Respiratory syncytial virus is unstable at $37°C$ and can be stored at $4°C$ for only a few hours without loss of infectivity; approximately 90% of its infectivity is lost following slow freezing. The virus can be preserved only when it is rapidly frozen in the presence of protein, serum, or hypertonic sucrose and stored at $-70°C$.

The respiratory syncytial viruses can be differentiated into 4 types on the basis of minor differences in the surface V-antigens that are detectable only by sensitive neutralization tests. All respiratory syncytial viruses share a common complement-fixing (CF) Ag that does not cross-react with that of other paramyxoviruses.

Host Range and Culture. Only man and the chimpanzee appear to develop disease from respiratory syncytial virus infections. However, inapparent infections can be produced in ferrets, monkeys, and many other mammals.

Respiratory syncytial virus can be isolated and propagated best in continuous human cell lines, of which HEp-2 cells are the most sensitive. Multiplication is slow and is detected by the appearance of large syncytial cells that contain dozens of nuclear and cytoplasmic inclusion bodies. Unlike most other paramyxoviruses, respiratory syncytial virus cannot be propagated in embryonated eggs.

C.   Picornavirus Group

The picornaviruses are the smallest of the RNA viruses, hence the name "pico (small) RNA virus." All members of the group are naked icosahedral viruses, 20 to 30 nm in diameter, and all contain single-stranded RNA; there is no common group Ag. The group was subdivided into 2 subgroups, the *enteroviruses* and *rhinoviruses*, primarily on the basis of their principal habitat in the body and their sensitivity to acid pH. The enteroviruses, which are found mainly in the gastrointestinal tract, are stable at pH 3.0; the rhinoviruses are found primarily in the nose and are inactivated at pH 3.0.

1. Enterovirus

The enterovirus group is subdivided into 3 "genera": (1) *poliovirus*, (2) *coxsackievirus*, and (3) *echovirus*. Poliovirus, the first of these viruses to be recognized, will be discussed in Chapter 13, which deals with neurotropic diseases. The other 2 groups of viruses were discovered during the course of intensive epidemiologic studies of poliomyelitis. The foundation of modern virology was laid in 1949, when Enders, Weller, and Robbins showed that poliovirus could be isolated and propagated in cultures of nonneural cells. They were awarded the Nobel Prize for their discovery.

a. **Coxsackievirus.** The coxsackieviruses were discovered in 1948 when a new virus was isolated from the feces of 2 children in Coxsackie, N.Y., during unsuccessful attempts to grow poliovirus in neonatal mice. Subsequently, the coxsackieviruses were subdivided into groups A and B on the basis of their effects on suckling mice: Group A coxsackieviruses cause flaccid paralysis and death within a week, whereas the group B viruses produce spastic paralysis that develops more slowly.

Antigenic Composition. There is no single Ag common to all group A and B coxsackieviruses. There are at least 24 group A and 6 group B serotypes that are distinguished by type-specific Ags on the virion surface. Although there is no common group A Ag, heterotypic cross-reactions have been observed between some of the group A viruses. All group B viruses possess a common group Ag, which is also shared with one group A virus.

Host Range and Culture. Man appears to be the only natural host for the coxsackieviruses. Both group A and group B serotypes are readily isolated and propagated in suckling mice. All coxsackie B viruses, but only a few coxsackie A serotypes, grow well in human or monkey kidney cell cultures. Some of the group A viruses that formerly could be propagated only in neonatal mice have been found to multiply in diploid strains of human fibroblasts. The cytopathic effects caused by coxsackieviruses are similar to those caused by other enteroviruses. The cells first become granular and then rounded. Cell degeneration proceeds rapidly, and within 24 to 48 hours after the effect first becomes apparent, the cells are completely lysed and released from the surface of the culture flask.

b. Echovirus. The echoviruses, like the coxsackieviruses, were discovered accidentally during epidemiologic studies of poliovirus. The viruses were isolated from the feces of apparently healthy individuals. Since they were not known to be associated with any specific disease, they were called "orphan" viruses. Subsequently, they were named *e*nteric *c*ytopathic *h*uman *o*rphan (ECHO) viruses because they were found in the intestinal tract of man and caused cytopathic changes in cell cultures.

Antigenic Composition. There are at least 34 serotypes of echoviruses. They do not share a common group Ag, but some immunologic cross-reactions have been observed between certain serotypes. In addition, some echoviruses cross-react with certain other enteroviruses.

The similarity between the coxsackieviruses and echoviruses prompted the adoption of the proposal that all new serotypes be assigned an enterovirus type number rather than attempting to subclassify them as coxsackieviruses or echoviruses. The designations of agents that have already been described were retained: These include poliovirus types 1, 2, and 3; the 24 types of group A coxsackieviruses; the 6 types of group B coxsackieviruses, and the 34 types of echoviruses.

Host Range and Culture. Man is the only known natural host for the echoviruses. However, monkeys develop a viremia and brain lesions following the intraspinal or intracerebral inoculation of some serotypes. The echoviruses can be isolated and propagated only in cell cultures. Primary human or monkey kidney cells are usually used, but some serotypes grow better in diploid strains of human fibroblasts. The echoviruses cause cytopathic effects that are like those of other enteroviruses except that they develop more slowly and are usually less complete.

2. Rhinovirus

The goal of the long search for "the" common cold virus appeared to have been reached when the first rhinovirus (nose virus) was isolated in 1956. Since then more than 100 serologically distinct viruses possessing the properties of rhinoviruses have been isolated, and the end probably is not in sight.

Structure and Antigenic Properties. The rhinoviruses that have been examined appear to resemble the enteroviruses morphologically (Fig. 9–2). However, the rhinovirus RNA has a higher molecular weight than the RNA of the enteroviruses. There are at least 100 serotypes of rhinoviruses, each possessing a type-specific Ag; there are other Ags that show variable patterns of cross-reactivity. However, no common Ag is found in all serotypes.

Host Range and Culture. Rhinoviruses related to human types have been isolated from natural infections in a number of domestic animals; chimpanzees can be infected experimentally with human isolates.

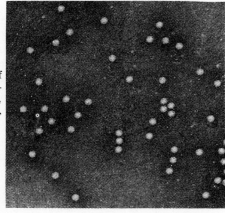

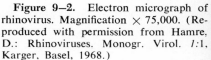
Figure 9—2. Electron micrograph of rhinovirus. Magnification × 75,000. (Reproduced with permission from Hamre, D.: Rhinoviruses. Monogr. Virol. *1*:1, Karger, Basel, 1968.)

The rhinoviruses are more difficult to grow in tissue culture than enteroviruses. Some serotypes (H strains) grow readily only in cells of human origin; other strains will multiply in both monkey and human kidney cell cultures and have been designated "M" strains. Diploid strains of human embryonic lung fibroblasts also support the growth of rhinoviruses; their use has alleviated the special cultural conditions required for isolation in primary cell cultures. The cytopathic effects observed in tissue cultures are similar qualitatively to those produced by enteroviruses but develop more slowly and may be localized and incomplete.

D.   Coronavirus Group

1. Human Respiratory Virus

In 1965, investigators at the Common Cold Research Unit in England reported the isolation of another common cold virus. The virus was obtained from nasal washings collected from a schoolboy suffering from a typical common cold. Attempts to isolate a rhinovirus or other known respiratory agents had failed. However, colds could be induced in human volunteers by the intranasal inoculation of the original specimen. Organ cultures consisting of small bits of human embryonic trachea were inoculated with throat washings from the volunteers who developed URT infections. Culture fluids collected up to 8 or 9 days later induced colds in volunteers. Sera from the volunteers were titrated for Abs against the viruses known to cause respiratory infections, but no rise in titer was detected. Electron microscopy of infected organ cultures revealed a virus morphologically indistinguishable from the mouse hepatitis and avian bronchitis viruses. It was concluded that a new human respiratory virus, now classified as a coronavirus, had been isolated.

Structure and Antigenic Properties. The coronaviruses superficially resemble the influenza viruses. The pleomorphic enveloped particles are 70 to 120 nm in diameter; the loosely wound nucleocapsid probably is helical. However, the surface projections are distinctive pedunculated or petal-shaped structures rather than the spikes typical of influenza virus. In electron micrographs, the virions resemble a crown or solar corona (Fig. 9–3), hence the name coronavirus. On the basis of morphology, the human isolates, called human respiratory virus, are grouped with the viruses of avian infectious bronchitis and murine hepatitis. Several serotypes have been isolated from man. Some types cross-react antigenically with mouse hepatitis virus but not with avian infectious bronchitis virus.

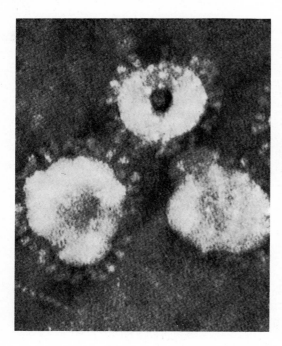

Figure 9–3. Electron micrograph of coronavirus. Magnification × 300,000. (Reproduced with permission from Bradburne, A. F., and Tyrell, D. A.: Coronaviruses of man. Progr. Med. Virol. *13:*373, Karger, Basel, 1971.)

Antigenic relationships between some of the human serotypes also have been demonstrated.

Host Range and Culture. The human serotypes of coronavirus, with a few exceptions, grow only in human cells; the avian viruses replicate only in avian cells, and the mouse virus in mouse cells. Although some human strains have been adapted to grow in mice, these viruses are probably species-specific in nature.

Most human coronaviruses can be isolated only in fragments of human trachea, but some have been isolated in diploid strains of human embryonic fibroblasts; some also can be propagated in human transformed cell lines.

The cytopathic effect develops slowly and usually does not involve the entire cell sheet. Infected cells become elongated and "stringy" in appearance; the cytoplasm becomes vesiculated, and the cells eventually degenerate.

E. Adenovirus Group

1. Adenovirus

The adenoviruses were discovered in 1953 during a search for a type of cell culture that could be used to isolate the common cold virus. It became apparent that prolonged culture of tonsil and adenoid tissue *in vitro* would activate viruses that were present as latent infections in healthy individuals. During an epidemic of influenza-like illness in army recruits, several similar agents were isolated in cultures of human cells inoculated with throat washings. These "new" viruses were officially designated adenoviruses to indicate the original tissue location of this group of agents.

The adenoviruses cause only a small proportion of the respiratory illnesses in man. However, some human adenoviruses produce cancer following inoculation into infant hamsters, mice, or rats. These viruses also can transform rodent cells to the malignant state *in vitro*. Although there is no evidence that adenoviruses are oncogenic in man, they provide an excellent system for studying the mechanism of viral tumorigenesis (Chapter 24).

Structure and Antigenic Properties. The adenoviruses are medium-sized (70 to 80 nm in diameter) naked viruses that contain double-stranded DNA. The virions have a dense central core (the nucleoid) surrounded by an outer icosahedral capsid composed of 252 capsomeres. Of these, 240 are called *hexons* because each is surrounded by 6 neighboring capsomeres. The hexons are the major morphologic subunits of the capsid. The capsomeres situated at the 12 vertices of the icosahedron are designated *pentons* because each is bounded by 5 neighbors. A *fiber* containing a terminal knob projects from the base of each penton (Fig. 9–4).

At least 31 serotypes of adenovirus have been isolated from man. The human isolates have been divided into subgroups on the basis of (1) their ability to agglutinate rhesus monkey or rat erythrocytes, (2) their oncogenic potential for hamsters, and (3) the molecular weight and guanine-cytosine content of their DNA. All adenoviruses possess a common group-specific Ag associated with the hexon, as well as subgroup-specific determinants on the penton. Type-specific Ags are associated with both the fiber and hexon; type-specific Abs against the fiber inhibit hemagglutination, whereas those against the hexon neutralize infectivity.

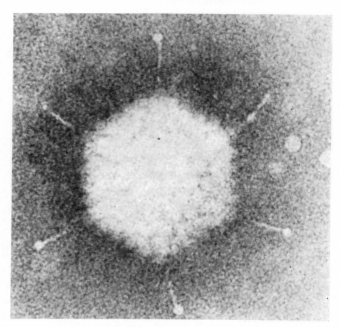

Figure 9—4. Electron micrograph of adenovirus. Magnification $\times$ 500,000. (Reproduced with permission from Valentine, R. C., and Pereira, H. G.: Antigens and structure of the adenoviruses. J. Mol. Biol. *13:*13, 1965.)

Host Range and Culture. Adenoviruses have been isolated from many animal species. With the exception of the human virus isolates which are oncogenic for certain rodents, most are highly species-specific. The host range is reflected in their specificity for cell cultures of their natural host or a closely related species. Primary cultures of human embryonic kidney or amnion and a number of continuous cell lines of human origin support the growth of human adenoviruses. The viruses will multiply in monkey kidney cells only if the cells are also infected with a latent simian virus (SV_{40}) that provides a missing gene product for adenovirus. Adeno-viruses grow slowly in cell cultures, and the typical cytopathic effects may not become apparent for 2 to 4 weeks. The cells, which become rounded and greatly enlarged, usually clump to form grape-like clusters. Nuclei of infected cells may contain characteristic inclusion bodies that are com-posed of aggregates of virions.

F. Diplornavirus Group

All viruses that possess a double-stranded RNA genome are classified as diplornaviruses. The first double-stranded RNA virus recognized, reovirus, was isolated from man. Similar viruses have since been found in plants and insects as well as in a number of ruminants, ungulates, and other mammals. The existence of viruses of similar structure in animals, plants, and insects appears to be a phenomenon unique to the diplornavirus group.

On the basis of capsid structure, the diplornaviruses are divided into 2 subgroups: (1) *reoviruses,* which possess a double capsid, and (2) *orbiviruses,* which have a single capsid. The reovirus subgroup includes the prototype reovirus and Colorado tick fever virus isolated from man, as well as viruses isolated from plants, insects, and other animals. No orbiviruses have been isolated from human beings.

1. Reovirus

The term reovirus (*r*espiratory *e*nteric *o*rphan virus) was coined to denote their dual respiratory and enteric trophism and their isolation in the absence of known disease. The first recognized reovirus was isolated from feces and was classified as an echovirus. However, it became apparent that the virus possessed physical and biological properties that set it apart from other known enteric or respiratory agents.

Structure and Antigenic Composition. Reoviruses are naked icosahedral particles 70 to 75 nm in diameter (Fig. 9–5). The genome consists of 10 loosely linked segments of double-stranded RNA that are surrounded by 2 protein layers. The outer layer appears to contain 92 "holes"; the holes are surrounded by capsomeres composed of either 5 or 6 structural units. The inner protein layer and the RNA genome make up the subviral particle (SVP). The SVP contains the RNA-dependent RNA polymerase that initiates virus replication.

All reoviruses share a group-specific soluble Ag. By hemagglutination-inhibition or neutralization tests, 3 distinct serotypes can be distinguished.

Host Range and Culture. The reoviruses are widely distributed in

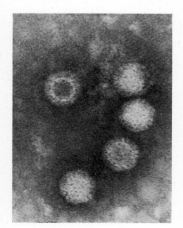

Figure 9–5. Electron micrograph of reovirus. Magnification × 96,000. (Reprinted with permission from: Spendlove, R. S.: Unique reovirus characteristics. Progr. Med. Virol. *12:*161, Karger, Basel, 1970.)

nature and have been isolated from both domestic and wild animals. It has not been proved that animals play a role in natural human infections; however, the extent of animal infections is such that they cannot be ignored as a possible reservoir of human infections.

The reoviruses can be isolated and propagated in primary cultures of epithelial cells from many animal species as well as continuous human cell lines. Infected cells undergo cytopathic changes that are slow to develop and are rather nondescript in appearance. However, distinctive acidophilic inclusion bodies are present in the perinuclear region of the cytoplasm and may eventually encircle the nucleus completely.

References

ANDREWES, C., and PEREIRA, H. G.: *Viruses of Vertebrates.* 3rd ed. Baltimore: Williams & Wilkins Co., 1972.

BRADBURNE, A. F., and TYRELL, D. A. J.: Coronaviruses of man. Progr. Med. Virol. *13:*373, 1971.

COHEN, A.: *Textbook of Medical Virology.* Oxford: Blackwell Scientific Publications, 1969.

FENNER, F., MCAUSLAN, B. R., MIMS, E. A., SAMBROOK, J., and WHITE, D. O.: *The Biology of Animal Viruses,* 2nd ed. New York: Academic Press, 1974.

GINSBERG, H. S.: Adenoviruses. Amer. J. Clin. Path. *57:*771, 1972.

HAMRE, D.: Rhinoviruses. Monogr. Virol. *1:*1, 1968.

KNIGHT, V.: *Viral and Mycoplasmal Infections of the Respiratory Tract.* Philadelphia: Lea & Febiger, 1973.

PHILIPSON, L., and PETTERSSON, U.: Structure and formation of virion proteins of adenoviruses. Progr. Exp. Tumor Res. *18:*1, 1973.

TOOZE, J. (ed.): The Adenoviruses. In: *The Molecular Biology of Tumor Viruses.* New York: Cold Spring Harbor Laboratory, 1973.

VERWOERD, D. W.: Diplornaviruses: A newly recognized group of double-stranded RNA viruses. Progr. Med. Virol. *12:*192, 1970.

WARD, T. G.: Viruses of the respiratory tract. Progr. Med. Virol. *15:*126, 1973.

WEBSTER, R. G., and LAVER, W. G.: Antigenic variation in influenza virus: Biology and chemistry. Progr. Med. Virol. *13:*271, 1971.

WENNER, H. A.: The enteroviruses. Amer. J. Clin. Path. *57:*751, 1972.

WOOD, H. A.: Viruses with double-stranded RNA genomes. J. Gen. Virol. *20* (Suppl.): 61, 1973.

Chapter 10

Viral Respiratory Syndromes

Viral respiratory infections can be inapparent or can present symptoms ranging from mild, self-limiting infections represented by the common cold to severe and even fatal pneumonias. The relative frequencies of the different clinical syndromes caused by the major respiratory viruses are presented in Table 10–1.

A.   The Common Cold

The common cold is a syndrome caused by viral infection of the mucous membranes of the upper respiratory tract (URT). More specifically, the term refers to afebrile, acute coryza or rhinitis of viral origin. The main differences between the common cold and other viral or bacterial respiratory tract infections is the absence of fever and the relative mildness of constitutional symptoms. In many cases, severe systemic viral infections begin with symptoms of the common cold.

1. Etiologic Agents

Over 100 antigenically different viruses can cause the common cold syndrome. The *rhinoviruses* account for 20 to 40% of acute coryza in young adults and 8 to 10% in children. The *coronaviruses* also appear to cause a substantial proportion of minor URT diseases, since up to 98% of a given population tested had Abs to one or more of the human

TABLE 10—1

Clinical Syndromes

Virus	Coryza	Pharyngitis (Conjunctivitis; Otitis)	Croup	Bronchitis	Other
Influenza A, B	++^{a}			++	++++
Influenza C	++			+	
Parainfluenza 1, 3	+++	++	+++	+	+++
Parainfluenza 2	+		++++		
Parainfluenza 4	++++				
Respiratory syncytial	+++		++	++++	+
Reovirus 1	+				
Adenovirus 1, 2, 5	+	++			+
Adenovirus 3, 4, 7, 14, 21	++	++++		+	+
Coxsackie A 2, 3, 4, 6, 8, 10	+	++++	+		++
A 21, 24	++++	+			
Coxsackie B 2, 3, 4, 5	+	+	+	+	++++
ECHO 4, 5, 7, 8, 9, 11, 19, 20, 25	++	++	+		++
Rhinovirus	++++	+		+	
Coronavirus	++++	+	+		

^{a} The relative frequency of the different clinical syndromes resulting from infection with some of the different viruses responsible for the common respiratory infections is indicated by + to ++++.

Modified from Jackson, G. G.: Nonbacterial pharyngitis, pp. 357–363. In P. B., Beeson and W. McDermott (eds.), *Cecil-Loeb Textbook of Medicine.* 13th ed. Philadelphia: W. B. Saunders Co., 1971.

respiratory viruses. The *parainfluenza* and *respiratory syncytial viruses,* which cause severe respiratory infections in children, usually produce only common colds in adults. Although the *adenoviruses* and *influenza viruses* may be associated with more severe infections, some individuals infected with these agents develop only acute coryza or rhinitis. *Coxsackievirus A* 21, 24 and *B* 4, 5, as well as *echovirus* types 11, 20, and possibly others, also cause the common cold. These mild illnesses probably represent the most common clinical manifestation of coxsackievirus and echovirus infections in infants and children and are frequently described as "summer grippe." These same agents less frequently cause other more severe illnesses, such as aseptic meningitis, epidemic myalgia, herpangina, myocarditis neonatorum, and various exanthems. *Reoviruses* have been isolated from children with mild respiratory infections as well as from some children with pneumonia and intestinal, hepatic, and central nervous system disease. However, the relationship of these viruses to clinical illness remains uncertain. During human volunteer studies, most of the subjects inoculated intranasally with reovirus showed no signs of illness; some developed variable symptoms, and no clear-cut clinical picture of the infections could be established.

2. Clinical Symptoms

The portal of infection for these respiratory viruses is the nasopharynx. The incubation period is short, usually 1 to 3 days, during which time the virus proliferates in the nasal mucosa.

The major clinical symptoms of the common cold differ appreciably from person to person, but for any given individual they tend to be repetitive. The occurrence of symptoms that 100 young adults described as characteristic of a naturally acquired cold is shown in Table 10–2. Sneezing, headache, and malaise are the initial signs of infection and are followed by a chilly sensation, sore throat, and nasal congestion. Fever of any significant degree is absent, and the constitutional symptoms, if present, usually last only 1 to 2 days. As the cold progresses, the nasal

TABLE 10–2

The Syndrome of the Common Cold

Symptoms	Frequency
Severe	
Nasal discharge	100
Nasal obstruction	99
Moderate	
Sore or dry throat	96
Malaise	81
Postnasal discharge	79
Headache	78
Cough	76
Mild	
Sneezing	97
Feverishness	49
Chilliness	43
Burning eyes and mucous membranes	28
Muscle aching	22

From Jackson, G. G.: The common cold, pp. 358–361. In P. B. Beeson and W. McDermott (eds.), *Cecil-Loeb Textbook of Medicine.* 13th Ed. Philadelphia: W. B. Saunders Co., 1971.

discharge, which at the onset is clear and watery, may become muco-purulent. These symptoms usually run their course within 5 to 7 days. However, a cough may appear as a prominent symptom during the acute illness and may persist for several weeks. As the symptoms recede, virus excretion ceases.

The results from human volunteer experiments indicate that a fair number of individuals who were infected, as evidenced by virus isolation, were asymptomatic throughout the course of the infection.

3. Pathogenesis

Virus appears to be confined to the respiratory tract. The pathologic changes in the mucous membranes of the respiratory passages include edema, hyperemia, transudation, and exudation. During the acute phase of infection, serum globulins become more abundant in nasal secretions, and substances of cellular origin accumulate. Picornaviruses cause more metaplasia and degeneration of cells from the nasal turbinates than the other causes of the common cold. All tissue damage is rapidly repaired.

4. Immunity

Specific immunity develops following infection with any of the etiologic agents of the common cold. In human volunteers, resistance against reinfection with the same strain of rhinovirus has been shown to persist for a month to several years. Even if specific Ab does not prevent reinfection, it usually results in an attenuated illness. However, because of the large number of viruses that can cause the common cold and the highly specific protection provided by Ab, reinfection with a different virus or even different strains of the same virus is likely to occur.

5. Diagnosis

Diagnosis of the common cold usually is made on the basis of the characteristic clinical symptoms. It is important to recognize or exclude the possibility that the patient may have a more severe disease. Prodromal symptoms of other infections, as well as allergic, vascular, and neoplastic processes, can mimic the common cold.

Virus isolation provides the only satisfactory method for establishing a definitive diagnosis. Serologic tests employing the patients' paired sera are not practical because of the large number of virus types that can cause the common cold. In most instances, etiologic diagnoses are made only for epidemiologic purposes.

6. Epidemiology

The common cold is worldwide in its distribution, and, during a given outbreak, the same virus often can be demonstrated even in isolated areas. Colds are most frequent in infants and children; the incidence of infection in adults declines significantly after middle age.

Although the common cold is spread by respiratory droplets and possibly by fomites contaminated with infected secretions, other factors also appear to be involved in disease transmission. There is support for the idea that colds increase following marked changes in temperature, humidity, or air pollution. However, the popular belief that cold weather, wet feet, and chilling increase susceptibility to common colds is not supported by the results from human volunteer experiments. The importance of person-to-person contact is indicated by epidemiologic studies performed in isolated areas; the incidence of URT infections remains low until contact is made with "the outside world," at which time there is a dramatic increase in the incidence of the common cold.

In the USA, 3 waves of common colds usually occur each year; one appears in the fall, another in midwinter, and a third in the spring. It has been established that asymptomatic carriers shed virus and can participate in the spread and perpetuation of infection.

7. Treatment and Prevention

Therapy is confined to nonspecific remedies such as aspirin and decongestants. At present, there are no drugs that are effective against the viruses that cause the common cold. Antibiotics effective against bacteria are useless and should not be given unless there are bacterial complications.

B. Acute Febrile Pharyngitis, Pharyngoconjunctival Fever, and Acute Respiratory Disease

Acute febrile pharyngitis is an illness of only a few days' duration that is characterized by a mild sore throat, fever, and cough, and sometimes by mild cervical lymphadenitis.

Pharyngoconjunctival fever resembles the foregoing illness but is accompanied by conjunctivitis, which may be unilateral; gastrointestinal symptoms occasionally develop, particularly in children.

Acute respiratory disease (ARD or recruit fever) is an influenza-like illness that lasts about a week and is characterized by fever, malaise, mild sore throat, cough, hoarseness, and rhinitis. The disease, which seldom occurs in civilian populations, appears almost exclusively in young adults shortly after their arrival in recruit camps.

1. Etiologic Agents

Acute febrile nonbacterial pharyngitis can be caused by almost any of the respiratory viruses, including *adenoviruses, coxsackieviruses, parainfluenza* viruses, *respiratory syncytial virus, echoviruses,* and occasionally *rhinoviruses.*

Pharyngoconjunctival fever is caused by *adenovirus* types 3 and 7, and less often by types 3, 14, and 21. Pharyngitis and conjunctivitis may also be present in patients with influenza, measles, and herpangina as well as a number of nonviral diseases.

Acute respiratory disease in recruits is caused by *adenovirus* types 4 and 7 and less often by types 3, 14, and 21.

2. Clinical Symptoms

The incubation period for adenovirus infections that result in pharyngoconjunctival fever, ARD, and febrile pharyngitis is 5 to 10 days. In the case of respiratory syncytial virus and parainfluenza virus infections, the incubation period is 4 to 6 days, and for the coxsackieviruses, echoviruses, and rhinoviruses, 2 to 5 days.

Febrile pharyngitis and *pharyngoconjunctival fever* often are preceded by symptoms of the common cold. Fever has a gradual onset and reaches a maximum of 103 to 104°F on the second or third day; fever may be high for 5 to 6 days. Nontender submandibular lymphadenopathy is commonly present. Conjunctivitis, when present, is mild to moderate and may persist longer than respiratory symptoms. The acute follicular conjunctivitis is nonpurulent; there is marked erythema, suffusion, and narrowing of the palpebral fissure. There is usually no involvement of the cornea or uveal tract.

Acute respiratory disease is a more severe illness than pharyngitis or pharyngoconjunctival fever. Fever reaches a maximum of 103 to 104°F on the second or third day. Pharyngitis, which is the most prominent localized manifestation of the disease, develops 4 to 5 days after infection, increases in severity for 2 or 3 days, and then gradually decreases. Malaise and headache are constant features of the disease, and bronchitis and laryngitis are frequent. Virus persists in the nose, throat, and feces for at least a month after recovery.

3. Pathogenesis

Little information is available on the pathogenesis or the pathologic changes produced as a result of these viral infections of the URT, mainly because of their relative mildness. The age and immunologic status of the host determine to a considerable degree the response to infection.

Depending upon the route of infection, virus multiplies initially in the pharynx, conjunctivae or small intestine. Examination of tissues from rare fatal cases of infantile pneumonia reveals massive necrosis of the bronchial and tracheal epithelium. The nuclei of infected cells contain basophilic inclusion bodies similar to those produced by adenovirus in cell cultures. Adenoviruses have been isolated from fragments of mesenteric lymph nodes as well as from tonsils and adenoids. It is apparent that these viruses frequently become latent in lymphoid tissue following a primary infection and may persist for long periods of time.

Although certain adenoviruses can induce tumors in animals, there is no evidence that these viruses are oncogenic in man.

4. Immunity

Neutralizing and complement-fixing (CF) Abs are detectable about a week after infection. Of particular importance is the development of a local IgA response.

In contrast to the short duration of immunity to most respiratory viruses, neutralizing (i.e. protective) Ab against adenoviruses can be detected at least 8 to 10 years after infection, perhaps as a result of viral persistence in the body. As a consequence, second attacks of illness due to the same type are rare. There is evidence that infection with some adenovirus types provides protection against other types within the same immunologic group.

5. Diagnosis

Pharyngitis caused by adenoviruses must be differentiated from similar illnesses caused by bacteria for which specific therapy is available. For example, it is essential to diagnose and treat β-hemolytic streptococcal infections promptly to prevent the development of rheumatic fever or glomerulonephritis.

When conjunctivitis is prominent, the differential diagnosis of *pharyngoconjunctival fever* includes influenza, measles, and herpangina, as well as leptospirosis, inclusion conjunctivitis, and ocular trauma.

The differential diagnosis of ARD should include influenza and other viral respiratory diseases, URT infections caused by *Mycoplasma pneumoniae,* and purulent sinusitis.

Virus isolation and serologic studies are not performed routinely in the case of URT infections. If a specific diagnosis is required, nasal washings or throat swabs, anal swabs, or fecal specimens for virus isolations, as well as acute and convalescent serum samples for serologic studies, should be submitted to the laboratory. Serologic tests, including CF and neutralization tests, are useful for determining the group to which the virus belongs. Since primary infection with any of the possible viruses involved in these illnesses most likely occurs during childhood, a 4-fold or greater rise in Ab titer must be demonstrated.

6. Epidemiology

Epidemics and sporadic cases of pharyngitis and pharyngoconjunctival fever occur throughout the world. There are at least 2 routes by which naturally occurring respiratory illness caused by adenoviruses may be transmitted. When the conjunctival sac is exposed to adenovirus, conjunctivitis is the most common symptom; however, there may also be respiratory involvement. Thus, during outbreaks of pharyngoconjunctival fever, infections may occur after ocular irritation commonly experienced in swimming pools. Volunteers who inhale a virus aerosol develop ARD or pneumonia. Ingestion of adenovirus does not usually initiate disease, but the virus multiplies in the gastrointestinal tract, and specific immunity develops.

Epidemic ARD is confined primarily to recruit centers. Under the crowded conditions in recruit camps, aerosols containing large amounts of infectious virus are generated by the sneezing and coughing of infected recruits. Inhalation of these virus-rich aerosols could account for the high incidence of severe adenovirus infections observed in these populations. In contrast, the occurrence of serious adenovirus infections in children most likely reflects a lack of specific resistance to the virus rather than an overwhelming inoculum.

7. Treatment and Prevention

Specific treatment is not available for adenovirus infections; aspirin and cough syrup may help alleviate the symptoms.

Swimming pools should be avoided during outbreaks of pharyngoconjunctival fever, and care should be exercised to prevent person-to-person spread by way of discharges from infected eyes.

Immunization with vaccines consisting of enteric-coated live adenovirus types 4 and 7 has been shown to be safe and highly effective in preventing respiratory illness. Because of the low incidence and sporadic nature of adenovirus infections in civilian populations, the use of these vaccines is limited to military recruits. Based on the results of the field trials in 1970 and 1971, it was established that vaccination of recruits with both adenovirus types 4 and 7 was required for effective protection against ARD. It was estimated that 26,979 ARD hospitalizations were prevented, with a saving of 7.53 million dollars.

Another potentially fruitful approach to adenovirus vaccines that is under investigation is the use of immunogenic virion subunits containing no viral nucleic acid. Such a vaccine would eliminate the problem of the potential oncogenicity of adenovirus DNA.

C. Herpangina

Herpangina is a mild infectious disease characterized by fever, malaise and small papular, vesicular, and ulcerative lesions in the palate and the faucal areas. The disease is one of the most frequent causes of summer illness in early childhood but may not be recognized unless it occurs in epidemic form. Although the disease occurs most often in children, it is also observed in young adults.

1. Etiologic Agents

In 1950, the group A coxsackieviruses were suggested as etiologic agents of herpangina. Since 1950, this disease has been recognized with increasing frequency and is one of the most common manifestations of certain types of *group A coxsackievirus* infection. Although serologically distinct from one another, several serotypes of coxsackievirus A commonly cause herpangina. In addition, herpangina-like illnesses may occasionally be caused by *echoviruses* and certain *group B coxsackieviruses*.

2. Clinical Symptoms

The incubation period for herpangina is about 4 to 6 days. Children between the ages of 1 and 7 years are most commonly afflicted. The disease is characterized by a sudden elevation in temperature (102 to 105°F), severe sore throat, nausea, and vomiting. In infants, convulsions may occur, whereas older children usually develop only a sore throat. The fever reaches a peak during the first 24 to 48 hours after symptoms appear. Minute papules or petechiae develop on the soft palate and in the tonsillar pillars; 12 to 24 hours later, superficial ulcers with grayish bases surrounded by red areolae are present at these sites (Fig. 10–1). The lesions increase in size and number for 2 to 3 days and heal within 4 to 5 days. The systemic symptoms also begin to recede within 4 to 5 days, and total recovery occurs within a week.

3. Pathogenesis

The pathogenesis of herpangina in man is not known. The illness is not fatal; therefore, autopsy tissues are not available for examination.

4. Immunity

Immunity to each type of coxsackievirus appears to be long-lasting. However, typical herpangina caused by serologically distinct virus types can occur in the same or a subsequent season. Most adults living in urban areas possess Abs to more than one type of group A coxsackievirus; the spectrum of type-specific immunity increases with age.

5. Diagnosis

A clinical diagnosis of herpangina often can be made on the basis of the typical appearance of pharyngeal lesions. However, not all infected individuals develop the ulcers characteristic of this disease.

The differential diagnosis must include a primary infection with herpes simplex virus, which usually produces larger and more painful ulcers than

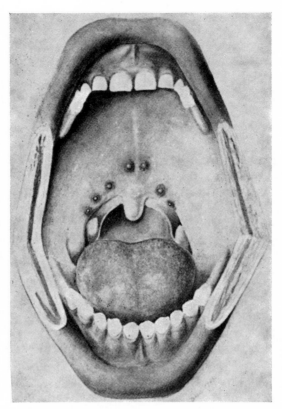

Figure 10–1.   Herpangina lesions. Reprinted with permission from Huebner, R. J.: *Herpangina*, pp. 75–76. In P. B. Beeson and W. McDermott (eds.), *Cecil-Loeb Textbook of Medicine*. 12th ed. Philadelphia: W. B. Saunders Co., 1967.

are seen in herpangina; ulcers due to herpes simplex are primarily in the anterior part of the mouth rather than in the pharynx. Bacterial pharyngitis and the oropharyngeal lesions of certain viral exanthems, such as measles or chickenpox, may be confused initially with herpangina until typical lesions appear. It is also difficult, if not impossible, to clinically separate herpangina without pharyngeal lesions from abortive or nonparalytic poliomyelitis.

The laboratory diagnosis can be established by recovering a group A coxsackievirus from vesicle fluid, pharyngeal washings, or stool in combination with a 4-fold or greater rise in serum Ab titer.

6. Epidemiology

Herpangina occurs most frequently during the summer months. Most illnesses occur in early childhood; up to 10% of children examined at random in pediatric clinics in the USA have been found to harbor herpangina strains of coxsackievirus during July, August, and September.

Within a household or other closed populations, nearly all susceptible contacts are rapidly infected; however, only about a third of the infected individuals manifest the typical pharyngeal lesions. A variable number of family contacts develop mild febrile illness without throat lesions. In addition, a large proportion of group A coxsackievirus infections are asymptomatic and are detected only by epidemiologic studies involving serologic examinations and virus isolation.

7. Treatment and Prevention

Treatment is confined to topical symptomatic measures. The use of anesthetics such as Benadryl Elixir or Butacaine for gargling will soothe the painful pharyngeal lesions. A fluid or soft diet is recommended.

D. Bronchitis, Croup, and Bronchiolitis

Acute bronchitis is an inflammation of the bronchial membranes. It is most often caused by viruses but can be caused by bacteria or external irritants. *Croup (laryngotracheobronchitis)* is an inflammation of the larynx or trachea that is characterized by difficult and noisy respiration and a hoarse cough. *Bronchiolitis* is an inflammation of the bronchioles.

1. Etiologic Agents

Acute bronchitis usually is caused by *respiratory syncytial virus,* the *parainfluenza* and *influenza viruses,* or the *adenoviruses.* Bronchitis may occasionally complicate the common cold, especially in infants.

The *parainfluenza viruses* account for one-third to one-half of all cases of severe *croup* in children. *Respiratory syncytial virus* causes most of the remaining cases, but group A and group B *coxsackieviruses,* as well as some *echoviruses,* also have been isolated from patients with croup. During influenza epidemics, *influenza virus* is the main cause of severe croup.

Bronchiolitis in infants is most often caused by *respiratory syncytial virus. Influenza virus* (during epidemics) and the *parainfluenza viruses* also can cause bronchiolitis. Although croup is the most distinctive syndrome caused by the *parainfluenza viruses,* these agents cause bronchitis, bronchiolitis, and pneumonia almost as frequently as they cause croup.

2. Clinical Symptoms

Acute bronchitis is usually preceded or accompanied by symptoms of URT infection. The patient has malaise, general aching, and frequently a headache; occasionally there is a mild sore throat and a nasal discharge. A dry, unremitting cough is the most important sign. After 1 to 2 days, it becomes productive and looser and is accompanied by mucopurulent sputum. The cough may be associated with substernal soreness. Fever is usually present but is moderate, rarely rising above 101°F.

In the absence of complications, acute bronchitis is a self-limited disease and seldom lasts more than 5 to 6 days. However, cough and expectoration may persist for 1 to 2 weeks or longer if the patient has preexisting chronic respiratory disease. Patients with chronic bronchitis or emphysema may have severe dyspnea, hypoxia, and increased carbon dioxide retention during episodes of acute bronchitis. An episode of bronchial obstruction may be precipitated in individuals with bronchial asthma; some allergic patients have attacks of asthma only in association with acute bronchitis.

Croup causes an alarming clinical picture in children. Initially, the mucous membranes of the nose and throat are involved, causing symptoms of URT infection for 2 to 3 days. The inflammatory process descends into the lower respiratory tract and produces bronchial changes accompanied by laryngeal and tracheal involvement. The onset is heralded by an abrupt rise in temperature; fever is variable but may reach 101 to 102°F. The first attack often occurs upon waking. There may be an arrest of respiration and the child becomes cyanotic as it struggles for breath. When the laryngeal spasm is suddenly released, air is drawn into the lungs with a high-pitched "whooping" sound. In young children, the attack may be accompanied by convulsions or tetany. Patients usually recover even when the initial symptoms are quite severe. Only a small proportion of cases proceed to bronchiolitis or pneumonia.

Acute bronchiolitis is observed mainly in infants 6 months of age or less. The onset is marked by a sharp rise in temperature after 2 to 3 days of URT infection. The temperature is variable and may be moderate or reach 102 to 104°F. Bronchiolitis is characterized by a dry, persistent cough and progressive dyspnea. Respiration is difficult and shortness of breath and cyanosis may be evident from the onset of symptoms; convulsions may occur in the young child. The chest is distended and breathing is rapid and shallow; expiration is often noisy. In the absence of complications, recovery is uneventful. The fever may drop rapidly within 48 hours or gradually during 4 to 5 days. The mortality is variable and can be as low as 1% or as high as 25% during different epidemics.

Complications include convulsions, heart failure, bacterial pneumonia, otitis, and dehydration. The more serious complications may be fatal, and the course of illness may be quite rapid. It has been suggested that some cases of "crib death" may be caused by viral respiratory disease.

3. Pathogenesis

In bronchitis, croup, and bronchiolitis, the mucous membranes of the nose and throat are involved initially; paranasal and eustachian tube obstruction also may occur. In bronchitis, there is an excessive secretion of thick and tenacious mucus that contains a mixture of mononuclear cells, desquamated bronchial cells, and some neutrophils. Bronchial biopsy shows edema of the submucosa accompanied by capillary dilation and mononuclear infiltrates. The paucity of neutrophils is an aid in distinguishing bronchitis of viral etiology from bacterial bronchitis.

If more extensive changes occur in the lower respiratory tract, the larynx may become inflamed and edematous, resulting in the croup syndrome; the accumulation of mucus causes additional obstruction of the airways. In young infants, bronchiolar obstruction can result in focal areas of atelectasis. Suppurative changes resulting from secondary bacterial infection may alter the pattern of the illness and complicate the effects produced by the virus alone.

The pathogenesis of respiratory infections is influenced to a considerable extent by the age and physical condition of the host. Bronchiolitis occurs most often in infections in early infancy and is less likely to be seen with increasing age. Immunologically compromised patients and individuals with preexisting allergies are most likely to develop serious infections.

4. Immunity

Immunity to parainfluenza, respiratory syncytial, and influenza viruses is relatively weak and depends mainly upon the production of IgA Abs in the respiratory tract. Reinfection with the same virus may occur, but the disease is usually mild and limited to the URT. Second attacks of illness caused by adenoviruses of the same type are rare.

5. Diagnosis

The diagnosis of acute viral bronchitis, croup, and bronchiolitis usually can be made on the basis of clinical symptoms. The main problem is to determine whether pneumonia is present. The chest x-ray, which is normal in uncomplicated bronchitis, is useful in detecting pneumonia. As with most other viral respiratory infections, the same virus can cause different clinical pictures. The specific agent involved in each case can be determined only by the diagnostic laboratory. However, except for epidemiologic studies and persistent infections, an etiologic diagnosis is seldom requested.

Since respiratory syncytial virus and, to a lesser extent, parainfluenza virus may be inactivated by freezing, respiratory secretions or nasopharyngeal washings submitted for virus isolation should be delivered to the laboratory as soon as possible without freezing. If the specimen must be frozen for transport, it should be frozen quickly in a stabilizing medium. Virus isolation provides the only definitive diagnosis for infections with parainfluenza virus because the serologic responses are not always type-specific. In contrast, a 4-fold or greater rise in the serum-neutralizing or CF Ab titer to respiratory syncytial virus, influenza, or adenovirus is regarded as diagnostic.

6. Epidemiology

Infections caused by parainfluenza virus types 1 and 3 are endemic and occur throughout the year. These viruses also cause epidemics during the winter, particularly in nurseries, orphanages, and other similar institutions.

Parainfluenza virus type 2 is less prevalent and more episodic in its occurrence than types 1 and 3; infections with type 4 are quite sporadic. Respiratory syncytial virus epidemics occur at intervals of 8 to 16 months and appear simultaneously in geographically separated locations. Usually there are sharp, well-defined limits to each epidemic. Although respiratory syncytial virus is detected less frequently during interepidemic periods, it has been isolated from respiratory illness during every month of the year. The adenoviruses play a minor role in respiratory infections among civilians; the epidemiology of these infections is discussed in section B. Influenza virus will be discussed in section E.

7. Treatment and Prevention

No specific treatment is available. Close observation and careful assessment of respiratory competence are essential in infants and young children, since a significant proportion of these patients may develop more extensive lower respiratory tract involvement. Bronchiolitis and the croup syndrome may cause respiratory insufficiency requiring urgent and decisive management; tracheotomy and mechanical assistance with ventilation may be necessary in occasional patients. A warm draft-free environment and vapor therapy are useful in reducing laryngeal stridor and bronchial and bronchiolar obstruction. Vaporization is indispensable after tracheotomy and also helps to relieve cough and dyspnea. Since oxygen in high concentrations dries the mucosa, it should not be administered routinely but only as required to reduce cyanosis. Perfusion may be necessary for rehydration. Antibiotics should not be administered in the absence of bacterial complications.

No commercial vaccines are presently available.

E. Influenza

Influenza is an acute respiratory infection of specific viral etiology; it is characterized by sudden onset of fever and prostration and is ordinarily benign.

1. Etiologic Agents

Influenza is caused by 3 antigenically distinct groups of *influenza virus,* designated A, B, and C. The terms influenza and "flu" should be restricted to those illnesses with laboratory or *bona fide* epidemiologic evidence of infection with one of the influenza viruses.

2. Clinical Symptoms

Infection with influenza virus may be asymptomatic, may cause only a slight fever, or may result in the typical prostrating illness that occurs during epidemics of influenza. Asymptomatic infection is the most common form of the disease. Clinical differentiation of infections caused by influenza A and B between epidemics is not possible; influenza C is particularly hard to recognize clinically because of its relative mildness.

The following description depicts a typical, uncomplicated influenza A virus infection. The incubation period of influenza is usually 2 to 3 days. Mild prodromal symptoms of malaise, chilliness, and cough are sometimes present, but more often the subject suddenly feels acutely ill. The most common initial symptom is severe generalized or frontal headache. A rapid rise in temperature (101 to 104°F) is accompanied by diffuse muscular aches, intense fatigue, and stabbing retroorbital pain. Respiratory symptoms may be entirely absent; if present, they are most prominent when the systemic manifestations and fever begin to subside. Patients almost invariably develop a cough that is brief and spasmodic and usually nonproductive. Sneezing and a watery nasal discharge or a stuffy nose occur in most cases. Conjunctival burning and itching watery eyes are also frequently observed.

Uncomplicated influenza, although acute and prostrating, is brief. Recovery is usually complete in 2 to 3 days, and it is uncommon for any symptoms to persist beyond 7 to 10 days. However, convalescence may be prolonged by postinfection asthenia and depression.

The most frequent complications of influenza are secondary bacterial infections of the paranasal sinuses, middle ear, bronchi, and lungs. At present, the most serious complication is staphylococcal pneumonia, which tends to run a fulminating and often fatal course.

The rapidly fatal *primary influenza pneumonia,* described during the 1958 epidemic, has been rare in more recent epidemics. These pneumonias were characterized by severe dyspnea, cyanosis, leukopenia, and scanty, grossly bloody sputum. Although staphylococci were isolated from the sputum of some patients, appropriate antibacterial therapy was ineffective. Influenza virus was cultured from the lungs, suggesting that the virus, rather than the bacteria, played the major role in producing the lung damage

Most patients who develop primary influenzal pneumonia have valvular heart disease, preexisting lung diseases, or are pregnant.

Another serious, sometimes fatal, complication of influenza is influenzal encephalopathy or postinfluenzal encephalitis. Even relatively mild influenza infections also can provoke cardiac involvement including pericarditis. Young children with influenza may develop laryngotracheitis and have difficulty in clearing the respiratory tract secretions.

3. Pathogenesis

The primary lesion of influenza involves necrosis of the ciliated epithelium of the respiratory tract. In uncomplicated cases, epithelial damage is confined to the upper and middle portion of the tract. Studies have shown that the laryngeal, tracheal, and bronchial mucosae present an acute inflammatory reaction, with desquamation of the ciliated cells and an exudate of mononuclear subepithelial cells; the basal layer remains intact. On about the fifth day of illness, regeneration begins in the basal layer with the development of undifferentiated transitional epithelium; after two weeks, ciliated cells are again present. There are no residual lesions in uncomplicated influenza.

When influenza is complicated by bacterial pneumonia, the pathologic findings vary, depending upon the nature of the secondary invader. Primary influenza virus pneumonia, however, presents a characteristic picture. The findings at autopsy include the following: (1) pulmonary hemorrhages, (2) marked edema of the alveolar septa and spaces, (3) hyaline membranes lining the alveolar ducts and alveoli, (4) bloody fluid in the trachea and bronchi, (5) hyperemic tracheal and bronchial mucosae, and (6) absence of ciliated epithelium in trachea, bronchi, and bronchioles. Although viremia is a transient and inconstant feature of influenza, the virus has been isolated from heart, kidney, and other extrapulmonary tissues. This observation suggests that virus and virus products may enter the circulation and account for some of the systemic manifestations of the disease.

4. Immunity

Specific immunity to influenza virus develops rapidly after infection but is effective for only 1 to 2 years. Resistance to reinfection reflects the levels of secretory IgA Ab rather than neutralizing Ab in serum. Recurrence of infection with the same antigenic type of virus may occur, especially under conditions of heavy exposure, such as those found in military barracks and dormitories. Resistance to one strain, however, does not protect against newly emerging variants. An individual's immune response to a second infection with an influenza virus is determined by his previous experience. New variants usually share enough antigenic determinants with earlier strains to elicit an anamnestic response to Ags present in previously encountered strains. After repeated infections with successive variants exhibiting minor antigenic differences, the dominant Abs present are usually those against the strain that was first encountered. This phenomenon has been called "the doctrine of original antigenic sin."

5. Diagnosis

In the context of an epidemic, influenza is easily recognized; however, the clinical diagnosis of cases at the beginning of an interepidemic outbreak may be difficult.

Radiologic findings of the lungs in uncomplicated influenza are most often normal, but pleural effusion is revealed in 10 to 20% of the cases. Accentuated bronchovascular markings, basilar streaking, small areas of patchy infiltration, atelectasis, and, less frequently, nodular densities also may be observed. The blood leukocyte count may be normal, or there may be a leukopenia 2 to 4 days after the onset of illness.

The differential diagnosis of influenza includes other viral as well as bacterial respiratory infections that can mimic the onset of influenza. Some adenovirus and respiratory syncytial virus infections are especially difficult to distinguish from influenza.

The definitive diagnosis of influenza depends upon isolation of the virus from throat washings or sputum or the demonstration of at least a 4-fold increase in specific Abs in serum.

Virus isolation is best accomplished by the intraamniotic inoculation of chick embryos with throat washings obtained during the first to the third day of illness. Tissue cultures of primary human or monkey cell cultures also may be used but are less satisfactory. Fluorescent Ab staining of exfoliated nasal epithelial cells has been used recently to establish a specific and rapid diagnosis.

Serologic diagnosis can be made most reliably by CF or hemagglutination-inhibition (HI) tests using acute and convalescent serum samples. Differentiation of Abs against individual strains within each serotype can be accomplished by the HI test, the strain-specific CF test, or the neutralization test.

6. Epidemiology

Influenza A viruses cause epidemics every 2 to 4 years, whereas influenza B and C viruses are associated chiefly with localized outbreaks or sporadic epidemics. There is no evidence that pandemics (worldwide epidemics) of influenza B or C have occurred.

The factors involved in the periodicity of influenza A epidemics are most likely due to the decline in immunity during interepidemic periods and the periodic emergence of new strains of virus. When a major antigenic change in the virus occurs, the antigenic variation may be so extreme that the existing immunity is inadequate to prevent infection with the new virus. Under these conditions, the new strain may become dominant and may replace the older virus in the population. People of all ages throughout the world would be susceptible to such a strain, and a pandemic could occur.

Because of the short incubation period of influenza, epidemics start abruptly once progressive spread begins, reach a peak in 2 to 3 months, and then rapidly subside. The attack rate is variable but exceeded 50% of urban populations in the 1958 epidemic; an additional 25% were asymptomatically infected as evidenced by serologic studies. Crowding seems to be a major factor predisposing to epidemics. Illness usually is observed first among schoolchildren, then young adults, and finally in the elderly, less exposed members of the population. Since infection of the aged is more frequently followed by bacterial pneumonia than infection in younger persons, a second wave of increased mortality may coincide with infections in this age group when influenza is no longer apparent in the community at large.

Minor outbreaks of influenza occur almost every winter when new young susceptibles and individuals who escaped the previous outbreak encounter the virus. Following a pandemic, the frequency and extent of outbreaks is reduced as a result of widespread immunity to the new virus. As more members of the population become immune, inapparent or mild infections become more frequent and probably serve to maintain the virus in the community.

7. Treatment and Prevention

There is no specific treatment for influenza. Codeine sulfate affords relief from incapacitating cough and irritability and is more effective than aspirin for symptomatic treatment of headache and myalgia. Aspirin often increases discomfort by causing excessive sweating and chills. Fluid should be given in abundance; high-fat foods are not well tolerated and should be avoided. Bed rest and gradual return to full activity are recommended. Treatment of primary influenza virus pneumonia usually is unsatisfactory; oxygen therapy with positive-pressure breathing devices may be useful.

Clinical trials have shown some benefit from amantadine (Symmetrel) hydrochloride, which inhibits the cellular penetration of influenza virus. This drug is effective as a chemoprophylactic agent but is not effective for treating clinical influenza. Antibiotics do not affect the course of uncomplicated influenza, and routine antibacterial prophylaxis is unnecessary and inadvisable. It has been demonstrated that suppression of certain of the normal microbial flora of the respiratory tract as a consequence of antibiotic therapy favors bacterial superinfection. Specific antibiotic therapy should be reserved for diagnosed secondary bacterial infections.

Inactivated *influenza virus vaccines* have been employed for more than 25 years. Polyvalent vaccines, containing a mixture of formalinized egg-grown influenza A and B viruses, are the standard preparations presently used in the USA. Some of the vaccines contain only the current strain of influenza A_2 and the post-1971 influenza B virus; other vaccines contain, in addition, A_0 and A_1 strains, which are representative of earlier isolates. These vaccines induce a broader immunization that could be protective should the A_0 and A_1 strain Ags reappear in new variants.

Hybrid influenza virus strains for possible use in living attenuated virus vaccines have been obtained by genetic recombination; however, the stability of the recombinants remains to be established. To ensure the safety of the vaccine, the attenuated parent virus should contain multiple detectable mutations, so that the attenuated vaccine strains can be identified after recombination with a new variant. A live attenuated influenza virus vaccine administered intranasally is already in use in the Soviet Union and is reportedly effective in preventing the disease.

Preliminary trials of influenza virus vaccines emulsified with mineral oil and Arlacel A have been conducted in the U.S. armed forces. Although these vaccines stimulate high levels of Ab, they should not be considered for routine use, since mineral oil is indigestible and produces permanent granulomas. Field trials are under way in which peanut oil is being used as an adjuvant with highly purified virus.

The use of immunogenic viral subunits, either alone or with adjuvant, also is being investigated. The results of these studies indicate that the subunit vaccine provides significant protection against infection with fewer side effects than vaccine containing intact virus.

The protection provided by the commercially available influenza vaccines is limited by the following factors: (1) Inactivated vaccine given parenterally stimulates mainly serum Abs, which are much less effective in preventing infection than local secretory IgA Abs; (2) the resistance that is induced is transient and persists for only a few months to a year. Immunization of the general population is not feasible; however, the U.S. Public Health Service strongly recommends routine yearly immunization for high-risk groups, including those with chronic cardiac or pulmonary disease, diabetes mellitus, or Addison's disease, as well as pregnant women and persons over 65 years of age. The vaccine also may be useful in reducing morbidity in individuals essential for community well-being, such as physicians and policemen, and in closed populations in military camps and institutions.

The influenza virus vaccine is administered subcutaneously; however, the effectiveness of intranasal administration is being investigated. Although the seroconversion rate is low after intranasal spray, the secretory IgA Ab response is marked; the protection seems comparable to that attained after parenteral vaccination, and there are fewer side effects.

Although the presently available influenza vaccine contains purified virus and is generally safe, it should not be given to individuals allergic to egg proteins and should be administered only advisedly and in small doses to infants and young children.

F. Viral Pneumonias

Viral pneumonias are acute diseases with involvement of the lungs, marked by a high fever and cough but with relatively few physical signs. For almost 20 years the descriptive term "primary atypical pneumonia" was applied to all illnesses possessing these characteristics. It was not until 1962 that the filterable agent most frequently involved in these illnesses was found to be *Mycoplasma pneumoniae* rather than a virus.

True viral pneumonias are not associated with a rise in "cold hemagglutinins" or streptococcal MG agglutinins but are essentially indistinguishable clinically from mycoplasma pneumonia. Other nonfilterable agents, including *Coxiella burnetii* and species of *Bedsonia,* also have been isolated from infections diagnosed as primary atypical pneumonia. It has been suggested that the term be dropped; however, because of the difficulties in establishing a rapid and precise etiologic diagnosis, practicing physicians most likely will continue to employ the term "atypical pneumonia" as a provisional diagnosis in many cases.

1. Etiologic Agents

Primary bronchopneumonia may be caused by a number of viruses, including *influenza virus* A, B, and C, several types of *adenovirus* or, in infants and children, *respiratory syncytial virus, parainfluenza virus,* and occasionally the *rhinoviruses.* Less frequently, pneumonia may result from infection with *coxsackieviruses* (particularly group B), various types of *echovirus,* and even more rarely, *reoviruses.* In addition, pneumonia may develop in adults experiencing a primary *varicella-zoster* infection, in immunologically compromised children infected with *measles virus,* and occasionally in children and adults infected with *mumps virus.* In recent years, there has been an increase in the incidence of fatal *cytomegalovirus* pneumonia in patients receiving immunosuppressive therapy.

There are still some cases of pneumonia in which an etiologic diagnosis cannot be made, suggesting that other causes of pneumonia remain to be discovered.

2. Clinical Symptoms

The incubation period for the viral pneumonias is variable and may last from 5 to 15 days, depending on the virus involved. At onset, the illness is characterized by malaise and chills, fever of 100 to 104°F, and occasionally pharyngeal redness and coryza. The most outstanding feature is a dry, persistent cough, which may become productive and cause thoracic pain. However, physical signs may be absent or moderate. Chest x-ray is required for a clinical diagnosis and often reveals abnormalities from the onset. The illness usually is mild but prolonged. The systemic symptoms often disappear within 3 to 10 days but may persist longer; however, the x-ray abnormalities last a month or more in 20% of patients.

Age of the patient is often an important factor in determining the clinical aspects of viral pneumonia. Although viral pneumonia in the newborn child is very rare, the neonate may develop a diffuse involvement of the respiratory tract following a nosocomial infection. Involvement of the lower respiratory tract is characterized by a sudden deterioration of the general physical condition of the infant. The complexion is grayish, and there is an acceleration and inversion of respiratory rhythm together with the appearance of diffuse bilateral rales. In contrast to the symptoms observed in older children and adults, cough may be infrequent and the temperature may be either normal or subnormal. Although recovery usually occurs by 1 to 2 weeks, the outcome may be fatal, particularly in premature infants.

3. Pathogenesis

During the acute phase of severe cases of viral pneumonia, the lesions observed include bronchial and bronchiolar inflammation, interstitial pneumopathy, and sometimes edematous or hemorrhagic alveolitis. In fatal pneumonias, alternating zones of atelectasis and emphysema have been observed. In approximately half of such cases, a hyaline membrane was present within the alveoli.

The lesions that develop in the lower respiratory tract may reduce the oxygenation of the blood substantially, resulting in shortness of breath, tachypnea, and, ultimately, cyanosis. Respiratory alkalosis may develop with reactionary hyperventilation. The hyperventilation may cause some dehydration and hemoconcentration. In very serious cases, respiratory obstruction and alveolar blockage induce hypoventilation and acidosis. Respiratory alkalosis and acidosis may be successive. Hypoventilation accompanied by acidosis is a grave sign that is observed more frequently in young children than adults. Death can occur from either vascular collapse or heart failure.

There appears to be a relationship between respiratory allergy and viral respiratory infection. It has been observed that asthmatic attacks often occur during a respiratory infection and that allergic subjects are more likely to develop respiratory obstruction than normal individuals. It has not been established whether the respiratory infections aggravate pre-existing allergic reactions or whether the viral disease sensitizes the respiratory mucosae.

Some chronic respiratory diseases in later life may result from severe pulmonary infections in childhood. For example, chronic disease following adenovirus infection of the lower respiratory tract in infancy may result in persistent airway obstruction with hyperinflation. There may be recurrent attacks of pulmonary infection, particularly during the first 3 to 4 years of life (Fig. 10–2).

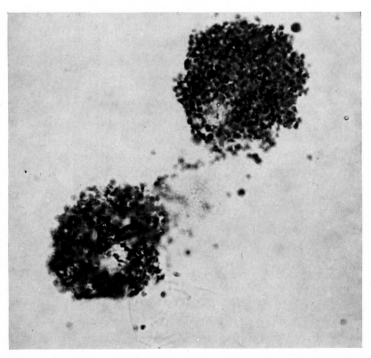

Figure 10–2. Four-year-old female who developed a unilateral hyperlucent lung following an adenoviral infection at age 8 months. Plain chest film (upper left) shows a hyperlucent lung. Bronchogram (upper right) reveals a typical "pruned tree" appearance of bronchiolitis obliterans. Pulmonary angiogram (lower left) and lung scan (lower right) confirm that there is a marked decrease in perfusion of the left lung. (Reprinted with permission from Chernick, V., and Macpherson, R. I.: Respiratory syncytial and adenovirus infections of the lower respiratory tract in infancy. Clin. Notes Resp. *10*(2):3, Fall 1971.)

4. Immunity

Pneumonia resulting from a second infection with any given virus is rare, since specific humoral and local neutralizing Abs are produced following the initial infection. Although specific immunity to most of the viruses involved may not prevent reinfection, previous immunization undoubtedly accounts for the fact that respiratory symptoms in adults are usually moderate, and subclinical infections are common. These facts also explain, in part, the relative frequency of viral pneumonias during the first years of life and their rarity in adults.

5. Diagnosis

As in the case of influenzal pneumonia (section E), the other viral pneumonias are distinct from most bacterial pneumonias but are difficult to distinguish from those caused by *Mycoplasma pneumoniae* and certain of the *Bedsonia* and rickettsiae. The diagnostic dilemma is compounded by the fact that many different viruses may cause identical patterns of pulmonary disease and the same agent can produce pneumonitis of varying severity.

Viral pneumonias are generally less severe than bacterial pneumonias and are associated with pulmonary infiltration of lesser density. Physical signs are absent or moderate. The blood count most often is normal, although a leukocytosis may occur in serious cases. The absence of an increase in neutrophils suggests a viral rather than bacterial etiology. The x-ray picture is variable, depending on the severity of disease. Most often, there is a nonhomogeneous, hazy opacity in an inferior lobe; it is bilateral in 20 to 50% of the cases. The opacities characteristically are progressive and become increasingly apparent over a period of 10 days to 2 weeks. Pleural effusion is rare. It is impossible to establish a relation between a specific virus and any particular radiologic picture.

To establish an etiologic diagnosis, the virus may be isolated from freshly collected throat washings, sputum, or feces, depending on the agent involved. A significant increase in specific Ab to the virus isolate confirms the diagnosis.

6. Epidemiology

Pneumonia due to adenovirus infection is rare in civilian adults but is observed in military recruits, usually as an extension of ARD. Sporadic and epidemic cases of highly fatal adenovirus pneumonia occur in infants. Pneumopathy caused by respiratory syncytial virus occurs most commonly in infants during epidemics in the late winter and early spring. Parainfluenza virus pneumonia also is observed mainly in children but occurs throughout the year; epidemics occur primarily in hospitals and densely populated institutions. Primary influenza pneumonia is observed only during epidemics. Fatal cases of pneumonia caused by coxsackieviruses and echoviruses are rare but have occurred in infants and young children.

7. Treatment and Prevention

In the absence of specific antiviral therapy, treatment for the viral pneumonias is symptomatic and is designed to (1) relieve the patient's discomfort, (2) maintain good hydration, (3) reduce pulmonary obstruction, (4) prevent or correct hypoxia and acidosis, and (5) prevent or control complications, including secondary infections and sequelae.

Codeine derivatives are used to suppress severe coughs and relieve thoracic pain. No attempt is made to control fever unless it is very high; large doses of aspirin favor acidosis and should be avoided. Humidification of room air and vapor therapy are widely used to reduce bronchial and bronchiolar obstruction by decreasing the density and viscosity of secretions. Intravenous perfusion is sometimes required to maintain hydration, especially in children. Oxygen therapy is indicated only if cyanosis develops. Antibiotics should not be administered unless a bacterial infection is indicated.

No vaccines are commercially available. Vaccines containing living adenovirus types 4 and 7 are used to prevent acute respiratory infections in military recruits.

G. Epidemic Myalgia (Bornholm Disease, Epidemic Pleurodynia, Devil's Grip)

Epidemic myalgia is an acute viral disease characterized by sudden onset of severe paroxysmal pain in the upper part of the abdomen or lower thorax. The pain is aggravated by breathing and movement.

The disease was first described by Daae and Homann in Norway in 1872. Following extensive observations during an epidemic of the disease on the island of Bornholm, Sylvest published a monograph in 1933 and applied the name Bornholm disease to the syndrome. The diagnostic confusion with pleurisy led to the pseudonym epidemic pleurodynia; the excruciating pain associated with the disease led to the synonym devil's grip. Epidemic myalgia describes the illness more precisely and is the preferred term.

1. Etiologic Agents

A viral cause of epidemic myalgia was postulated for many years, but all efforts to demonstrate such an agent failed until 1948, when a *group B coxsackievirus* was isolated from a 14-year-old boy suffering from the disease. Subsequently, it was established that all group B coxsackieviruses can cause epidemic myalgia; this disease is the most typical manifestation of infections by these viruses. Other enteroviruses, including various types of *group A coxsackieviruses* and *echoviruses,* occasionally cause an identical clinical picture.

2. Clinical Symptoms

The incubation period for epidemic myalgia is 2 to 4 days. The onset is sudden and usually begins with a violent, sharp pain in the thorax; less frequently, the pain occurs progressively. In about 25% of the cases, the acute illness is preceded by 1 to 10 days of fever, anorexia, malaise, stiffness, and URT infection. Fever is a constant finding during the initial attack and usually fluctuates from 100 to 103° F but may occasionally exceed 104°F. The most characteristic manifestation of the disease is intense pain in the lower portion of the thorax. Breathing is painful and, as a result, is rapid and shallow. Pain and spasm of anterior abdominal muscles occur in about half the cases, usually in combination with the chest pain. There is often a pronounced headache and pain in the neck, shoulders, and scapulae. Nausea and vomiting, diarrhea, shivering, and pharyngeal pain may occur. After the initial attack, the patient may suddenly feel well; however, several successive recurrences of severe pain may occur at intervals of 2 to 8 days. The acute phase of the illness usually lasts 3 to 7 days, but additional relapses may occur. Weakness, discomfort, and tenderness may persist for several weeks. Despite the severity of the attacks, virtually no deaths have been attributed to uncomplicated epidemic myalgia. Other clinical manifestations of infection by the virus may accompany epidemic myalgia or may occur as complications of the disease. The most frequently reported complication is an orchitis lasting 3 to 7 days that occurs in 2 to 3% of adult males with epidemic myalgia. No aftereffects or secondary atrophy of the testicles have been reported. Aseptic meningitis also may precede or accompany epidemic myalgia.

3. Pathogenesis

The specific pathologic process of epidemic myalgia in man is unknown, since the disease is rarely fatal and no autopsy examinations have been reported. The presence of virus in stool, muscle biopsy material, and throat washings suggests a generalized infection.

4. Immunity

Acquired immunity to group B coxsackieviruses is type-specific and long-lasting. However, since all antigenic types of the virus can cause epidemic myalgia, recurrences theoretically are possible.

5. Diagnosis

The diagnosis of epidemic myalgia usually can be made on the basis of the characteristic clinical symptoms once the existence of an epidemic is apparent. However, during the initial stages of an epidemic or when sporadic cases occur, the disease may be confused with serious and even life-threatening conditions. Depending upon the age of the patient and the site of the pain, epidemic myalgia must be differentiated from pulmonary infarction, acute pericarditis, myocardial infarction, angina, pancreatitis, pleurisy, spontaneous pneumothorax, pneumonia, and appendicitis.

Laboratory confirmation of epidemic myalgia is essential to confirm the clinical diagnosis. The virologic diagnosis is made by demonstrating group B coxsackievirus in throat washings taken during the acute illness or in feces for up to a month after infection. The diagnosis is confirmed by demonstrating a 4-fold increase in specific serum Ab.

6. Epidemiology

Outbreaks of epidemic myalgia have been described at all latitudes and in all races. The illness occurs in all age groups but is most common in young adults and children. In temperate zones, it occurs during the summer and early autumn, usually as minor epidemics limited to several households or a community.

Epidemics of Bornholm disease frequently are associated with epidemics of other clinical manifestations of group B coxsackievirus infections, such as acute lymphocytic meningitis and, less frequently, acute infantile myocarditis. Acute myocarditis due to group B coxsackievirus is confined almost exclusively to newborns. Many group B coxsackievirus infections are asymptomatic.

The spread of coxsackieviruses depends directly or indirectly on a human source. The viruses can be found in the throats and feces of patients or healthy carriers. Infection, therefore, may occur by way of respiratory droplet transmission or by the fecal-oral route. In the community or family, children appear to be the principal agents for spreading infection. No natural reservoir other than man has been discovered for the Group B coxsackieviruses.

7. Treatment and Prevention

Treatment is aimed at relieving pain. Aspirin has little effect and may cause excessive sweating; stronger analgesics may be used in severe forms of the disease. Cortisone treatment is contraindicated since it aggravates experimental coxsackievirus infections.

No vaccines are available.

References

BRADBURNE, A. F., and TYRRELL, D. A. J.: Coronaviruses of man. Progr. Med. Virol.
   13: 373, 1971.

BEESON, P. B., and McDERMOTT, W. (eds.): *Cecil-Loeb Textbook of Medicine.* 13th ed. Philadelphia: W. B. Saunders Co., 1971.

COHEN, A.: *Textbook of Medical Virology.* Oxford: Blackwell Scientific Publications, 1969.

DAVENPORT, F. M., and MONTO, A. S.: Practical considerations in the diagnosis of myxovirus infections. Amer. J. Clin. Path. *57:* 777, 1972.

DEBRÉ, R., and CELERS, J.: *Clinical Virology.* Philadelphia: W. B. Saunders Co., 1970.

FENNER, F., McAUSLAN, B. R., MIMS, C. A., SAMBROOK, J., WHITE, D. O.: *The Biology of Animal Diseases,* 2nd ed. New York: Academic Press, 1974.

FENNER, F., and WHITE, D. O.: *Medical Virology.* New York: Academic Press, 1970.

HAMRE, D.: Rhinoviruses. Monogr. Virol. *1:* 1, 1968.

HOPE-SIMPSON, R. E., and HIGGINS, P. G.: A respiratory virus study in Great Britain: Review and evaluation. Progr. Med. Virol. *11:* 354, 1969.

KNIGHT, V.: *Viral and Mycoplasmal Infections of the Respiratory Tract.* Philadelphia: Lea & Febiger, 1973.

LENNETTE, E. H., and SCHMIDT, N. J. (eds.): *Diagnostic Procedures for Viral and Rickettsial Infections.* 4th ed. New York: American Public Health Association, 1969.

MELNICK, J. L.: Classification and nomenclature of animal viruses. Progr. Med. Virol. *13:* 462, 1971.

PEREIRA, H. G.: Influenza: Antigenic spectrum. Progr. Med. Virol. *11:* 46, 1969.

SCHILD, G. C. (ed.): Influenza vaccines. Proc. of Symposium, Royal Institution, London, on 27th April 1972. Postgrad. Med. J. *49:* 151, 1973.

WINTROBE, M. M., THORN, G. W., ADAMS, R. D., BENNETT, I. L., JR., BRAUNWALD, E., ISSELBACHER, K. J., and PETERSDORF, R. G. (eds.): *Principles of Internal Medicine.* 6th ed. New York: McGraw-Hill Book Company, 1970.

Chapter 11

Properties of Viruses Associated with Skin Lesions

Maculopapular eruptions and exanthems are among the most frequent manifestations of infections by many viruses; they may constitute the main symptoms of the disease or may be minor manifestations of disease associated with neurologic, respiratory, or other major syndromes. Measles, rubella, and chickenpox are among the most common diseases of childhood and are well-defined clinical entities. Other cutaneous infections present ill-defined symptoms, and diagnosis can be made only by isolating and identifying the virus. In still other diseases, such as roseola (exanthem subitum), the clinical symptoms are characteristic and presumably caused by a virus, but no agent has been isolated.

Infections that result in predominantly cutaneous manifestations are caused by viruses in at least 6 of the major virus groups.

A. Paramyxovirus Group

1. Measles Virus

Although measles was long assumed to be of viral etiology, the causative virus was not isolated until 1954, when J. F. Enders and co-workers developed techniques for propagating the virus in human kidney tissue cultures. Following isolation of the virus, serologic procedures of basic importance in studying measles infection also became available. The basic research of Enders ultimately led to the development of the attenuated strains of virus presently used in live-virus vaccines against measles.

Structure and Antigenic Properties. The measles virion is spherical and measures 100 to 150 nm in diameter. The internal nucleocapsid, which contains single-stranded RNA, is surrounded by a thick lipoprotein envelope containing short spike-like projections. Hemolytic activity and a hemagglutinin for monkey erythrocytes are associated with the virion. Apparently, the virus contains no neuraminidase, since hemagglutination is maximal at 37°C and is not followed by elution of the virus from the agglutinated cells. Measles virus is highly temperature-sensitive; it is rapidly inactivated at 37°C or by refrigeration. Specimens for virus isolation must either be inoculated into tissue cultures shortly after collection or frozen at −70°C.

Only one serotype of measles virus has been isolated. Although they are morphologically similar, there is no antigenic relationship between measles virus and the other paramyoxviruses that infect man. However, an antigenic relationship has been demonstrated between the viruses of measles, rinderpest (which infects cattle), and canine distemper. These three closely related viruses are classified in the medipest subgroup within the paramyxovirus group.

Host Range and Culture. Man is the only natural reservoir for measles virus. Although monkeys are susceptible, they are not infected in their natural habitat. Monkeys acquire the virus only after capture and contact with human beings infected with measles virus. The virus can be adapted to the newborn mouse and hamster.

Measles virus can be cultured in a number of cell systems, either on primary isolation or after adaptation. Primary cultures of human and monkey kidney cells are the most satisfactory; human amnion cells are less sensitive. The propagation of measles virus in human and monkey mononuclear leukocytes supports the suggestion that these cells may play a role in the transport of virus during the incubation period of the disease. After initial isolation in primary cell cultures, measles virus will multiply in continuous cell lines of human or monkey origin and in primary dog kidney cells. The virus can be adapted to other cell systems such as chick embryo fibroblasts, which were used to develop the attenuated Edmonston vaccine strain. Strains adapted to human amnion cells will subsequently grow in the amniotic cavity of the chick embryo.

The cytopathic effects produced by measles virus include the formation of syncytia and multinucleate giant cells, as well as the formation of spindle-shaped fibroblast-like cells. Both types of cytopathic effects may occur in the same culture; initially, the changes are focal but, as virus spreads contiguously from cell to cell, the entire cell culture is destroyed. Numerous acidophilic inclusion bodies can be observed in the cell cytoplasm and nuclei of stained preparations. Chromosomal breaks are regularly demonstrated by standard karyotyping techniques.

B. Togavirus Group

1. Rubella Virus

The first clinical description of rubella appeared in Germany in the early 1800s, hence the name "German measles." Although a viral etiology of the disease was suspected, efforts to isolate the agent were unsuccessful until 1962, when rubella virus was isolated in cell cultures. The availability of specific diagnostic tools during the 1964 epidemic led to a marked advance in knowledge of the epidemiology and control of this disease.

Structure and Antigenic Properties. The rubella virion is roughly spherical and is about 60 nm in diameter; however, pleomorphic forms have been observed. It is composed of an internal helical nucleocapsid of approximately 30 nm surrounded by a lipoprotein envelope with numerous short projections at the surface. The virus contains a hemagglutinin for red blood cells from day-old chicks, adult geese, or pigeons. The virus is relatively labile, but infectivity can be preserved by storage at $-70°C$.

Only one serotype of rubella virus has been recognized; there is no antigenic relationship to other known viruses.

Host Range and Culture. In nature, rubella appears to be limited to man. However, inoculation of monkeys and ferrets results in subclinical infection; a chronic infection may develop in newborn ferrets. Virus administered to pregnant rabbits may cause congenital abnormalities in the offspring. These abnormalities include cataracts and other malformations of the eye, necrotic lesions in the liver and spleen, and interstitial pneumonitis. Infection of the Japanese quail results in a febrile reaction and alterations in the genital system. These experimental models may be useful in delineating further the pathogenesis of congenital rubella in man.

Rubella virus can be propagated in a wide range of cell types from several animal species; however, visible cytopathic effects are not produced in all cells. One of the procedures used for detecting rubella virus depends upon the interference phenomenon, i.e., the capacity of rubella virus to interfere with the subsequent multiplication of a cytopathogenic challenge virus. Primary green monkey kidney cells are inoculated with the specimen, incubated for 7–10 days, and challenged with an enterovirus such as echovirus 11. If typical enterovirus cytopathic effects fail to develop, the specimen is presumptively considered to be positive for rubella virus; serologic tests with known positive antiserum can be used to confirm the diagnosis. A number of continuous cell lines in which the virus multiplies and produces a cytopathic effect are now available; these include RK-13 (rabbit kidney), SIRC (rabbit cornea), BHK-21 (baby hamster kidney), and Vero (green monkey kidney). The cytopathic effect begins in isolated microfoci, spreads slowly, and seldom involves the entire culture. The hemadsorption technique has been used to detect virus multiplication before typical cytopathic effects appear in BHK-21 cells but apparently is unsatisfactory in many other cell systems.

C. Herpesvirus Group

The members of the herpesvirus group are morphologically indistinguishable. The virion is made up of three parts: The core that contains the DNA is surrounded by the capsid, which is enclosed in an envelope composed of one, two, or more concentric membranes (Fig. 11–1). The core is 75 nm in diameter, is usually spherical, and is comprised of the nucleoid

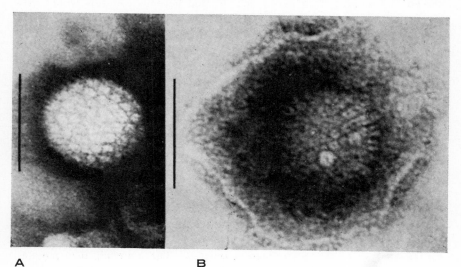

A   B

Figure 11–1. Electron micrograph of herpes simplex virus. *A*, "Naked," and *B*, enveloped virion. Phosphotungstic acid negative contrast; 100 μm (bars). (Reprinted with permission from Goodheart, C. R.: Herpesviruses and cancer. J.A.M.A. *211:* 91, 1970.)

(primary body) and an area of low electron density. The icosahedral capsid has a diameter of 100 to 110 nm and is made up of 162 elongated hollow capsomeres, of which 150 are hexagonal and 12 pentagonal. The diameter of the virion ranges from 145 to 200 nm due to variation in the size of the envelope. At the periphery, the envelope is condensed as a membrane 4 to 5 nm thick from which protrude periodic structures 8 to 10 nm long and 8 nm thick.

The herpesviruses are divided into subgroups A and B on the basis of their behavior in cell cultures. The viruses in group A are readily released from infected cells and include herpes simplex virus types 1 (oral) and 2 (genital) of man, as well as herpesviruses of monkeys, several domestic mammals, and fowl. The group B viruses are strongly cell-associated and infectious virus is released with difficulty. Included in group B are varicella-zoster (V-Z), cytomegalovirus, and Epstein-Barr virus, all of which infect man; a number of other animal herpesviruses have also been described.

Varicella-zoster and herpes simplex virus will be discussed in this chapter; the other viruses associated with disease in man will be covered in subsequent chapters.

1. Herpes Simplex Virus

Herpes simplex virus (HSV) was first isolated in 1919, when it was shown that a virus from herpes labialis and herpetic keratitis would produce specific lesions on the cornea of a rabbit. A year later, it was reported that the disease had been transmitted from an experimentally infected rabbit back to the cornea of a blind man. Subsequently, it was observed that many normal adults possess neutralizing Ab against HSV and that recurrent herpes characteristically occurs in individuals with neutralizing Abs. The virus was later isolated from many forms of HSV infections, both primary and recurrent. With recovery, the infection becomes latent or hidden but can be activated later by fever, colds, sunburn, and many factors that alter the physiology of the host.

Antigenic Properties. There are two serotypes of HSV. Type 1 herpes simplex can be differentiated from type 2 on the basis of several minor antigenic differences and also by the G + C content of the DNA, as well as by cultural characteristics. Herpes simplex type 2 has been found in association with carcinoma of the cervix; this aspect of the infection will be discussed in Chapter 24. The types can be differentiated into strains by the analysis of Ab neutralization kinetics. The antigenic determinants of strains may undergo slight changes even during recurrence in a single individual.

There are some cross-reactions between HSV and other members of the group; of particular importance with respect to diagnosis are the antigenic determinants shared with V-Z virus.

Host Range and Culture.   Man is the natural host for HSV.   However, most strains are pathogenic for conventional laboratory animals, including rabbits, mice, guinea pigs, hamsters, cotton rats, day-old chicks, and owl monkeys, depending upon the route of inoculation.

The virus grows well in embryonated chicken eggs and a wide variety of tissue culture cells.   Rabbit kidney cells are commonly used for the initial isolation of the virus.   Human embryo and baby hamster kidney cells also are highly susceptible.   Various continuous cell lines and some strains of human diploid cells are less susceptible.   Monkey kidney cells support the growth of HSV with difficulty, although they are susceptible to other members of the herpesvirus group.   Diagnostic laboratories usually inoculate more than one cell type or animal with each specimen to insure isolation of the agent.

The cytopathic effects characteristic of HSV infections can take two forms: The cells become rounded, swollen, and clumped; multinucleated giant cells are formed.   Both forms usually are observed on primary isolation.   The nuclei of infected cells contain inclusion bodies that give unfixed preparations a refractile appearance.

2. Varicella-Zoster Virus

Varicella-zoster virus is the etiologic agent of varicella (chickenpox) and zoster (shingles).   The identity of the agents involved in these two diseases was suggested as early as 1888, when outbreaks of varicella were observed after contact of susceptible children with zoster patients.   Following isolation of the viruses from each syndrome, the antigenic and biologic identity of the agents was confirmed.   It is now apparent that clinical zoster results from the activation of latent V-Z virus that has persisted in the host after primary infection manifested as chickenpox.   The two names formerly used to describe the virus, namely varicella and herpes zoster, have been combined to coin the currently accepted term varicella-zoster virus.

Antigenic Properties.   There is only one serotype of V-Z virus. Isolates from cases of varicella and zoster are serologically indistinguishable.

Host Range and Culture.   Man appears to be the only natural host of V-Z virus.   However, there is one report of a naturally acquired disease resembling chickenpox in young anthropoid apes.   Therefore, it is possible that nonhuman primates are susceptible to V-Z virus.

The virus can be propagated in primary or secondary human or monkey cell cultures; human diploid cell strains or cell lines also may be employed. The virus cannot be grown in embryonated eggs.

Cytopathic effects are focal and slow to develop. The virus remains cell-associated; extension of individual lesions occurs by the direct passage of virus to contiguous cells. Infected cells become rounded, swollen, and refractile. Multinucleate giant cells may develop, and radiating cytoplasmic processes extend from infected cells. Acidophilic inclusions are observed in the nucleus and occasionally in the cytoplasm of stained cultures.

D. Poxvirus Group

The poxvirus group includes the largest and structurally most complex viruses that infect man. They are classified as complex viruses because the nucleocapsids do not conform to either helical or icosahedral symmetry. The group is subdivided into 5 subgroups on the basis of antigenic relatedness and the ability of the viruses in each subgroup to recombine. There is extensive cross-neutralization between viruses in each subgroup but none between viruses in different subgroups. However, all poxviruses contain a common nucleoprotein (NP) Ag that can be extracted from the core.

There are 6 poxviruses that can infect man: variola virus, vaccinia virus, and cowpox virus are classified in subgroup I; contagious pustular dermatitis virus and milkers' nodule virus are placed in subgroup II; and molluscum contagiosum virus belongs to subgroup V.

1. Variola, Vaccinia, and Cowpox Viruses

Smallpox has been recognized as a life-threatening disease for many centuries and was the first disease against which active immunization was widely practiced. The first vaccine used contained variola virus from lesions of smallpox patients. Material from a smallpox lesion was inoculated by incision or puncture into the skin. Although the illness that developed was usually milder than naturally acquired smallpox, variolation was sometimes fatal. This dangerous vaccine was replaced by Jenner's cowpox vaccine taken from cowpox lesions. Jenner's procedure was based on an observation common at that time, namely that milkmaids who became infected with cowpox developed resistance to smallpox. The cowpox virus was passed from arm to arm for many years with the occasional introduction of new material from infected cows; later the "lymph" used as vaccine was produced by serial passage of the virus in calves, sheep, or rabbits. In the course of time, the virus underwent minor antigenic changes, and the laboratory strains presently used can be differentiated from fresh isolates of cowpox virus. For this reason, strains recently isolated from cowpox are called cowpox virus and the vaccine strains used to immunize against smallpox are called vaccinia virus.

Structure and Antigenic Properties.   Variola, vaccinia, and cowpox viruses are morphologically indistinguishable. The virions measure about 300 $\times$ 200 $\times$ 100 nm and appear brick-shaped when purified virus is viewed in the electron microscope (Fig. 11–2A). However, in ultrathin sections of infected tissue, the particles are ellipsoid. An outer membrane composed of tubular strands of lipoprotein encloses a layer of soluble protein Ags, surrounding the dense dumbbell-shaped nucleoid (core) and the lateral bodies (Fig. 11–2B). The nucleoid contains the high molecular weight double-stranded DNA genome in association with an inner membrane.

The viruses in the variola-vaccinia subgroup differ from each other by only 1 or 2 of the 20 or more Ags that can be detected by immunodiffusion tests. Serologic tests used in the diagnosis of smallpox depend upon a complex soluble Ag (LS) that contains heat-labile (L) and heat-stable (S) components. The LS Ag is present in both the virion and extracts of infected tissue or fluid from smallpox vesicles. It is distinct from the high molecular weight structural Ag that induces the formation of neutralizing Ab. Hemagglutinins are produced in infected cells but are not an integral part of the virion; i.e., purified poxvirus does not agglutinate red blood cells.

Host Range and Culture.   Man is probably the only natural host and reservoir of variola virus. Monkeys infected experimentally develop a mild generalized disease with a rash. The virus also can be serially passed in suckling mice inoculated intracerebrally. Although lesions can be produced in rabbits, serial passage is achieved with difficulty. Vaccinia and cowpox viruses readily infect cows and sheep, as well as a number of laboratory animals.

Inoculation of embryonated chicken eggs is the most reliable laboratory test for this group of viruses. Variola virus grows readily on the chorioallantoic membrane and produces small dome-shaped pocks that are easily differentiated from the large centrally depressed lesions of vaccinia and cowpox.

The growth of the poxviruses in cell cultures reflects their host range *in vivo.* Vaccinia and cowpox readily produce cytopathic effects in many types of cells, including chick embryo fibroblasts, monkey kidney cells, and a number of continuous cell lines. Variola virus also grows in various mammalian tissue cultures, but cytopathic changes appear more slowly than those produced by vaccinia virus. Although the poxviruses are DNA viruses, they replicate in the cytoplasm and produce characteristic cytoplasmic inclusions called Guarnieri bodies; the inclusions are composed of a dense aggregation of many virus particles. Virus particles are also referred to as "elementary bodies" or Paschen bodies. The cytoplasmic inclusion bodies observed in specimen material are useful for establishing a diagnosis of infections caused by members of the poxvirus group.

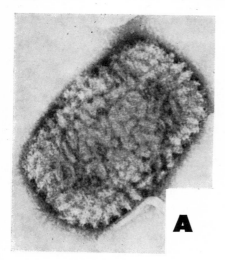

Figure 11–2A. Electron micrograph of purified poxvirus (variola-vaccinia-cowpox group), phosphotungstate stain (superficial penetration). Note the short surface filaments. × 150,000.

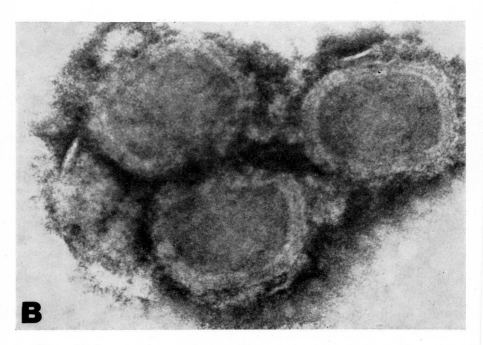

Figure 11–2B. Poxvirus (variola-vaccinia-cowpox group) from specimen material, phosphotungstate stain. The deep penetration of stain permits observation of three concentrically laminated zones around the core. × 150,000. (Reprinted with permission from Long, G. W., *et al.:* Experience with electron microscopy in the differential diagnosis of smallpox. Appl. Microbiol. *20:* 497, 1970.)

2. Contagious Pustular Dermatitis (Orf) and Milkers' Nodule (Paravaccinia) Viruses

Structure and Antigenic Properties. The virions of contagious pustular dermatitis and milkers' nodule are indistinguishable morphologically. They are slightly narrower and less brick-shaped than those of the variola-vaccinia subgroup; the tubular strands of the surface membrane are spirally arranged, giving the virus a "ball of yarn" appearance (Fig. 11–3). These

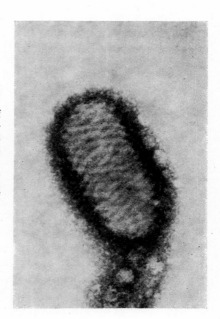

Figure 11–3. Electron micrograph of milkers' nodule virus from specimen material, phosphotungstate stain (superficial penetration). Note the cylindrical shape and spiral arrangement of surface filaments. × 150,000. (Reprinted with permission from Long, G. W., *et al.:* Experience with electron microscopy in the differential diagnosis of smallpox. Appl. Microbiol. *20:* 497, 1970.)

viruses are antigenically related but share no immunogenic Ags with variola or vaccinia. Neither contagious pustular dermatitis nor milkers' nodule virus produces a hemagglutinin.

Host Range and Culture. Sheep and goats are the natural hosts of contagious pustular dermatitis virus; the disease affects mainly the mouth and lips of young lambs and kids, but adults also can be infected. Man may develop localized skin lesions as a result of contact with infected animals.

The cow is the principal natural host of milkers' nodule virus, which causes a cowpox-like disease on the teats and udders. The virus may be spread to milkmaids or farmworkers and causes lesions on the hands.

Orf virus grows poorly, if at all, in most routine laboratory animals or in embryonated eggs but can be cultured in the scarified skin of lambs. Laboratory strains can be propagated in primary human amnion cells as well as in sheep, goat, or bovine cells. The virus causes focal areas of cellular degeneration and destruction after 5 to 18 days of incubation.

Milkers' nodule virus does not produce lesions in chick embryos or other laboratory animals but can be propagated in cultures of bovine tissue or primary human amnion. Cytopathic effects may not appear for 10 to 12 days on primary isolation, but, on second passage, cytotoxicity may be evident in 2 to 3 days.

3. Molluscum Contagiosum Virus

Structure and Antigenic Properties. Morphologically the molluscum contagiosum virus resembles the members of the variola-vaccinia subgroup. A soluble, heat-labile Ag has been prepared from skin lesions; this Ag is distinct from Ags produced by other members of the poxvirus group.

Host Range and Culture. Man is the only known natural host for molluscum contagiosum virus. The virus has not been cultured in experimental animals or in chick embryos. Although cytopathic effects have been observed in some primary human cell cultures and in HeLa cells (a continuous human cell line), the virus cannot be serially passed.

E.   Papovavirus Group

The papovaviruses are divided into two subgroups: (1) papillomavirus and (2) polyomavirus. The papillomavirus virion is larger than polyomavirus and contains a higher molecular weight DNA genome. The papovaviruses are of special interest to viral oncologists because they are tumorigenic either in their natural hosts or in other animal species. The only known member of the group that is of human origin is the human papilloma or wart virus. However, papovaviruses have also been observed in association with progressive multifocal leukoencephalopathy, which may be a late sequela of Hodgkin's disease. In addition, papovavirus-like particles have been observed in cells from patients with lymphocytic leukemia and lymphosarcoma. The neurotropic and oncogenic papovaviruses are discussed in Chapters 21 and 23.

1. Human Papillomavirus (Wart Virus)

Structure and Antigenic Properties. The human papillomavirus is a naked icosahedral particle that contains a cyclic double-stranded DNA genome. The capsid is about 53 nm in diameter and contains 72 capsomeres in an outer shell that surrounds a dense core (Fig. 11–4).

Little is known about the antigenic properties of the wart virus, since the only source of material is tissue excised from patients. Antiserum prepared against partially purified virus contains Abs that fix complement and agglutinate virus particles. Virus extracted from one form of wart

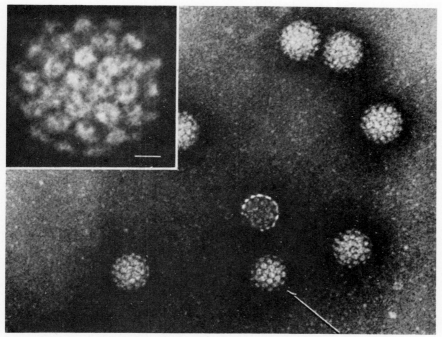

Figure 11—4. Electron micrograph of human papillomavirus, negatively stained with phosphotungstate. The virus particles are intact and well preserved (arrow) with the exception of one damaged particle. Bar indicates 0.1 μm. Inset is higher magnification of particle at arrow. Bar indicates 100 Å. (Reprinted with permission from Noyes, W. F.: Structure of the human wart virus. Virology 23: 65, 1964.)

will produce clinically different types of warts when inoculated in different sites on the body. Although this observation indicates that a single serotype can produce different clinical forms of warts, it does not preclude the existence of more than one serotype of human papillomavirus.

Host Range and Culture. Man is the only known host for human papillomavirus. It has been serially passaged from person to person but has not been transmitted to laboratory animals. Many attempts have been made to propagate the virus in tissue cultures; however, reports of apparent replication of the virus *in vitro* await confirmation.

F. Picornavirus Group

1. Enterovirus

Various types of group A and B coxsackieviruses, as well as some echoviruses, may cause maculopapular or vesicular rashes. The properties of these viruses are described in Chapter 9.

References

ANDREWS, C., and PEREIRA, H. G.: *Viruses of Vertebrates*. 3rd ed. Baltimore: Williams & Wilkins Company, 1972.

JOKLIK, W. K.: The poxviruses. Annu. Rev. Microbiol. *22:* 359, 1968.

KAPLAN, A. S.: Recent studies of the herpesviruses. Amer. J. Clin. Path. *57:* 783, 1972.

LENNETTE, E. H., and SCHMIDT, N. J.: *Diagnostic Procedures for Viral and Rickettsial Infections*. 4th ed. New York: American Public Health Association, 1969.

MELNICK, J. L. (ed.): Proceedings of the Second International Congress for Virology. Internat. Virol. II. New York: S. Karger, 1972.

PLUMMER, G.: Comparative virology of the herpes group. Progr. Med. Virol. *9:* 302, 1967.

ROIZMAN, B., Spear, P. G. and Keiff, E. D.: Herpes simplex viruses I and II: A biochemical definition. Perspect. in Virol., *VIII:* 129, 1973.

Chapter 12

Viral Diseases of the Skin

A. Measles (Rubeola)

Measles is an acute, highly contagious febrile illness characterized by a maculopapular rash, ocular symptoms, and catarrhal inflammation of the respiratory tract.

1. Etiologic Agent

Measles is caused by the *measles virus,* which is antigenically distinct from rubella virus, the etiologic agent of rubella (German measles).

2. Clinical Symptoms

The incubation period for measles is 9 to 12 days. Natural infection invariably results in recognizable illness; inapparent infections rarely, if ever, occur. The early prodromal manifestations of disease are high fever (103 to 105°F), malaise, myalgia, headache, conjunctivitis, excessive lacrimation, and photophobia. These symptoms are accompanied or followed by upper respiratory tract (URT) symptoms, including sneezing, hacking cough, and nasal discharge. One to two days before the onset of the rash, Koplik's spots appear on the inside of the cheek (Fig. 12–1). The lesions described by Koplik are small red macules or ulcers with a bluish-white center; they constitute a valuable diagnostic sign.

The rash first appears as a blotchy erythema behind the ears or on the face, spreads downward over the trunk and finally involves the extremities;

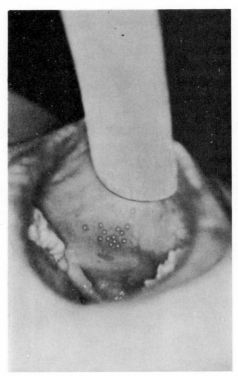

Figure 12—1.   Koplik's spots on the buccal mucosa during the prodromal phase of measles. (Reprinted with permission from Eli Lilly and Co., *Physicians Bulletin*, 1959, series of slides distributed by Lilly entitled "Current Advances and Concepts in Virology.")

the feet and hands are often spared (Fig. 12–2). The eruption consists of discrete reddish-brown macules that become slightly elevated and tend to coalesce (Fig. 12–3). After 3 to 4 days, the lesions fade in the same order in which they appeared. The skin becomes brownish, and there is fine, powdery desquamation of granular skin. Fever and malaise usually persist until the rash reaches a maximum and then subside. In adults, the fever may follow rather than precede respiratory signs; in addition, the rash tends to be more prominent, and complications are more frequent.

Measles is usually a benign, self-limited disease; however, viral involvement of the respiratory tract may lead to croup, bronchitis, or bronchiolitis. Children suffering from leukemia may develop an interstitial pneumonia characterized by the presence of giant cells containing intranuclear and intracytoplasmic inclusion bodies. Giant-cell pneumonia may occur in the absence of rash, in which case measles may not be suspected; this form of the disease is usually fatal. However, most of the severe or fatal cases of

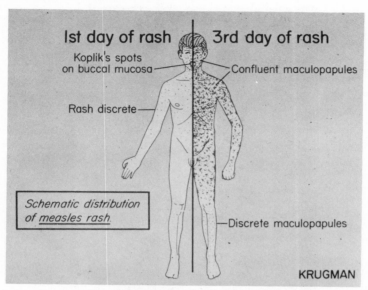

Figure 12—2. Schematic distribution of measles rash. (Reprinted with permission from Krugman, S., and Ward R. (eds.): *Infectious Diseases of Children and Adults.* St. Louis: C. V. Mosby Co., 1973.)

measles in normal individuals result from superimposed bacterial infections that can cause otitis media and pneumonia.

Serious complications directly caused by the measles virus are rare. However, a demyelinating encephalomyelitis appears in about one of every thousand cases of measles and is fatal in approximately 10% of the patients; about half of those who survive suffer permanent residual CNS damage, including mental changes, epilepsy, and paralysis. Measles infection of pregnant women results in fetal death in about 20% of the cases; however, no teratogenic effects, such as those caused by rubella virus, have been demonstrated. Less serious complications include myocarditis, which occurs in about 20% of patients and results in transient changes in the electrocardiogram but rarely causes irreversible cardiac dysfunction.

3. Pathogenesis

Measles virus enters by the respiratory route, multiplies in the epithelium of the respiratory tract and is disseminated by way of the blood to distant sites. During the prodromal period and for 1 to 2 days after the rash appears, the disease is highly contagious; virus is present in conjunctival and respiratory secretions, and in the blood and washed leukocytes as well as in lymphoid tissue. Virus may persist in the urine up to 4 days after the onset of rash.

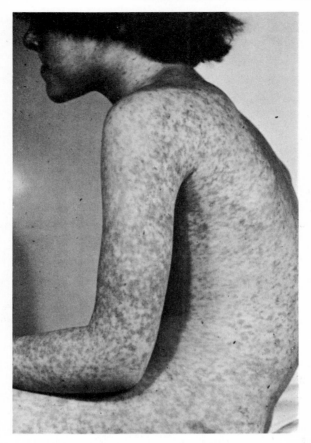

Figure 12–3. Full-blown, coalescing skin eruption in measles. (Reprinted with permission from Eli Lilly and Co., *Physicians Bulletin,* 1959; series of slides distributed by Lilly entitled "Current Advances and Concepts in Virology.")

The skin and mucous membrane lesions may be caused by virus infection of these areas or by the action of immune complexes consisting of virus and Ab. Koplik's spots arise from inflammatory mononuclear cell infiltration of submucous glands and focal necrosis of vesicular lesions of the mucosa. Rash results from the proliferation of capillary endothelium in the corium and exudation of serum and occasionally erythrocytes into the epidermis; epithelial cells become vacuolated and necrotic, and vesicles are formed. Large multinucleate giant cells are characteristic of measles virus infection. They are present in hyperplastic lymphoid tissues, skin lesions, and Koplik's spots as well as in the respiratory tract. Necrosis and sloughing of respiratory epithelium may promote secondary bacterial infection. Changes in the brain of patients with encephalitis include diffuse focal hemorrhage, lymphocytic infiltration, and demyelinization.

There is mounting evidence that measles virus may persist in the body for many years and may be of etiologic significance in some of the chronic "slow virus" diseases (Chapter 22). Measles virus appears to be the cause of subacute sclerosing panencephalitis, a rare chronic degenerative brain disorder that may develop over a period of years following a typical uncomplicated case of measles. Elevated levels of measles virus Ab have been detected in the serum and spinal fluid of patients with multiple sclerosis. Although many viruses have been suggested as the etiologic agent of this disease, only measles virus Ab titers have consistently been found to be higher in patients with multiple sclerosis than in normal individuals. In addition, measles virus Ag has been detected in the endothelium of glomeruli and peritubular capillaries in biopsy tissue and kidneys removed from patients with systemic lupus erythematosus; the significance of the virus in the pathogenesis of this disease remains to be established.

4. Immunity

There is only one antigenic type of measles virus, and an unmodified attack of measles results in lifelong immunity to exogenous reinfection. Antibody can be detected in the blood about two weeks after infection, and IgG persists in a relatively high titer even in older persons. Although cases of recurrent measles in otherwise normal individuals have been reported, it appears likely that either the primary or recurring illness was incorrectly diagnosed. However, some immunologically impaired patients may be subject to repeated infections with measles virus, as well as with other systemic viruses that usually confer lasting immunity in normal persons.

5. Diagnosis

Uncomplicated measles during childhood can be diagnosed on the basis of the characteristic clinical picture; in adults, the disease may be more severe and difficult to diagnose. Even before the rash appears, the diagnosis is suggested by the appearance of Koplik's spots on the buccal mucosa and pronounced catarrhal symptoms with a high fever (Fig. 12–4). Typical giant cells with inclusion bodies are often present in stained preparations of nasal secretions or sputum, particularly in giant-cell pneumonia.

An etiologic diagnosis may be required in the absence of Koplik's spots or in modified or atypical cases of measles. Virus can be isolated, with some difficulty, by inoculating appropriate cell cultures with nasopharyngeal washings, conjunctival secretions, blood, or urine obtained during the prodromal stages or 1 to 2 days after the rash appears.

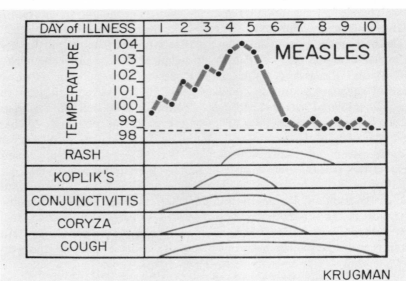

Figure 12–4. Clinical manifestations of measles. (Reprinted with permission from Krugman, S., and Ward R. (eds.): *Infectious Diseases of Children and Adults*. St. Louis: C. V. Mosby Co., 1973.)

Attempts to isolate virus thereafter are usually futile. Immunofluorescence techniques have been used successfully to identify specific virus Ag within cells obtained from nasal or conjunctival swabs. Increases in serum Ab can be detected by neutralization, complement-fixation (CF), or hemagglutination-inhibition (HI) tests.

6. Epidemiology

Measles is endemic throughout the world except in isolated populations. It may occur at any time of the year but is most common in the late winter or early spring. Prior to the development of an effective vaccine, the disease occurred in epidemic cycles every 2 to 3 years, presumably because new susceptible populations were emerging continuously. There is no evidence that subclinical infections, infectious carrier states or animal reservoirs maintain the virus between epidemics. Thus it appears likely that virus is periodically introduced into susceptible populations by infected individuals entering the community from other areas. It is possible that widespread immunization against measles could ultimately eradicate the disease.

Measles is primarily a disease of childhood. Before active immunization became widespread, 90% or more of the population had neutralizing Ab against the virus by 10 years of age. Since the disease is highly contagious, most nonimmunized individuals become infected upon primary exposure to the virus. In isolated areas where measles is not endemic, introduction of the virus results in infection of nonimmune adults as well as children. The morbidity and mortality are very high during these epidemics because of the high susceptibility of affected adults to secondary bacterial infection and other complications.

7. Treatment and Prevention

There is no specific therapy for measles. In the absence of complications, treatment is symptomatic: Aspirin may reduce fever, headache, and myalgia; codeine sulfate is effective when the cough is severe. Bright light does not present an ocular hazard, but a darkened room may reduce the symptoms of photophobia. Bacterial superinfections should be vigorously treated with appropriate antibiotics. However, the incidence of serious bacterial infections is not sufficient to justify routine prophylactic use of antibiotics.

The administration of pooled human gamma globulin within 5 days of exposure will prevent or attenuate measles, depending upon the amount given. Passive immunization may be considered for children under 3 years of age, adults over 60, chronically ill patients, pregnant women, and individuals with impaired immune mechanisms.

Highly effective *live attenuated measles vaccines* are available. The measles vaccine may be given alone or in combination with rubella. Immunization appears to protect about 98% of those vaccinated and is effective for at least 4 to 5 years. The maximum duration of immunity remains to be determined. Vaccination is recommended for all healthy children over 9 months of age who have not had the disease. Maternal Ab passively protects infants during the first 6 to 9 months of life but suppresses the effectiveness of attenuated virus vaccines given during this period; the vaccine is also relatively ineffective in patients who have received gamma globulin during the preceding 4 to 6 weeks. Vaccination is contraindicated for pregnant women, individuals with leukemia or other widespread malignant processes, patients being treated with immunosuppressive drugs or irradiation, and persons with allergies to eggs or other products in the vaccines.

Vaccination with killed measles virus is no longer recommended. Some subjects who received killed measles vaccine in past years developed severe, atypical measles upon subsequent infection with wild-type measles virus; other individuals experienced intense localized hypersensitivity reactions when revaccinated with attenuated virus.

B.   Rubella (German Measles)

Rubella is a benign exanthematous disease of children and young adults. It was first reported to be a distinct disease entity early in the 19th century and has subsequently been recognized as one of the most common infectious diseases of childhood. The disease attracted little attention until 1941, when Gregg, an Australian ophthalmologist, reported an epidemic of congenital cataracts in infants whose mothers had rubella during early pregnancy. It is now known that contraction of rubella during the first trimester of pregnancy may lead to infection of the fetus and cause congenital abnormalities in virtually any organ.

1. Etiologic Agent

The etiologic agent of rubella is the *rubella virus,* a member of the togavirus group.

2. Clinical Symptoms

Postnatal Rubella. The clinical patterns of rubella present a spectrum ranging from inapparent infection to a characteristic clinical picture of lymphadenopathy, rash, and low-grade fever (Fig. 12–5). The incubation period is 17 to 20 days. In adolescents and adults, mild prodromal symptoms may accompany the onset of adenopathy; these include malaise, headache, low-grade fever, mild sore throat, and mild coryza. These symptoms may precede the rash by 1 to 5 days. In young children, the

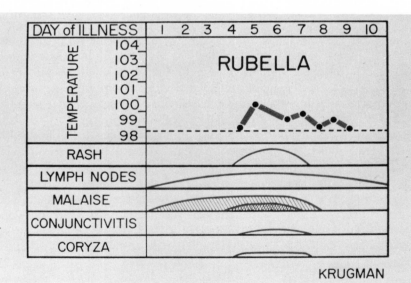

Figure 12–5. Clinical manifestations of rubella. (Reprinted with permission from Krugman, S., and Ward, R. (eds.): *Infectious Diseases of Children and Adults.* St. Louis: C. V. Mosby Co., 1973.)

prodrome is usually absent, and the rash may be the first sign of disease. In some cases, there may be lymph node involvement without skin lesions.

The rubella rash is variable and has no characteristic features. It may be only a transient blush, but usually the lesions persist for 2 to 3 days. Initially, small pink macules and papules appear on the forehead and spread within 24 hours to the neck, trunk, arms, and finally the legs (Fig. 12–6). The lesions are usually discrete but may coalesce and simulate

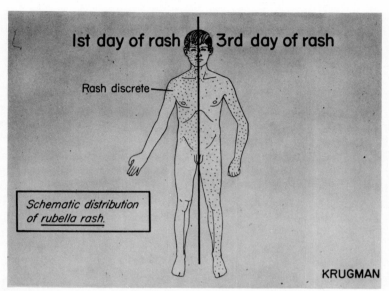

Figure 12–6. Schematic distribution of rubella rash. (Reprinted with permission from Krugman, S., and Ward, R. (eds.): *Infectious Diseases of Children and Adults.* St. Louis: C. V. Mosby Co., 1973.)

measles or scarlet fever. The rash on the face often clears by the time a full-blown rash appears on the legs. Desquamation and discoloration of the skin are rare. Fever is usually absent or low-grade in children and seldom exceeds 102°F. On rare occasions, rubella in adults may simulate measles. Such patients may experience a fever of 105°F, conjunctivitis, cough, photophobia, and generalized debilitation. Recovery is almost always prompt and uneventful. Secondary bacterial infections rarely occur.

Polyarthralgia and polyarthritis may occur as complications of rubella in adult females; they occur less often in males and are rare in children. Pain and swelling, usually in the small joints, are most pronounced during the exanthematous period. Severe symptoms usually disappear in a few days to 2 weeks but may persist several months. Paresthesia, usually numbness and tingling, often accompanies and may outlast the joint symptoms.

Postinfectious encephalitis and thrombocytopenic purpura are rare but serious complications of rubella. Encephalitis occurs in approximately 1 out of 5,000 patients and is fatal in about 20% of those afflicted. In contrast to other viral encephalitides, rubella encephalopathy is not associated with demyelinization. The fact that the onset of symptoms coincides with the appearance of rubella-neutralizing Ab has resulted in speculation that this complication may have an immunologic component. The prognosis for thrombocytopenia is generally excellent, but fatalities due to CNS hemorrhage may occur on rare occasion.

Congenital Rubella. About 10 to 15% of living infants born to mothers with apparent or inapparent rubella during the first trimester of pregnancy present evidence of infection recognizable at birth or during the first year of life. The consequences of *in utero* infection are varied and unpredictable. The spectrum includes spontaneous abortion, stillbirth, and live birth with moderate to severe abnormalities, as well as completely normal infants. Virtually every organ system may be affected either transiently, progressively, or permanently.

The congenital rubella syndrome was originally considered to consist only of neurologic and developmental defects, cardiovascular defects, hearing loss, and eye lesions, including pearly cataracts (Fig. 12-7), glaucoma, chorioretinitis, microphthalmia, and corneal clouding. Following the 1964 epidemic of rubella, additional abnormalities were encountered in association with previously recognized manifestations. The expanded congenital

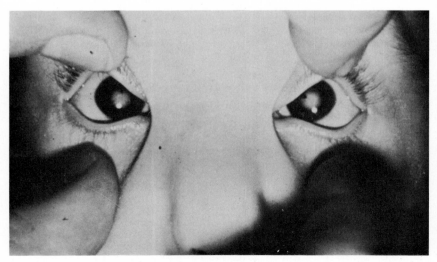

Figure 12—7. Congenital rubella. Typical pearly, bilateral rubella cataracts. (Courtesy of Dr. Louis Z. Cooper.)

rubella syndrome includes thrombocytopenic purpura, hepatosplenomegaly, metaphyseal bone lesions, interstitial pneumonia, anemia, and intrauterine growth retardation. Any combination of anomalies may occur in an individual infant. Many infants lack evidence of disease at birth, but symptoms may become apparent within a few weeks to a year.

3. Pathogenesis

Postnatal rubella infection is transmitted by the respiratory route. The virus multiplies in the URT and spreads to the blood by way of the cervical lymph nodes. Virus is present in throat washings, blood, and feces for several days before the rash appears. Virus may persist in the pharynx for 1 to 2 weeks but is rarely found in the blood after the first day of the exanthem. There is suggestive evidence that the rash is immunologically mediated and is not associated with direct viral action. Since the appearance of the rash coincides with the development of detectable humoral Ab and a decrease in circulating virus, it is possible that immune complexes are involved.

Although lymph nodes show edema, hyperplasia, and loss of follicles, there are no histologic changes pathognomonic for rubella. The onset of disease is attended by a leukopenia that results from decreased levels of both lymphocytes and neutrophils; there is a marked lymphocytosis 4 or 5 days later.

Congenital rubella results from the transplacental transmission of virus during the viremic stage of maternal infection. Greatest risk of fetal damage follows infection in the first 12 weeks of pregnancy, but there is risk up to the 16th week. Organogenesis occurs during the second through the sixth week after conception, and infection is a maximum hazard to the heart and eyes during this period. Deafness may be the only overt manifestation when the infection occurs after the first 8 weeks of pregnancy. Recent studies indicate that rubella infection during the first trimester results in fetal abnormalities, abortion, or stillbirth in approximately 30 to 35% of the cases.

The mechanism of rubella embryopathy may be explained in part by the chronic nature of the infection and the inhibition of mitosis that occurs. Results from studies on tissues obtained at autopsy reveal that many body organs are underdeveloped and have fewer cells than normal. Although only a small percentage of cells are infected *in utero,* the infected cells are characterized by a slower growth rate when cultured *in vitro.* Accordingly, mitotic inhibition *in vivo* would undoubtedly result in derangement of growth and differentiation. Examination of lymphocytes cultured from children with the rubella syndrome also reveals an increased number of chromosomal breaks. Rubella virus is relatively noncytocidal, and cells are chronically infected rather than destroyed. Chronic infection may contribute to the acute illness seen in the newborn and also to the progressive effects occasionally observed during infancy.

4. Immunity

Immunity to rubella is lifelong following either apparent or inapparent postnatal infection. Antibody is first detected at about the time the rash appears and reaches a peak level 21 to 28 days later. The presence of any demonstrable level of naturally acquired Ab in the serum seems to protect against disease. However, there is some evidence that asymptomatic mucosal reinfection may occur in some individuals in the presence of Ab.

The serum of newborn infants with congenital rubella contains passively acquired antirubella IgG as well as IgM produced by the fetus. Both IgM and IgG are synthesized after birth, and high levels of Abs of both immunoglobulin types can be detected at 4 to 6 months of age. In contrast, normal infants possess only passively acquired IgG at birth, and antirubella titers gradually decline as maternal Ab is lost. Most infants with congenital rubella have normal immunoglobulin levels by 1 year of age; however, some children may present persistent dysglobulinemia characterized by low levels of IgG with or without an elevation of IgM. Impaired cell-mediated immunity has also been observed in some cases of congenital rubella. These children fail to respond to various skin test Ags, and their lymphocytes do not undergo blast transformation when exposed to mitogens such as phytohemagglutinin.

5. Diagnosis

Except during epidemics, it is almost impossible to diagnose rubella on the basis of clinical symptoms. Many viruses, including echoviruses, coxsackieviruses, adenoviruses, paramyxoviruses, and reoviruses, may cause rubelliform rashes. Other fevers accompanied by a rash, such as exanthema subitum, as well as toxic rashes, may also be confused with rubella. It may even be difficult to differentiate rubella from mild or attenuated cases of measles; conversely, severe rubella may simulate measles or scarlet fever.

A diagnosis of rubella can be confirmed only by virus isolation or serologic procedures. Nasopharyngeal swabs collected within 4 days following appearance of the rash and inoculated directly into cell cultures yield virus in 85 to 90% of cases. In practice, feces are also cultured for virus in the event that the disease is caused by an enterovirus or other enteric agent. The final identification of rubella virus may take 2 weeks or longer, but often a presumptive diagnosis can be made within a week.

Serologic procedures used in the diagnosis of rubella include HI, neutralization, CF, and immunofluorescence tests. In patients with clinical rubella, neutralizing and HI Abs are detectable within 24 to 48 hours after the onset of rash, and peak titers are reached in 6 to 12 days. In rubella without a rash, these Abs are detectable about 14 to 21 days after exposure. The promptness of these responses makes the serodiagnosis of rubella difficult unless acute phase blood is obtained within a few days after the rash. However, the range of retrospective diagnosis may be extended by examining the CF Ab response, which develops somewhat more slowly than the HI Ab response. It may be possible to demonstrate a rise in the titer of CF Ab in sera obtained too late to show an increase in HI Ab. In some patients, the HI Ab titer drops significantly within 6 weeks after infection. Therefore, a 4-fold or greater *decrease* in Ab in paired sera may also be considered highly suggestive of recent rubella. In addition, the serum can be examined for rubella IgM HI Ab; a 4-fold or greater decrease in rubella HI Ab after treating the serum with 2-mercaptoethanol provides evidence of a primary Ab response.

Much effort has been expended to develop rapid procedures for the diagnosis of suspected cases of rubella in pregnant women and in persons with whom they have been in contact. Direct immunofluorescent staining of infected cells from throat swabs has been found to be as sensitive as virus isolation in diagnosing rubella in children; however, the procedure is less reliable in adults. Indirect fluorescent Ab techniques have been used to detect rubella-specific IgM in serum. This procedure is more sensitive for diagnosis than the demonstration of virus Ag in infected cells and is recommended as the method of choice when early diagnosis is urgent.

Resistance or susceptibility to rubella is usually determined by testing a single serum sample for HI Ab; any detectable Ab indicates resistance.

6. Epidemiology

Rubella occurs throughout the world and has its highest incidence in the springtime. The seasonal character of the disease is useful in diagnosis since many of the skin diseases with rubelliform rashes are caused by enterovirous infections which occur most frequently in the summer and fall. Rubella is endemic in many areas but also occurs in explosive epidemics at irregular intervals. The disease is most common in children of elementary and high school age; however, a small but significant number of persons reach adulthood without contracting the infection. In the USA, approximately 20 to 30% of women of childbearing age have no detectable rubella Ab.

Individuals with inapparent as well as apparent infections are a source of rubella virus. Patients are contagious for a few days before, during, and after the rash appears. Virus is shed from the pharynx and is transmitted by close person-to-person contact. A chronic carrier state does not occur following recovery from rubella acquired postnatally. In contrast, congenital rubella is characterized by chronic shedding of virus for months after birth. These infants are a particular hazard for susceptible hospital personnel. It is, therefore, important that only seropositive or postmenopausal nurses be assigned to congenital rubella patients. Similarly, the serologic testing of young women working in a rubella diagnostic laboratory is essential.

7. Treatment and Prevention

No effective treatment for either postnatal or congenital rubella has been developed. Early diagnosis of auditory and ocular abnormalities should be followed by attempts to correct the defects. Every effort should be made to prevent the shunting of infants into institutions for the retarded without adequate trials and testing in an education-rehabilitation program.

Gamma globulin has been administered to pregnant women exposed to rubella virus during the first trimester of pregnancy, but there is no convincing evidence that it is effective for preventing fetal infection. Passive immunization may only mask the symptoms of disease in the mother and confound the decision about the need for a therapeutic abortion.

Several *live attenuated rubella virus vaccines* have been licensed for use in the USA. Although vaccine-induced immunity appears to be effective in preventing disease, the degree of protection is much lower than that produced by natural infection with wild-type virus. In most individuals studied, Ab has persisted for 3 years or more after vaccination, but maintenance of adequate protection has sometimes been proved to result from asymptomatic infection by wild-type virus. In some cases, Ab titers in vaccinated subjects may decrease slowly to the point where they are inadequate to protect against infection. Immunized persons with inapparent infections constitute a danger to susceptible individuals who, after contact, may develop clinical disease. Spread of wild-type virus from an immunized child to its pregnant nonimmune mother is probably not common but is an ever-present danger.

Some adults, especially women, develop a rash, malaise, arthralgia, and arthritis following immunization with derivatives of the rubella high passage virus (HPV-77) vaccine. Vaccination with the Cendehill strain rubella vaccine also has caused joint manifestations, but they have been less frequent and generally milder than those associated with the HPV-77 strain. The incidence of complications is directly related to age; in children, vaccination seldom causes any adverse reactions.

The HPV-77DK$_{12}$ vaccine, which is produced in dog kidney cells, should not be given to individuals allergic to dog dander and HPV-77DE$_5$ produced in duck embryo cells is contraindicated for patients allergic to eggs. No living vaccine should be administered to persons with impaired immunologic functions.

In anticipation of a rubella epidemic in the early 1970's, a nationwide immunization program was begun in 1969 and was directed towards the vaccination of all children between the age of 1 year and puberty. The program was based primarily on the concept of "herd immunity." It was anticipated that immunizing one "herd," i.e., prepubertal children, would reduce the spread of rubella and protect a second "herd," namely, susceptible pregnant women. However, it has become apparent that the concept of immunizing one segment of a population to prevent infection in another segment may not be valid for rubella. During a rubella outbreak in 1971, involving 1,000 cases, rubella spread among nonimmune individuals despite a fairly high level of immunity in the 1- to 12-year-old group. Most of the cases occurred among unimmunized adolescents 12 to 18 years old, but 7 pregnant women became infected.

Since the principle of herd immunity does not seem to function in a population in which some of the members have not received rubella vaccine, alternatives may be considered. The only means of eliminating rubella would involve vaccination of all infants, followed by appropriate booster injections until the total population is immune. However, this is not a feasible program because of the impossibility of reaching and maintaining contact with the entire population. Therefore, a more practical approach would be to identify and vaccinate all susceptible females approaching the childbearing age.

The difficulty with a program aimed at immunizing postpubertal women is that the vaccine itself could represent a definite threat to the fetus if inadvertently administered during pregnancy. The potential fetal hazard presented by vaccination was evaluated by giving the vaccine to 35 women already certified for legal abortions. Rubella virus was subsequently recovered from the placenta in 6 cases and from the fetus in one case. Virus was also isolated from 13 of 22 uterine cervical swabs taken 9 to 25 days after vaccination of seronegative mothers; no virus was found in comparable specimens obtained from women with preexisting rubella virus Ab. These results indicate the need to observe strict precautions when postpubertal females are vaccinated. It has been suggested that all premarital and pregnancy laboratory studies include a test for rubella Ab. All seronegative patients who are not pregnant should be vaccinated and warned that it is imperative not to become pregnant for at least 3 months. Seronegative patients who are pregnant should be given the vaccine immediately after delivery.

C. Herpes Simplex

Primary herpes simplex is usually inapparent but may be a serious and even fatal systemic disease. The most common clinical form of the disease is characterized by localized clusters of vesicles on the mucous membranes or skin. *Recurrent herpes simplex* results from the activation of latent virus that persists in the tissues after recovery from a primary infection.

1. Etiologic Agent

The etiologic agent of herpes simplex is *herpes simplex virus* (HSV). Type 1 HSV is associated with most nongenital infections and type 2 with the majority of genital and neonatal herpetic infections. In addition, HSV type 2 has been found in association with carcinoma of the cervix (Chapter 24). Infections with HSV type 1 appear to be much more common than type 2 infections on the basis of results from serologic studies.

2. Clinical Symptoms

a. *Primary Herpes Simplex.* Primary herpetic infections may be inapparent, benign, or severe. Approximately 90% of the cases are subclinical, and the only evidence of infection is the appearance of specific Abs. Since most infections are inapparent, the incubation period has not been well defined; however, during several institutional outbreaks, it was observed to vary from 2 to 12 days, averaging about a week. In patients who develop mild or severe illness, fever and malaise are often prominent symptoms. Vesicles may develop at single or multiple mucosal or cutaneous sites.

Herpetic gingivostomatitis is the most common clinical form of primary herpetic infection. It is observed most frequently in children 1 to 4 years of age and less often in adults. The onset is usually gradual and is marked by fever (101 to 104°F), sore throat and mouth, malaise, and irritability. White plaques and edematous vesicles develop on the buccal mucous membranes, tongue, and oropharynx. As the vesicles ulcerate or erode, the mucosal surface becomes denuded, which results in intense pain and difficulty in swallowing. The gums are inflamed, particularly at the gingival margin, and bleed easily. The regional lymph nodes are enlarged and tender. Fever and pain usually persist for 6 to 8 days, and the ulcers gradually heal during the following week.

Herpetic vulvovaginitis, usually caused by HSV type 2, gives rise to extensive and painful lesions similar to those of gingivostomatitis. The vesicular stage may be followed by confluent ulcerations extending to the whole area surrounding the vulvular orifice and occasionally as far as the anus; the ulcerations are often covered with a yellowish-grey pseudomembrane. The inguinal nodes are consistently enlarged and tender. In contrast to genital infections in women, the lesions in men are usually few in number and discrete. The vesicles, most often on the penis and the prepuce, open quickly and exude a clear serous fluid, i.e., "weep." Genital herpes in both sexes may be transmitted venereally.

Herpetic keratoconjunctivitis is characterized by edema and inflammation of the conjunctiva and cornea. It may occur alone or may accompany herpetic lesions on the eyelid or elsewhere. Usually, only one eye is involved; preauricular lymphadenopathy is a constant finding on the affected side. Although the primary corneal opacities may be superficial, scar formation from repeated attacks may result in permanent visual impairment. In addition to the cornea, the lens, retina, and choroid may be involved, with the subsequent development of cataracts and pigmentary alterations in the peripheral retina.

Traumatic herpes simplex is characterized by the appearance of large vesicles and pustules around a cutaneous abrasion or burn. The lesions sometimes assume a radicular distribution similar to that observed in zoster (Section D).

Eczema herpeticum (Kaposi's varicelliform eruption) is a rare but sometimes fatal form of primary herpes simplex infection that occurs in individuals with eczema or neurodermatitis. A generalized pustular eruption develops over a period of days. Groups of vesicles appear in "crops," so that lesions in all stages of development are present simultaneously on a single area of the body; in this respect, the disease is similar to varicella (Section D). The disease may be mistakenly diagnosed as eczema vaccinatum, which occurs under similar conditions following vaccination for smallpox (Section E). The eponym "Kaposi's varicelliform eruption" has unfortunately been applied to both conditions.

Herpetic meningoencephalitis is a serious life-threatening manifestation of primary herpesvirus infection. The neurologic symptoms often indicate localized brain lesions in the temporoparietal region of the cerebal cortex. The mortality rate is high; patients who survive often have permanent psychic, psychomotor, purely motor, or epileptic sequelae. Occasionally, meningitis develops with no involvement of the brain, and, more rarely, encephalitis occurs in the absence of meningitis. It has been estimated that 5 to 7% of cases of aseptic meningitis may be caused by herpesvirus.

Neonatal herpes may develop in infants infected with HSV type 2 by contact with herpetic lesions during passage through the birth canal or by transplacental infection; the illness can vary from mild to severe disseminated disease. Generally, herpetic disease of the newborn occurs only in the absence of maternally acquired IgG. Premature infants, who are less well immunized, are more likely to develop the severe generalized form of the disease (visceral herpes) than full-term infants. *Visceral herpes* of the newborn is a fulminating infection, with fever, viremia, and necrotic lesions in the liver, spleen, lungs, adrenals, kidney, and brain. The few infants who survive almost invariably have permanent brain damage.

b. *Recurrent Herpes Simplex.* Although specific Abs develop following either apparent or inapparent primary herpes infections, herpesvirus may persist in a latent form and be reactivated later by various non-specific stimuli. In some individuals, the recurrent attacks appear after excessive exposure to sunlight or heat; others may be affected following febrile episodes, respiratory or gastrointestinal disturbances, trauma, or exertion. Menstruation, emotional disturbances, and pregnancy also may predispose to recurrent herpes.

The lesions of recurrent herpes are usually benign but painful and tend to occur repeatedly. The recurrences often involve the same site as the primary symptomatic or, presumably, subclinical infection. In most cases, the lesions resulting from reactivation of latent virus take the form of *herpes labialis,* i.e., fever blisters or cold sores (Fig. 12–8). The affected area(s) becomes erythematous and begins to burn, itch, or tingle several hours before the typical fragile, clear vesicles develop. The vesicles rupture soon

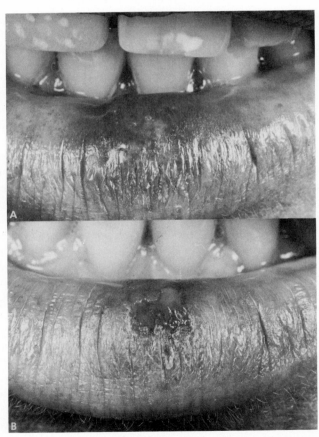

Figure 12–8.   Recurrent herpes labialis. *A,* Six hours after initial symptoms. *B.,* Third day.

after they appear and exude a serous fluid that forms a yellow crust as it dries. The eruptions heal without scarring within several days to a week unless they become secondarily infected with bacteria.

Recurrent generalized herpes and *recurrent meningoencephalitis* are rare but may occur in individuals who recover from eczema herpeticum or primary herpetic encephalitis. A more frequent form of severe recurrent infection occurs following primary herpetic *keratoconjunctivitis;* the most common complication is permanent stromal scarring with loss of visual acuity.

3. Pathogenesis

Herpes simplex can enter the host through the mucous membranes of the nasopharynx, conjunctivae, and genitalia or through abraded or traumatized skin. The virus multiplies at the portal of entry and is spread by either the hematogenous or neurogenic route. Evidence suggests that meningitis and extraneural visceral involvement result from hematogenous dissemination but that isolated encephalitis and some cases of ocular herpes are a consequence of neural spread. After resolution of the primary infection, the virus becomes latent. During the latent period, virus apparently persists intracellularly, since sufficient neutralizing Ab is present to inactivate extracellular virus. Recent evidence indicates that virus may persist within spinal ganglia between recurrent episodes. The virus has been isolated from trigeminal ganglia removed during routine autopsy and cultured *in vitro*. These results indicate that the virus probably is present in a high proportion of human trigeminal ganglia in the absence of overt herpes infections. The common denominator among the factors that precipitate recurrence may be an alteration in host cell physiology that permits virus multiplication; however, the precise mechanism of reactivation is not known.

In recurrent herpes simplex, humoral Ab prevents dissemination of virus but does not inhibit the development of local lesions. The virus can spread directly from cell-to-cell by the fusion of infected cells with adjacent uninfected cells. The lesions of primary and recurrent herpes are indistinguishable microscopically. Skin biopsies taken during the early vesicular stage show dermal congestion with swelling and ballooning degeneration of prickle cells of the epidermis. Vesicles or ulcerated areas contain degenerated epithelial cells as well as multinucleated giant cells. The nuclei of infected cells are enlarged and filled with homogeneous inclusion bodies that first stain blue and later red with hematoxylin and eosin; each of the many nuclei in giant cells often contains one or more inclusion bodies. The intraepidermal vesicles do not extend below the basement membrane and hence do not cause permanent scarring. During healing, the vesicle and corium are densely infiltrated with inflammatory cells.

In fatal cases of herpes encephalitis, there is perivascular infiltration and nerve cell destruction; intranuclear inclusion bodies may be observed in glial cells and, less frequently, in nerve cells.

Visceral herpes of the newborn is characterized by multiple areas of focal necrosis with mononuclear infiltration. All organs of the body, especially the liver and adrenals, may be involved.

The branch-like *dendritic lesion* is the classical sign of ocular herpes simplex infection. An acute florid conjunctivitis, often follicular, may precede the onset of herpetic keratitis by several days. Corticosteroid therapy appears to predispose to the enlargement and ulceration of primary dendritic lesions. At later stages, an epithelial ulcer may persist for weeks or months in the absence of detectable virus multiplication. The failure of the epithelium to regenerate over the corneal stroma is thought to result from a damaged basement membrane. The stroma underlying the epithelial ulcer develops pathologic changes that often spread, even if the epithelial lesion heals. The entire thickness of the corneal stroma is invaded by inflammatory cells, with development of edema, degeneration of the endothelium and stromal scarring. This chronic form of ocular herpetic infection, referred to as *disciform keratitis,* is thought to be a hypersensitivity reaction. In contrast, involvement of the iris in stromal keratitis may be due to direct invasion of the virus or to a toxic effect.

4. Immunity

Maternal IgG usually affords protection against HSV type 1 infection during the first 6 months of life. Although the majority of adults possess Ab to HSV type 1, the incidence of type 2 infection is considerably lower. As a consequence, passively acquired immunity to HSV type 2 is not common.

The primary immune response following either apparent or inapparent infection is characterized by the appearance of neutralizing Ab, which can be detected only in the presence of fresh complement; shortly thereafter, this Ab is replaced by complement-independent neutralizing Ab. The presence of serum Abs probably accounts for the attenuated clinical symptoms and absence of viremia during recurrent herpes. However, since reactivation of latent virus can occur in the presence of high levels of circulating Ab, it appears that cell-mediated immunity may play the dominant role in resistance to and recovery from recurrent infections. It has been suggested that an exaggerated hypersensitivity to viral Ag may contribute to pathogenesis.

5. Diagnosis

Virus isolation and serologic studies are used mainly to confirm the clinical diagnosis of primary herpes simplex. The history and clinical appearance of recurrent skin and eye infections are usually sufficient to establish the diagnosis. In instances of severe disease, a laboratory diagnosis may be required.

For virus isolation, specimens should be collected within the first 4 to 5 days of illness and inoculated into tissue cultures. Embryonated eggs and laboratory animals are now seldom used for primary isolation of the HSV but are useful for differentiating it from varicella-zoster (V-Z) virus, which replicates only in tissue cultures. Herpes simplex virus usually can be isolated from vesicle fluid, scrapings of ulcerations, and throat swabs or saliva. Direct examination of stained cells from the lesions or infected tissue culture cells reveals eosinophilic intranuclear inclusion bodies characteristic of the herpesvirus group; vaccinia and variola, with which some herpes infections may be confused, cause cytoplasmic inclusion bodies. Herpes simplex virus must be specifically identified by CF, neutralization, or immunofluorescence techniques to differentiate it from V-Z virus, which causes similar lesions.

Serologic studies using patients' paired sera are of value in the diagnosis of primary herpes infections only in instances in which a rise in specific Ab titer can be demonstrated. In recurrent herpes, high Ab levels may be present, but there is no consistent rise in titer. It is important to note that patients with a recent history of V-Z virus infection may respond to HSV infection with an increase in CF Abs to both viruses. In addition to infections with V-Z virus, vaccinia, and variola viruses, the differential diagnosis of herpes simplex includes herpangina, Vincent's angina (which responds dramatically to penicillin), and the secondary bacterial infection of eczema. Herpetic meningoencephalitis must be differentiated from bacterial and viral encephalitides and postinfectious encephalitis in order to institute the proper therapy as soon as possible.

6. Epidemiology

Man is the only known natural reservoir of HSV. It has been estimated that 70 to 90% of adults possess neutralizing Ab against HSV type 1; this agent is probably the most ubiquitous virus in man.

Primary infection with HSV type 1 usually occurs before the age of 5 years but is rare in infants under 6 months of age, who are passively protected by maternal Ab. There is a high infection rate during infancy in lower socioeconomic groups where crowded living conditions and poor sanitation exist. Herpes simplex is an endemic disease but may occur in minor epidemics within family groups, hospitals, and institutions. Patients with overt disease as well as convalescents and healthy carriers may shed the virus in vesicle fluid, saliva, and stools. The virus is believed to be spread from person-to-person by direct contact or indirectly from eating or drinking utensils contaminated with saliva.

In contrast to HSV type 1, HSV type 2 is transmitted venereally. With the exception of neonatal infections acquired at or before birth, genital herpes seldom is observed before adolescence (i.e., children are infrequently infected). The incidence of type 2 infection is lower than type 1 infection and correlates with veneral exposure. For example, the incidence among prostitutes is high, but it is negligible among nuns.

7. Treatment and Prevention

Herpes simplex virus type 1 infections were among the first of the viral infections to be successfully treated with chemotherapeutic agents. The majority of patients with primary herpetic keratitis, cutaneous infections, and even encephalitis respond dramatically when treated with iododeoxyuridine (IUdR) early in the course of the infection; many individuals are asymptomatic within a week. Topical application of the drug every two hours is particularly effective in preventing the sequelae associated with dendritic keratitis. Chronic infections that involve the corneal stroma do not respond to IUdR but may be reduced by judicious topical application of corticosteroids; steroid therapy is contraindicated with dendritic keratitis since it may increase the chance of ulceration and perforation. Combined IUdR and steroid therapy should be attempted only by an experienced ophthalmologist. Although IUdR is toxic when administered by perfusion, recent experience indicates that it may be useful in treating generalized herpes of the newborn, for which there is no effective treatment at present. Iododeoxyuridine is relatively ineffective for gingivostomatitis because it is rapidly washed away by secretions. Although the drug suppresses viral multiplication, it neither eliminates the virus (i.e., it is nonviricidal) nor prevents relapses; recurrent infections occur as frequently in IUdR-treated patients as in untreated patients. Some strains of HSV type 1 and most strains of HSV type 2 are resistant to IUdR. The emergence of drug-resistant or drug-dependent mutants may account for the decreased effectiveness of the drug during recurrent infections.

Preliminary results with cytosine arabinoside (Ara-C) and adenine arabinoside (Ara-A) suggest that these thymidine analogues are less toxic than IUdR and may be equally effective in treating herpetic infections. They appear to be particularly promising for use when IUdR-resistant mutants emerge and in cases of allergic or toxic reactions.

The prophylactic use of gamma globulin derived from hyperimmune serum is recommended when a newborn has been in contact with an infected individual; however, it is not effective for treating congenital infections.

No vaccines for HSV are commercially available. Some success in preventing recurrent infections has been reported following repeated intradermal and subcutaneous injections of an experimental inactivated vaccine.

The mechanism involved in the resistance that develops is not known, but it appears to be at the cellular level, since there is no consistent increase in circulating Abs.

The results from controlled studies indicate that the formerly popular practice of administering smallpox vaccine to prevent recurrent herpes labialis has no scientific basis and is no more effective than placebos.

D. Varicella (Chickenpox) and Zoster (Shingles)

Varicella is a highly contagious disease that occurs mainly in children. It is characterized by a disseminated vesicular eruption that develops in brief successive crops; when the disease occurs in adults, neonates, or immunologically compromised patients, the symptoms may be severe.

Zoster is a sporadic infectious disease characterized by unilateral inflammation of dorsal root ganglia or extramedullary cranial nerve ganglia. A unilateral vesicular skin eruption usually develops along the pathway of the involved nerves. The disease occurs mainly in adults and probably results from reactivation of virus that persists in latent form following recovery from chickenpox.

1. Etiologic Agent

Chickenpox and zoster are caused by a single serotype of virus, *varicella-zoster* (V-Z), a member of the herpesvirus group. The virus is distinct from herpes simplex virus, although the two share minor antigenic determinants.

2. Clinical Symptoms

Varicella. The incubation period from the time of exposure to the appearance of rash usually ranges from 13 to 17 days. There may be fever and malaise for 1 to 2 days before the rash appears, but more often these symptoms and the rash develop concurrently. The lesions, which appear in crops over a period of 1 to 5 days, are first observed on the trunk and later on the extremities. The typical chickenpox eruption begins as a maculopapule that evolves within a few hours into a fragile, teardrop-shaped vesicle surrounded by a red border. Within a day, the erythema diminishes and the vesicle collapses in the center, forming an umbilicated pustule. The lesion becomes crusted, and after several days the scab falls off. There is no scarring in the absence of secondary bacterial contamination. However, because of intense itching, children usually scratch, and vesicles may become infected. New maculopapules continue to erupt and go through a similar evolution. Because of the appearance of new crops, lesions in various stages of development (maculopapule, vesicle, pustule, and scabs) are present simultaneously in a single area (Fig. 12–9). In regions of the world where smallpox occurs, it is essential that chickenpox be differentiated from mild cases of smallpox. The characteristics listed on Table 12–1 are useful for establishing a presumptive diagnosis.

Although chickenpox is usually a benign disease in childhood, it can be severe and sometimes fatal in adults, neonates, children with leukemia, and individuals on immunosuppressive therapy. In these patients, the rash often persists longer than usual and may become hemorrhagic. Primary

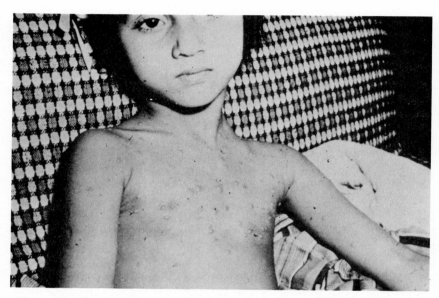

Figure 12—9. Varicella. Lesions in various stages of development on trunk. Minimal involvement of face and arms. (Courtesy of Center for Disease Control.)

TABLE 12—1

Comparison of Smallpox and Varicella Lesions

Smallpox

1. Single crop of lesions on a given area of skin.
2. Lesions first appear on the face and extremities.
3. Lesions on palms.
4. Cytoplasmic inclusions observed in skin scrapings from lesions.

Varicella

1. Lesions in all stages of development on a given area of skin.
2. Lesions first appear on trunk.
3. Palms not involved.
4. Nuclear inclusions observed in skin scrapings from lesions.

varicella pneumonia develops in about 15% of adults with chickenpox. The fatal disseminated form of the disease is seen most frequently in children being treated with steroids for leukemia or other diseases of the hematopoietic system. Postvaricella encephalitis is a rare but grave complication that can follow either mild or severe disease.

Zoster. The preeruptive stage of zoster may be preceded by 1 to 4 days of fever with pain and paresthesia over the area of the involved nerve. Subsequently, an erythematous rash appears, the individual lesions evolving as in chickenpox. The eruption is confined, for the most part, to the area of distribution of one or more spinal nerves or the sensory division of a cranial nerve. Infection of the ophthalmic division of the trigeminal nerve may result in damage to the cornea, as well as in skin eruptions on the forehead, eyelids, and nose. The corneal changes range from lesions with no stromal alterations to lesions with epithelial and stromal ulceration and opacity. The localized distribution of the lesions in zoster gives the eruption its characteristic unilateral band-like pattern (Fig. 12–10). Re-

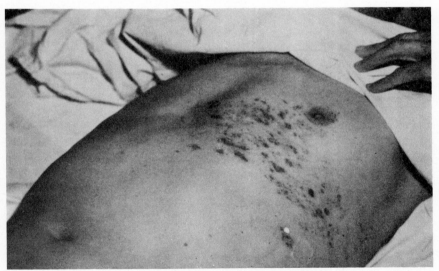

Figure 12–10.   Zoster skin lesions. The unilaterally located vesicles have ruptured. (Reprinted with permission from Eli Lilly and Co., *Physicians Bulletin*, 1959; series of slides distributed by Lilly entitled "Current Advances and Concepts in Virology.")

gional lymph node involvement is a constant finding. Some patients develop a generalized vesicular rash resembling varicella shortly after the localized lesions appear.

The course of zoster from onset to complete recovery is about 2 to 3 weeks. Adults over 40 years of age may not recover completely for 4 to 5 weeks. Postherpetic neuralgia is a serious and painful complication of zoster that may occur in elderly patients with arteriosclerosis. Frequently, there is an interval between the acute phase of the disease and the development of characteristic severe pain; pain may persist for weeks to months.

3. Pathogenesis

Varicella. Varicella is probably transmitted by the respiratory route. The appearance of successive crops of widely distributed skin lesions suggests that intermittent viremia may occur. Focal viral infection of blood vessels in the corium results in fluid accumulation and ballooning degeneration of cells in the basal and prickle layers of the epithelium. The resulting vesicles contain serum, epithelial and inflammatory cells, and multinucleate giant cells. Eosinophilic inclusion bodies identical with those seen in herpes simplex may be observed in the nuclei of infected cells. Virus is present in vesicle fluid for several days after eruption but is seldom detected in crusts or scales. In varicella pneumonia, the tracheobronchial mucosa, the alveolar septa, and the interstitium of the lung become edematous and are infiltrated with monocytic inflammatory cells and giant cells. The CNS changes observed in patients who develop encephalomyelitis include diffuse focal hemorrhage, lymphocytic infiltration, and demyelinization.

Zoster. The pathogenesis of zoster is not clear. The disease occurs in individuals with a history of varicella and apparently results from the reactivation of latent virus. The trigger mechanism is not known in some cases of zoster; in others, the disease develops following trauma, exhaustion, sunburn, injection of drugs, or immunosuppressive therapy, or is concomitant with diseases such as tuberculosis or malignancy. The cutaneous lesions of zoster are histopathologically identical with those of varicella. In addition, there is an acute inflammatory reaction of the dorsal nerve roots and ganglia. Often only a single ganglion is involved. Zoster most commonly involves areas of the skin innervated by the thoracic ganglia or, less frequently, the cervical ganglia or the ophthalmic branch of the gasserian ganglia. The affected spinal ganglion is infiltrated with mononuclear cells and presents scattered hemorrhagic areas. Intranuclear inclusions have been demonstrated in ganglia and in satellite cells. The inflammatory response may extend to the posterior horns or, less often, to the anterior horns of the spinal cord.

Virus is abundant in vesicle fluid and occasionally may be recovered from spinal fluid; V-Z virus has been detected in trigeminal nerves and ganglia by immunofluorescence and electron microscopy but it has not been isolated from these tissues.

4. Immunity

Immunity to exogenous reinfection with V-Z virus is long-lasting. However, the neutralizing Ab produced does not protect against reactivation of latent virus. There is some evidence to indicate that varicella convalescent Ab may differ qualitatively from zoster Ab. Two subclasses of IgG have been separated from sera of patients with V-Z virus infection. The two classes, "slow" and "fast" IgG, differ in their neutralizing activity, depending upon the clinical manifestation of the infection. In varicella infections, neutralizing activity was demonstrable in the "slow" IgG fraction, whereas in zoster, the neutralizing Ab was in the "fast" IgG fraction. The "slow" IgG fraction following chickenpox may not prevent the subsequent development of zoster. However, a second generalized exposure to V-Z virus in the form of zoster results in significant levels of efficient neutralizing Ab. This Ab may account for the fact that second attacks of zoster are rare.

In established V-Z virus infections, the virus most likely spreads by direct cell-to-cell transfer, and cell-mediated immunity probably plays an important role in recovery from infection.

5. Diagnosis

Varicella. Varicella can usually be diagnosed by the character of the rash and a history of recent exposure. In areas where smallpox is a possibility, differentiation from mild smallpox may be difficult when distribution of the lesions is atypical. A rapid presumptive diagnosis can be made by examining stained scrapings of early vesicles or biopsied tissue; the presence of characteristic multinucleated giant cells containing intranuclear inclusion bodies rules out smallpox or vaccinia. Differential diagnosis from smallpox and vaccinia also may be obtained by electron microscopic examination of vesicle fluid for typical virus particles. Complement-fixation and agar-gel diffusion tests are useful for demonstrating specific Ag in vesicle fluids. Atypical varicella occasionally must be differentiated from other generalized vesicular eruptions, including complicated herpes simplex, rickettsialpox, and some coxsackievirus infections. When a specific etiologic diagnosis is required, virus may be isolated in tissue cultures inoculated with fluid obtained from vesicles in an early stage of development. Varicella-zoster virus, in contrast to HSV, does not multiply in either embryonated eggs or laboratory animals. Serologic tests using patients' paired sera may be used to confirm a diagnosis of varicella when virus can no longer be isolated.

Zoster. The diagnosis of zoster is difficult before the appearance of the characteristic unilaterally distributed vesicles. During the preeruptive stage, the disease often is confused with more common causes of intense pain, such as pleurisy, a collapsed intervertebral disc, or appendicitis. If the eruption is atypical, zoster may be clinically indistinguishable from recurrent herpes simplex, which may also follow radicular lines. Since second attacks of zoster are rare, most reported cases of recurrent zoster are probably examples of HSV infection. A specific diagnosis can be established by isolating and identifying the etiologic agent.

6. Epidemiology

Varicella is one of the most common contagious diseases of childhood. The attack rate is 70% or more among susceptible individuals exposed to the virus; inapparent infections are rare. Although the disease is endemic in the USA, epidemics occur during the winter or spring every 2 to 5 years. Children 5 to 8 years of age are most commonly affected, but newborns, younger children, and adults who escaped infection during childhood also may develop the disease. Chickenpox presumably is spread by droplet transmission as well as by direct or indirect contact with skin lesions. The infectious period extends from 1 to 2 days before the rash up to about a week after lesions appear.

In contrast to chickenpox, zoster is a sporadic disease without a seasonal prevalence and occurs more commonly in adults than in children. If a zoster patient transmits the virus to a susceptible child, the child develops typical chickenpox and may initiate an epidemic. However, the incidence of zoster does not increase during epidemics of chickenpox. The increasing use of immunosuppressive drugs for tumor therapy and organ transplantation has led to a rise in the incidence of zoster, especially in the life-threatening disseminated forms of the disease.

7. Treatment and Prevention

Uncomplicated varicella and zoster are self-limiting diseases. Therapy is symptomatic and consists primarily of ointments, such as calamine lotion, to relieve the itching. In the acute phase of zoster, aspirin and codeine usually control the pain; no treatment is completely satisfactory for relieving severe postherpetic neuralgia. Treatment of ocular lesions includes atropine and cortisone, which should be administered by an ophthalmologist. Secondary bacterial infections should be treated with appropriate antibiotics.

Controlled studies are in progress to evaluate the reported effectiveness of Ara-A and Ara-C for treating severe cases of chickenpox and zoster. Since these drugs suppress the immune response, they should not be administered to exposed individuals to prevent chickenpox. Iododeoxyuridine appears to be ineffective against zoster when given in the usual doses; however, continuous local application may reduce the duration of pain. Although steroids are contraindicated during the incubation period of chickenpox, it has been demonstrated that pain following zoster may be diminished in duration by early therapy with steroids.

Passive immunization with pooled gamma globulin is not effective for preventing varicella or for treating generalized zoster or severe varicella.

However, it has been demonstrated that varicella can be prevented or attenuated by giving zoster (but not chickenpox) hyperimmune globulin to susceptible children within 72 hours after exposure. Immune zoster-globulin is in short supply and should be used only to protect high-risk patients (e.g., newborns, children with leukemia or immune deficiency diseases, and individuals on immunosuppressive drugs).

No vaccines are available for V-Z virus infections.

E. Smallpox

Smallpox (variola major) is a contagious febrile disease characterized by vesicular and pustular lesions. *Alastrim* (variola minor) is a form of small-pox that is clinically indistinguishable from mild cases of variola major but consistently has a lower mortality rate. *Vaccinia* is a disease of the skin induced by inoculating vaccinia virus for the prevention of smallpox.

1. Etiologic Agents

Smallpox is caused by *variola virus*. Alastrim is caused by a stable attenuated variant of variola virus that is antigenically indistinguishable from the virulent virus; the origin of the attenuated virus is unknown. Vaccinia is caused by *vaccinia virus,* which was originally obtained from cowpox lesions.

2. Clinical Symptoms

Smallpox may assume many different clinical forms, ranging from a minor febrile illness with no rash (*variola sine eruptione*) to a rapidly fulminating disease.

A typical moderate case of smallpox is diphasic; it can be divided into a preeruptive (prodrome) and an eruptive phase. After an incubation period of approximately 12 days, the illness begins with a vague syndrome consisting of fever (102 to 106°F), headache, abdominal pain, vomiting, backache, limb pains, and prostration. In a few patients, the prodromal symptoms include a transient erythematous or petechial rash. After 3 to 4 days, the fever subsides and there is marked clinical improvement.

When the eruptive phase begins, the patient is usually afebrile. Early manifestations include painful ulcers on the buccal mucosa and macules that appear first on the face and forearms and rapidly develop into papules. The papules increase in number and spread from the face and distal extremities to involve the trunk. A characteristic feature of smallpox is the fact that lesions in any one area are all in the same stage of development. Lesions are generally found on the palms of the hands, which are seldom involved in chickenpox (Fig. 12–11). Within 2 or 3 days after the appearance of the focal rash, the papules develop into vesicles that contain clear

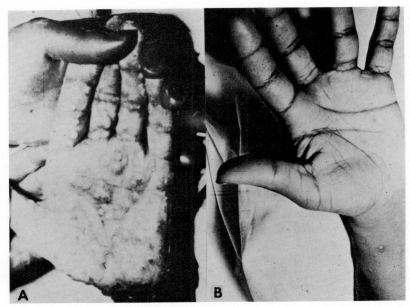

Figure 12–11. *A,* Variola major; extensive eruptions on palm. *B,* Varicella; minimal involvement of palm. (Courtesy of Center for Disease Control.)

fluid. Shortly thereafter, the vesicles become cloudy and pustular as a result of infiltration of pus cells and desquamated epithelial cells. Concomitant with pustule formation, there is a secondary rise in temperature proportional to the severity of the disease. The fever, which probably results from absorption of toxic products released by cell necrosis, persists until healing begins. About 8 to 9 days after onset of the eruption, the pustules umbilicate and begin to form crusts. The scabs drop off within 3 to 4 weeks after the beginning of the disease. Pitted scarring of the skin is more pronounced on the face and distal parts of the arms and legs, where the eruption is characteristically more severe (Fig. 12–12).

In naturally immunized or vaccinated individuals, the focal eruption may be absent or scant. Following the usual incubation period and prodrome, a rash resembling chickenpox may develop. Regardless of how mild an index case of smallpox may be, susceptible contacts may suffer severe disease. Incorrectly diagnosed or undiagnosed cases are frequently the cause of severe epidemics.

The case mortality rate for smallpox ranges from 2% in patients with a scant, discrete rash to 25% if the rash is semiconfluent to 50% if the rash is confluent. A case of severe variola major is illustrated in Fig. 12–13. The fulminating hemorrhagic type of smallpox results from an over-

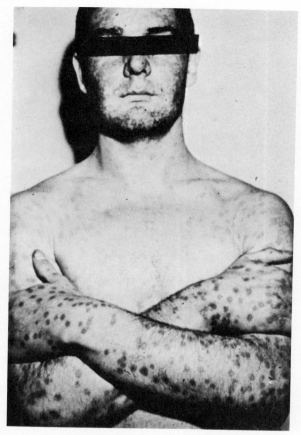

Figure 12—12. Variola major. Late disease, early scarring. (Courtesy of Armed Forces Institute of Pathology.)

whelming infection and is almost always fatal. After the usual incubation period, the patient develops a severe prodromal illness characterized by prostration, high fever, bone marrow depression, hemorrhagic skin lesions, bleeding from any or all orifices of the body, shock, coma, and death. The disease may progress from onset to death within 3 or 4 days without evidence of the typical focal eruption.

Alastrim resembles the mild to moderate forms of smallpox in that it has the same incubation period and a similar, but less severe, prodromal illness. The focal eruption is less extensive and is of shorter duration than the focal eruption in smallpox (Fig. 12–14); the case mortality of alastrim is less than 1%. The mildness of the illness makes it difficult to distinguish from chickenpox and benign forms of variola major.

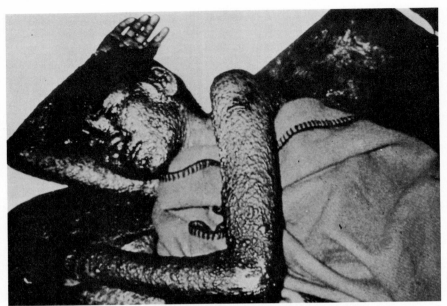

Figure 12—13. Variola major. Severe infection, 10th to 12th day. (Courtesy of Center for Disease Control.)

3. Pathogenesis

The portal of entry for variola virus is probably the URT. During the incubation period, the virus multiplies at an unknown site, most likely in regional lymphoid tissue. The fact that patients are not infectious during the incubation period suggests that there are no open lesions in the respiratory mucosa. A primary viremia occurs at the onset of fever and persists for the first 2 or 3 days of the prodrome. Virus localizes in the cells of the RES and undergoes a second phase of multiplication. Release of virus from these tissues causes an intense secondary viremia. From the bloodstream, virus is distributed to the mucous membranes and skin where it produces the typical focal lesions.

The first pathologic changes leading to skin lesions include capillary dilatation, plasma cell infiltration of the corium, and proliferation of the prickle-cell layer. Infected epithelial cells become swollen and vacuolated and undergo ballooning degeneration. Intercellular and intracellular edema lead to the formation of vesicles where the epithelial cells have been destroyed. The accumulation of epithelial cell debris and the infiltration of neutrophils into the vesicle fluid converts the lesion into a pustule. Infected epithelial cells contain acidophilic intracytoplasmic inclusion bodies, called Guarnieri bodies, which are surrounded by a clear unstained halo.

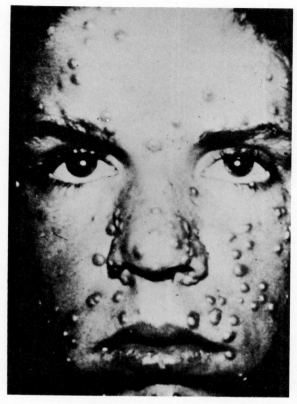

Figure 12–14. Alastrim (variola minor). Second week. (Courtesy of Center for Disease Control.)

4. Immunity

Active immunity following recovery from smallpox persists for many years and is probably lifelong. The immunity that develops following vaccination is of shorter duration but appears to be effective for at least 3 to 5 years.

Antibodies can be detected in the blood of smallpox patients as early as the fourth day of the disease, but they do not prevent progression of the focal lesions. The role of cell-mediated immunity has not been clearly defined, but it is probably important in suppressing cell-to-cell spread of virus within the lesions. Patients with hypogammaglobulinemia usually respond normally to vaccination and develop immunity, whereas those with defects in both cell-mediated immunity and humoral Ab production develop progressive, often fatal, disease.

5. Diagnosis

Typical cases of smallpox are easily diagnosed on the basis of clinical symptoms, particularly in endemic areas and during epidemics. *In countries where smallpox is not endemic, the first case may be difficult to diagnose.* This is particularly true if the patient has either a very mild form of the disease, as a result of previous vaccination, or the fulminating hemorrhagic type in which death may occur before the disease reaches the eruptive phase. Unless there is a history of exposure, a clinical diagnosis cannot be made during the prodromal phase. In the eruptive phase, the most useful clinical features in establishing the diagnosis are (1) the centrifugal distribution of the lesions; (2) the progressive appearance of lesions that spread from the face and arms to the legs and finally the trunk; and (3) the fact that all lesions in a given area of the body are in the same stage of development.

Laboratory procedures usually are required to establish or confirm the diagnosis of the first case of smallpox that appears in the community. A rapid presumptive diagnosis of smallpox can be made by either demonstrating intracytoplasmic inclusion bodies in stained smears of cells from papules and vesicles or by electron microscopic demonstration of poxvirus particles in vesicle fluid. These two procedures are not satisfactory after the vesicular stage of the disease has passed. Viral antigen in vesicles, pustules, and scabs may be demonstrated by fluorescent microscopy, agar gel diffusion, or CF tests. Serologic procedures, such as CF, neutralization, and HI tests, may be used to detect an increase in specific Abs during the eruptive phase.

Virus isolation is more time-consuming but is the most reliable way to establish a specific diagnosis. Isolation procedures are particularly important in differentiating smallpox from generalized vaccinia, which may occur following vaccination during an epidemic. Virus may be isolated from the blood during the preeruptive phase of severe disease, particularly the hemorrhagic type; in milder cases the viremia may last only a few hours, and often virus cannot be isolated. The focal lesions invariably contain virus at any stage of the disease. The specimens are inoculated onto the chorioallantoic membrane of the chick embryo or susceptible cell cultures. Virus isolates are identified by appropriate serologic tests.

6. Epidemiology

Man is the only natural host and reservoir of variola virus. Although smallpox affects monkeys, they do not appear to be an important source of virus in the absence of human cases.

Smallpox patients are not infectious during the incubation period or the prodrome but become highly infectious in the early eruptive phase. The virus may be spread by either direct or indirect contact. The buccal lesions, which appear before the skin eruptions, ulcerate and cause gross contamination of saliva and respiratory secretions. During this period, virus is spread by droplet transmission. Vesicles and pustules contain large amounts of virus and, when ruptured, provide a major source for dissemination. Virus is also present in exfoliating scabs, where it may persist in infectious form for long periods of time. Bedlinens and clothes contaminated with virus from open lesions or secretions may serve as an indirect source of infection; in this case, the virus is probably acquired by the inhalation of infected dust.

Smallpox has been eradicated in many parts of the world. No cases have been reported in the USA since 1949, and only sporadic outbreaks have occurred in Europe. However, the disease is still endemic in some parts of the world, principally Asia, Africa, and South America. Mass vaccination campaigns supported by the World Health Organization (WHO) have been successful in reducing the incidence in some endemic areas. Because of the possible importation of the disease, smallpox will remain a potential problem until global eradication is achieved.

7. Treatment and Prevention

Treatment. At the present time, there is no effective treatment for smallpox. Beta-thiosemicarbazone, which is effective prophylactically, is of no value in the treatment of established cases.

Vaccination. The commercially available *live vaccinia virus vaccine* is probably still more widely used than any other vaccine. Its effectiveness in preventing smallpox has been demonstrated beyond question during the 175 years since it was first popularized by Jenner.

Smallpox vaccine is prepared from vaccinia virus propagated in the skin of calves or sheep. The material is treated with 1% phenol to reduce bacterial contamination and is either lyophilized or stabilized with glycerol and stored at $-10°C$. At $-10°C$, the vaccine retains its infectivity for about a year. The lyophilized vaccine, however, can be preserved at $0°C$ or lower for about 5 years; in temperate zones, it retains its potency for approximately a year without refrigeration, but only for a month in the tropics. Once the vaccine has been reconstituted, it can be kept for only a few days in the refrigerator. Recently, a vaccine has been developed that eliminates these inherent disadvantages of the currently available vaccines. It consists of a trifurcated needle device precoated with freeze-dried vaccinia virus. The vaccine appears to be stable for long periods without freezing or refrigeration and can be administered percutaneously without rehydration.

The preferred site for vaccination is the outer aspect of the upper arm over the insertion of the deltoid muscle. Reactions are less likely to be severe in this area than on other parts of the body. Vaccine may be introduced by a variety of techniques, including multiple-pressure, multiple-puncture, and jet injector. The scratch method gives satisfactory results in persons being vaccinated for the first time but may not be effective for revaccination.

Interpretation of vaccination results should follow the recommendations presented in the 1972 report of the WHO Expert Committee on Smallpox Eradication. Following successful *primary vaccination,* a vesicle develops after 3 to 5 days; subsequently, the lesion becomes pustular and achieves its maximal size after 8 or 9 days (Fig. 12–15A). A scab is then formed, which separates at 14 to 21 days, leaving a typical vaccination scar.

Revaccination is considered to have been successful if, on examination after 6 to 8 days, there is either a pustular lesion or an area of definite induration or congestion surrounding an ulcer or a scab. This is termed a "major" reaction (Fig. 12–15B); all other responses to revaccination are termed "equivocal reactions" (Fig. 12–15C). Equivocal reactions, previously classified as accelerated (vaccinoid) or immediate (immune) responses, may be exhibited by persons with varying degrees of immunity. However, an equivocal reaction may also develop in individuals who are allergic to the vaccine or who have been vaccinated with an inactive vaccine. When equivocal reactions are observed in vaccinees who are likely to be exposed to smallpox, the procedure should be repeated at a different site with fresh vaccine.

Complications Resulting from Vaccination. A small but definite risk of serious complications is associated with smallpox vaccination. The risk of death from all complications is about 1 per million primary vaccinees and 1 per 100,000 revaccinees; the risk of death for infants under 1 year of age is approximately 5 per million primary vaccinations. Vaccination is contraindicated for individuals with immune deficiency diseases or conditions requiring the use of immunosuppressive drugs, steroids, or radiation therapy. In addition, pregnant women and individuals with eczema or persons in contact with eczematous patients should not be vaccinated.

Eczema vaccinatum may result when vaccinia virus is transferred from the inoculation site to preexisting skin lesions of either the vaccinated person or a contact (Fig. 12–16). Although many cases of eczema vaccinatum resolve satisfactorily, some progress and may prove fatal.

Progressive vaccinia (vaccinia necrosum) is a very rare and serious complication occurring in persons with impaired cell-mediated or humoral immunity. The initial lesion fails to regress and becomes progressively necrotic (Fig. 12–17). Foci may develop in other parts of the body, including the bones and internal organs. The disease is usually fatal.

Postvaccinal encephalitis is a rare complication that occurs most often during the second week after primary vaccination; it is extremely infre-

A. PRIMARY REACTION

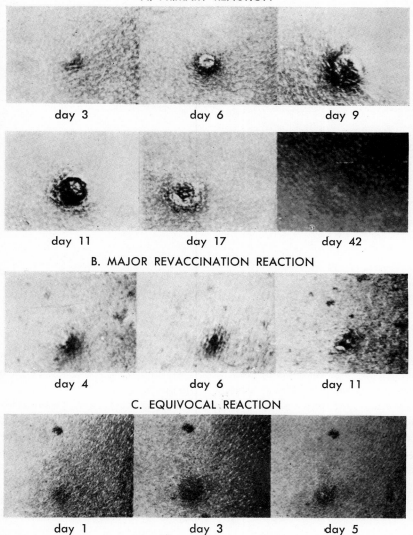

Fig. 12—15.   Typical responses to smallpox vaccination.

A, Primary reaction: day 3, papule with early vesiculation; day 6, vesicle; day 9, vesicle with early scab formation; day 11, scab; day 17, scab shed, leaving area of desquamation and discoloration; day 42, remaining scar.

B, Major revaccination reaction: day 4, papule with central scab; day 6, papule covered by scab; day 11, scab shed, leaving small area of desquamation.

C, Equivocal reaction: day 1, erythema and papule; day 3, papule larger, surrounding erythema fading; day 5, papule fading.

(Modified from Elisberg, B. L., McCown, J. M., Smadel, J. E.: J. Immunol. *77:* 340, 1956.

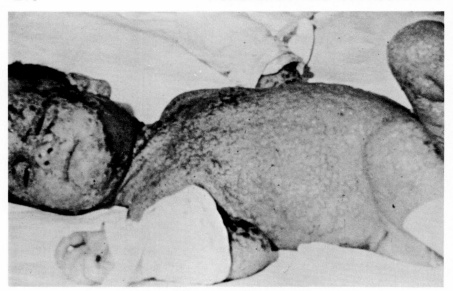

Figure 12–16. Eczema vaccinatum. Eight-month-old boy with eczema vaccinatum who acquired vaccinia from recently vaccinated sibling. (Courtesy of Center for Disease Control.)

quent after revaccination. There are no known predisposing factors. Although the etiology is not clear, the timing suggests that the encephalitis may be caused by Ag-Ab complexes. Most persons affected with postvaccinal encephalitis recover completely, but some die, and a few of those who recover have residual neurologic sequelae.

Autoinoculation or *accidental infection* of contacts may result when vaccinia virus is transferred from the vaccination site to mucous membranes or to abraded skin surfaces. Localized lesions develop at the infection sites in the absence of predisposing factors. Except in the rare instances in which ocular infection is followed by permanent scarring of the cornea, this complication has no serious consequences.

Generalized vaccinia may develop following a transient viremia. Vaccinial lesions begin to appear 5 to 10 days after vaccination and may be widely distributed over the body. There are no known predisposing factors; generalized vaccinia may occur in individuals with no detectable immunologic deficiencies and in the absence of preexisting skin lesions. This complication is not progressive and is never fatal.

Hypersensitivity reactions in the form of urticarial, morbilliform, and erythema multiform eruptions are sometimes seen and may be confused with generalized vaccinia.

Fetal vaccinia may follow maternal vaccination in the 3rd to 24th weeks of gestation. Most fetal infections result in stillbirths. Living infants may

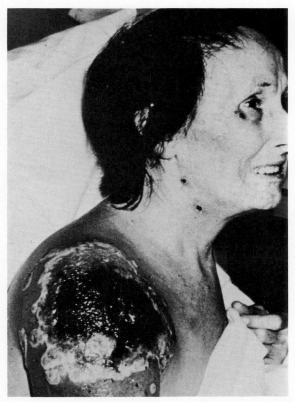

Figure 12–17. Progressive vaccinia. Sixty-two-year-old patient with chronic lymphocytic leukemia who was vaccinated as a therapeutic measure for herpes simplex. (Courtesy of Center for Disease Control.)

have extensive hemorrhagic lesions (Fig. 12–18). Depending upon the severity of the infection, the disease can be fatal or the infant may recover with no effects other than scarring.

Patients with eczema vaccinatum, progressive vaccinia, generalized vaccinia, or ocular vaccinia should be treated promptly with vaccinia immune globulin. The use of immune globulin has reduced the fatality rate of eczema vaccinatum from 40% to about 1%. Although globulin administered at the time of vaccination reduces the incidence of encephalitis, it is not effective in the treatment of the disease.

Vaccine Recommendations. In 1971, the U.S. Public Health Service recommended that smallpox vaccination in the USA be used selectively rather than as a routine procedure. It is recommended that the only individuals who should receive the vaccine are those who travel in endemic areas and those who might be early contacts of an imported case (health

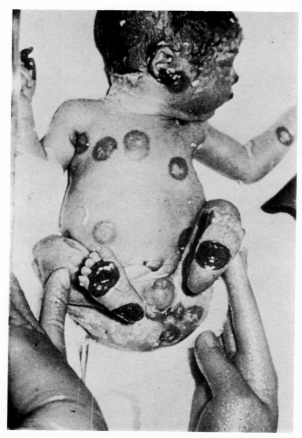

Figure 12—18.   Fetal vaccinia in a child born in the 28th week of gestation. (Courtesy of Center for Disease Control.)

service and hospital personnel, port and customs officials). This revision of the vaccination requirements was made on the basis of results from statistical and epidemiologic studies which indicated that the risks from the vaccine outweighed the current risk of exposure to the disease. The network of health services is extensive in the USA, and the smallpox surveillance program is well developed. Should the disease be introduced into the USA, it would be rapidly detected and contained.

F.   Contagious Pustular Dermatitis (Orf) and Milkers' Nodule

Contagious pustular dermatitis is a disease of sheep that is occasionally transmitted to man. Milkers' nodule is a benign infectious disease that man contracts from cows. Both diseases are characterized by painless dark red papules that become enlarged and may ulcerate.

1. Etiologic Agents

Contagious pustular dermatitis and *milkers' nodule viruses* are morphologically identical poxviruses that are distinguished mainly on the basis of their natural hosts. The relationship between the viruses is obscure. It has been shown that inoculation of sheep with bovine virus from milkers' nodule causes lesions identical to those of orf.

2. Clinical Symptoms

In man, the incubation period for both diseases is 4 to 11 days. The eruption begins as single or multiple lesions, usually on the hands or face. The initial lesions are small, reddish-blue macules or papules that enlarge to form vascularized bullae from which little fluid can be expressed. The surface gradually becomes white and sodden, a crust forms, and a granulomatous reaction may develop. The mature lesions are elevated or tumor-like and well demarcated from normal skin. Systemic manifestations are rare, except for occasional low-grade fever and mild regional lymph node involvement. Healing occurs spontaneously in 4 to 6 weeks with little or no scar formation.

3. Pathogenesis

These infections result in proliferation, ballooning, and reticular degeneration of epidermal cells. There is multilocular vesiculation and hyperplasia that can mimic malignancy of the epithelium. A granulomatous reaction is present in the dermis.

4. Immunity

Neutralizing and CF Abs have been demonstrated in the blood of recovered animals and man. A single attack seems to confer lasting immunity to reinfection.

5. Diagnosis

Diagnosis usually is on the basis of the characteristic lesions in individuals with a history of contact with sheep or cows. The diagnosis can be confirmed by virus isolation in tissue culture and by demonstrating a rise in titer of serum neutralizing Ab against the specific agent.

6. Epidemiology

Orf is a worldwide disease of sheep and goats that causes crusty, warty, or granulomatous lesions on the lips, nose, or eyelids. Milkers' nodule is a natural infection of cows and causes chronic small papulovesicular lesions on the teats. The diseases may be transmitted to sheepherders, dairy farmers, butchers, and veterinarians by direct contact with infected animals, animal products, or virus contaminated dried crusts shed from lesions into grazing pastures. Both viruses are resistant to drying and remain infectious for months to years in dried crusts.

7. Treatment and Prevention

Treatment of both diseases is symptomatic and is directed toward prevention or cure of secondary bacterial infection. Prevention of infection with these viruses in man involves control of the disease in animals. Vaccination with live vaccines and quarantine of infected pastures are effective in eliminating contagious pustular dermatitis in sheep. Flocks of sheep and herds of cattle in which the disease is widespread should be destroyed.

G. Molluscum Contagiosum

Molluscum contagiosum is a benign infectious disease of the skin characterized by the presence of small pearly nodules.

1. Etiologic Agent

The *molluscum contagiosum virus* has not been grown in the laboratory but has been classified morphologically with the group V (unclassified) poxviruses.

2. Clinical Symptoms

The incubation period of molluscum contagiosum is not known; on the basis of human volunteer studies, different investigators have reported it to range from 2 weeks to 2 months. The disease usually occurs in children or young adults. It is characterized by the formation of painless, pearly white, wart-like nodules limited to the epidermal layer of the skin and mucous membranes. The lesions appear most frequently on the face, trunk, and anogenital areas; the conjunctiva, lips, and buccal mucosa are rarely affected, and no lesions develop on the palms of the hands or soles of the feet. The lesions may vary in size and number, ranging from 1 mm to 1 or 2 cm in diameter. The nodules are umbilicated and contain a white core of curd-like material that contains numerous virus particles. The lesions usually persist for 6 months to a year or more, but spontaneous regression eventually occurs without scarring.

3. Pathogenesis

The nodules of molluscum contagiosum are characterized by epithelial cell proliferation, hyperplasia, skin thickening, and degeneration. Light microscopy reveals that infected cells are greatly enlarged and contain large intracytoplasmic, eosinophilic inclusion bodies that displace the nucleus to one side. These "molluscum bodies" consist of masses of virus particles embedded in a spongy protein matrix that may be divided into cavities.

4. Immunity

Convalescent human serum contains Abs against Ag extracted from skin lesions. Some sera possess CF Abs against a soluble, heat-labile Ag obtained from suspensions of nodules. The role of these Abs in immunity is not known, and the immune mechanisms that mediate regression remain to be elucidated.

5. Diagnosis

Molluscum contagiosum is diagnosed on the basis of the characteristic appearance of the lesions and histologic examination of the core, which is composed of clusters of cells containing the diagnostic giant eosinophilic inclusion bodies.

The virus has not been propagated in tissue cultures or experimental animals, and no satisfactory serologic tests are available for diagnostic use.

6. Epidemiology

Man is the only known natural host of molluscum contagiosum virus. The disease has a worldwide distribution and has occurred in epidemics within orphanages and family groups. The exact mode of transmission is not known, but the virus appears to be spread by direct contact or by infected fomites; outbreaks have occurred among wrestlers. Autoinoculation from suppurating lesions appears to be common and may account for spread of the virus from one part of the skin to another.

7. Treatment and Prevention

There is no effective antiviral treatment. Lesions can be removed surgically.

H. Warts (Verrucae)

Warts are epithelial tumors of the skin and adjoining mucous membranes.

1. Etiologic Agent

In man, warts are caused by *human papillomavirus*. One virus, or closely related strains of a single virus, appears to cause several different types of warts, depending upon the site of infection and host reaction.

2. Clinical Symptoms

The incubation period, determined by inoculation of volunteers, varies between 1 and 20 months and averages about 4 months. Single or multiple warts can occur at any site on the skin or mucous membrane adjacent to the skin. Warts may persist and spread, presumably by autoinoculation, for several years. Most lesions eventually regress spontaneously without scarring; however, they may recur even after treatment. The lesions are classified according to morphology and location.

Sessile or *common warts* (*verruca vulgaris*) are raised, gray or brown lesions with a rough surface. They are usually seen on the hands and around or under the fingernails; they also may occur on the feet, legs, face, and neck. They vary in size from 1 mm to 2 cm; clusters of lesions may become confluent.

Filiform warts are horny finger-like projections that are a few millimeters in diameter and several millimeters long. They usually occur on the bearded area of the face, the neck, and scalp. The lips and eyelids may also be involved.

Plantar warts are flat and have a horny surface; they are demarcated from normal skin by a hyperkeratotic ring. The mass of the lesion is beneath the skin surface and is conical, with the pointed end projected inward. Plantar warts occur principally beneath pressure points on the soles of the feet and are often quite painful. Some plantar warts are not visible from the surface and are recognized only by acute pain at a calloused pressure point. In contrast, "mosaic plantar warts," produced when a number of lesions coalesce, are relatively painless keratotic lesions that may not be recognized.

Flat warts (*verruca planae*) are only slightly elevated, smooth, skin-colored papules that are 1 to 5 mm in diameter. They usually occur in multiples on the face, neck, chest, and back of the hands.

Moist warts (*condyloma acuminatum*) are moist, soft, pink or white lesions that may be clustered together to produce cauliflower-like growths. They appear most frequently on the moist skin of the external genitalia and the perianal region and on the vulvar and vaginal or anal mucosae. However, they may also occur at other moist sites, such as the conjunctiva, margins of the mouth, and between the toes. Because of their location, moist warts may become macerated and malodorous. This is the only type of human wart that may become malignant.

3. Pathogenesis

The principal pathologic changes observed in warts occur in the epidermis. Depending upon the type and location of the lesion, varying degrees of hyperplasia of the prickle cell, granular, or horny layers may occur. Characteristic large vacuolated cells appear in the upper prickle cell and granular layers; the nuclei of these cells may be large and variable in size. Nuclear inclusion bodies are frequently observed in plantar warts but only occasionally in common warts.

4. Immunity

Low titers of specific IgM Abs against human papillomavirus can be detected in patients carrying warts; as the warts regress, serum IgG Abs develop. The role of the immune response in spontaneous regression and resistance is by no means clear. Following treatment of one wart, untreated lesions sometimes disappear. The increased incidence of warts in patients receiving immunosuppressive drugs after kidney transplantation suggests that the immune response is important in resistance.

5. Diagnosis

Most warts can be recognized by their appearance. The diagnosis may be confirmed by histologic examination. A persistent single moist wart on the genitalia should be biopsied to rule out a malignancy such as squamous cell carcinoma. In addition, some lesions of secondary syphilis may be confused with virus-induced genital warts. Mosaic plantar warts may not be apparent until the epidermal layers are successively removed to reveal the infected rounded white mass.

6. Epidemiology

Warts are quite common; their distribution is worldwide, and both sexes and all ages are affected. They are contagious, but the sources of infection and modes of transmission are frequently unknown. Minor abrasions may be important in establishing the infection. Autoinoculation apparently accounts for the appearance of satellite lesions around traumatized older warts.

7. Treatment and Prevention

Treatment of warts is empirical and depends upon the number, location, and type of lesion. Since most warts regress spontaneously, treatment should be conservative to avoid excessive local irritation and scarring. In general, therapy involves the physical destruction or removal of the lesions. If deemed necessary, most sessile, filiform, or flat warts can be eliminated by electrodesiccation or freezing with liquid nitrogen or dry ice. Weekly application of podophyllin in tincture of benzoin is recommended for moist warts. Plantar warts, which are especially hard to eliminate, may require daily application of salicylic acid or other caustic agents.

There are no known methods for preventing warts.

References

BARINGER, J. R., and SWOVELAND, P.: Recovery of herpes-simplex virus from human trigeminal ganglions. New Eng. J. Med. *288:* 648, 1973.

BEARDMORE, W. B.: A new form of smallpox vaccine. J. Infect. Dis. *127:* 718, 1973.

BRUNELL, P. A., and GERSHON, A. A.: Passive immunization against varicella-zoster infections and other modes of therapy. J. Infect. Dis. *127:* 415, 1973.

BUTEL, J. S.: Studies with human papilloma virus modeled after known papovavirus systems. J. Nat. Cancer Inst. *48:* 285, 1972.

COOPER, L. Z., and KRUGMAN, S.: The rubella problem. Disease-a-month, February 1969.

CRAIG, C. P., and NAHMIAS, A. J.: Different patterns of neurologic involvement with herpes simplex virus types 1 and 2: Isolation of herpes simplex virus type 2 from the buffy coat of two adults with meningitis. J. Infect. Dis. *127:* 365, 1973.

DUDGEON, J. A.: Maternal rubella and its effect on the foetus. Arch. Dis. Child. *42:* 110, 1967.

FORGHANI, B., SCHMIDT, N. J., and LENNETTE, E. H.: Demonstration of rubella IgM antibody by indirect fluorescent antibody staining, sucrose density gradient centrifugation and mecaptoethanol reduction. Intervirol. *1:* 48, 1973.

HAIRE, M., and HADDEN, D. S. M.: Rapid diagnosis of rubella by direct immunofluorescent staining of desquamated cells in throat swabs. J. Med. Microbiol. *5:* 231, 1972.

KLOCK, L. E., and RACHELEFSKY, G. S.: Failure of rubella herd immunity during an epidemic. New Eng. J. Med. *288:* 69, 1973.

LENNETTE, E. H., and SCHMIDT, N. J.: *Diagnostic Procedures for Viral and Rickettsial Infections.* 4th ed. New York: American Public Health Association, 1969.

LONG, G. W., NOBLE, J., JR., MURPHY, F. A., HERRMANN, K. L., and LOURIE, B. Experience with electron microscopy in the differential diagnosis of smallpox. Appl. Microbiol. *20:* 497, 1970.

LONGSON, M. (ed.): Acute necrotizing encephalitis and other herpes simplex infections. A symposium held at the University Hospital of South Manchester on 19 and 20 January, 1972. Postgrad. Med. J. *49:* 371, 1973.

MEYER, H. M., JR., PARKMAN, P. D., and HOPPS, H. E.: The clinical application of laboratory diagnostic procedures for rubella and measles (rubeola). Amer. J Clin. Path. *57:* 803, 1972.

MIMS, C. A.: Pathogenesis of viral infections of the fetus. Progr. Med. Virol. *10:* 194, 1968.

PAVAN-LANGSTON, D., and DOHLMAN, C. H.: A double blind clinical study of adenine arabinoside therapy of viral keratoconjunctivitis. Amer. J. Ophthal. *74:* 81, 1972.

RAWLS, W. E. Congenital rubella: The significance of virus persistance. Progr. Med. Virol. *10:* 238, 1968.

SEIGEL, M., FUERST, H. T., and GUINEE, V. F.: Rubella epidemicity and embryopathy. Results of a long term prospective study. Amer. J. Dis. Child. *121:* 469, 1971.

VAHERI, A., VESIKARI, T., OKER-BLOOM, N., SEPPALA, M., PARKMAN, P. D., VERONELLI, J., and ROBBINS, F. C.: Isolation of attenuated rubella-vaccine virus from human products of conception and uterine cervix. New Eng. J. Med. *286:* 1071, 1972.

WENSTEIN, L., and CHANG, T.: Rubella immunization. New Eng. J. Med. *288:* 100, 1973.

WHO Expert Committee on Smallpox Eradication: Second Report, Publication No. 493, World Health Organization Technical Report Series. Geneva: World Health Organization, 1972.

Chapter 13

Properties of Viruses Associated with Neurotropic Disease

Over 300 different viruses belonging to several virus groups (picornavirus, paramyxovirus, togavirus, herpesvirus, and rhabdovirus) are capable of invading the CNS. In the case of some viruses, infection of the CNS is a rare but serious complication resulting from the dissemination of virus from sites of infection in other organs and tissues of the body. Viruses enter the CNS by crossing the blood-brain barrier or passing along peripheral nerve roots. They can cause paralysis, meningitis, encephalitis or meningoencephalitis. Practically all cases of paralysis and encephalitis due to infectious agents are caused by viruses rather than by bacteria.

A. Picornavirus Group

1. Enterovirus

As discussed in Chapter 9, the picornavirus group is subdivided into the enterovirus and rhinovirus subgroups. Three "genera" are included in the enterovirus subgroup, namely, poliovirus, coxsackievirus, and echovirus.

a. Poliovirus. Poliovirus is responsible for an acute infectious disease that occasionally involves the CNS. Damage to motor neurons in the spinal cord may lead to flaccid paralysis.

Structure and Antigenic Properties. Polio virions possess a single-stranded RNA genome. The nucleocapsid has cubic symmetry, is non-enveloped, and measures about 38 nm in diameter (Fig. 13–1). Infectivity

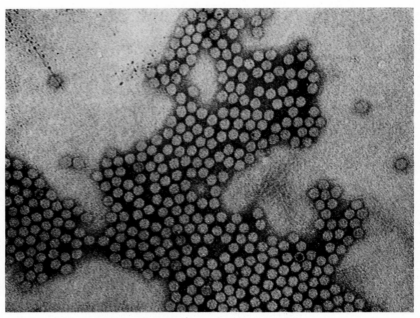

Figure 13–1. Electron micrograph of typical poliovirus particles. ×141,500. (Reprinted with permission from Mayor, H. D., and Jamison, R. M.: Morphology of small viral particles and subunit components. Progr. Med. Virol. *8:* 183, 1966, Karger, Basel.)

of poliovirus is stable to many physical (e.g., freezing) and chemical (e.g., ether or deoxycholate) agents.

Three distinct antigenic types of poliovirus exist that can be identified by Ab neutralizing tests for infectivity; there is almost no cross-neutralization. Inactivation of virions by formalin, heat, or ultraviolet light releases a soluble complement-fixing (CF) Ag. This Ag cross-reacts with heterotypic poliovirus Abs. In addition, two type-specific Ags called "N" (native) and "H" (heated) are detectable by precipitin or CF tests. The N Ag is associated with virus infectivity, whereas the H Ag is found in ruptured or incomplete virus particles.

Host Range and Culture. Man is the only natural host for poliovirus. Nonhuman primates are susceptible to paralysis following intraspinal or intracerebral inoculation. Poliovirus is pathogenic only for man and closely related species because of the requirement for specific attachment sites in the membrane of susceptible cells. Poliovirus is usually isolated and grown in rhesus monkey kidney cells. The virus multiples in the cytoplasm of cells and is rapidly cytocidal; the cytopathic changes produced include cell rounding, increased refractivity, nuclear pyknosis, and finally lysis (Chapter 2).

b. Coxsackievirus and Echovirus.   See Chapter 9 for discussion of these viruses.

B.   Paramyxovirus Group

1. Mumps Virus

Mumps is an acute contagious disease common among children and young adults (Chapter 18). The disease is characterized by nonsuppurative enlargement of one or both parotid glands; complications include orchitis in young males and meningoencephalitis.

Structure and Antigenic Properties.   Structurally, mumps virus is a typical paramyxovirus (Chapter 9) that contains hemagglutinin, neuraminidase, and hemolysin associated with the virus envelope. Virions are helical and range in size from 100 to 300 nm in diameter. There is only one serotype of mumps virus; however, mumps virus shares minor Ags with other paramyxoviruses.

Host Range and Culture.   The natural host of mumps virus is man. The virus can be grown in the amnion or yolk sac of embryonated chicken eggs and assayed by hemagglutination. Primary cultures of human or nonhuman primate kidney cells are used for virus isolation. Mumps virus is identified by hemadsorption-inhibition tests in infected cell cultures. Cytopathic effects of mumps-virus-infected tissue cultures include syncytial cell formation and acidophilic intracytoplasmic inclusions.

C.   Togavirus (Arbovirus) Group

This group includes well over 250 different viruses, of which about 65 have been shown to cause disease in man. These viruses characteristically require a suitable bloodsucking vector (invertebrate host) and an effective reservoir (vertebrate host) in their complex biological cycle. Recently, the name togavirus has been approved (Chapter 1) to designate those arboviruses (arthropod-borne viruses) that multiply in bloodsucking insects and are transmitted to vertebrates by insect bites. Togaviruses of medical importance in the USA are currently subdivided into the genus *alphavirus* (group A), the genus *flavovirus* (group B), and the California group (e.g., *California encephalitis viruses*) on the basis of shared Ags demonstrable by neutralization, hemagglutination-inhibition, or CF tests. The neutralization test is considered to be the most specific and is generally employed to differentiate the viruses within each group. Viruses classified as togaviruses are named either after a geographic location in which they occur (e.g., Eastern encephalitis virus) or after the disease they cause (e.g., phlebotomus fever virus). This classification scheme has resulted in some rather unusual and exotic names, such as O'nyong-nyong, Bunyamwera, and Chikungunya viruses.

1. Group A

Eastern Equine Encephalitis (EEE). This virus was first isolated from a horse that died from encephalitis in 1933, hence the name equine. Since then, EEE virus has been found to be responsible for disease in horses and man throughout the eastern and southeastern USA, as well as in parts of Central and South America.

Western Equine Encephalitis (WEE). Of the equine encephalitis in the USA, WEE is the most widespread. Although the virus was first isolated in states west of the Mississippi river, it is now known to occur in many states east of the Mississippi river as well. Of interest is the fact that human disease has been reported to occur only in the continental USA and Brazil. In contrast to EEE, the disease is rare on the Eastern coast of the USA.

2. Group B

Saint Louis Encephalitis (SLE). This viral infection was first recognized as a disease entity during an epidemic in St. Louis, Missouri, in 1933. It has subsequently been found to occur frequently in the USA either in widespread epidemics or as sporadic cases in areas where the virus is endemic.

3. California Group

California Encephalitis Virus (CEV). In 1943, a new virus was isolated from pooled homogenates of mosquitoes (*Culex tarsalis*) and ticks (*Dermacentor andersoni*). The virus could be transmitted to rabbits and various rodents but not to birds. However, birds serve as hosts for other togaviruses (e.g., EEE, WEE, and SLE viruses). Two years later, a significant Ab response to CEV was detected in 3 cases of human encephalitis that occurred in a region where infected mosquitoes were found. During the following years, isolations of the virus were made from mosquitoes and ticks in various parts of the USA. The disease is especially severe in children, but the number of subclinical cases always exceeds the number of clinical cases.

Structure and Antigenic Properties. All togaviruses are spherical and contain an electron-dense core surrounded by a lipoprotein envelope (Fig.

13–2). The nucleocapsid has 32 capsomeres and a diameter of 35–40 nm. The peplomeres in the viral envelope contain the virus hemagglutinin.

Host Range and Culture.   Most togaviruses multiply in embryonated chicken eggs or in tissue cultures of chicken, duck embryo, or mammalian origin. The natural vertebrate host of most togaviruses is a wild bird or mammal; several host species are usually involved in the biological cycle of the virus. The most susceptible laboratory animal is the mouse or day-old chick. All togaviruses replicate in the cell cytoplasm and acquire their lipoprotein envelope by budding through cell membranes (e.g., vacuolar or plasma membranes). Virus multiplication can be detected by the cytopathic effects produced, virus-specific immunofluorescence, or hemadsorption tests. Togavirus infectivity titers can be easily quantified by plaque assay in cultures of chick embryo cells as well as kidney cells of hamster or nonhuman primate origin.

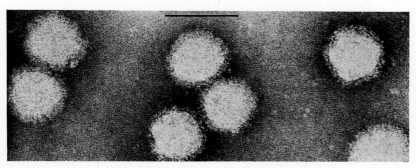

Figure 13–2.   Negative-stained virions of group A (genus alphavirus) togaviruses. ×240,000. (Reprinted with permission from Simpson, R. W., and Hauser, R. E.: Basic structure of group A arbovirus strains Middleburg, Sindbis, and Semliki Forest examined by negative staining. *Virology 34:*358, 1968.)

D.   Herpesvirus Group

1. B Virus (Herpesvirus simiae)

A herpesvirus has been recovered from rhesus and cercopithecus nonhuman primates that causes a meningoencephalitis in man following bites by apparently healthy monkeys or contact with infected materials (e.g., tissue culture fluids) derived from monkeys.

Structure and Antigenic Properties.   Morphologically, the virus resembles other herpesviruses (Chapter 11). Virus particles measure about 110 nm. Antiserum made against herpes simplex virus has weak neutralizing activity against B virus, whereas B virus antiserum neutralizes herpes simplex virus and B virus equally well.

Host Range and Culture.   The virus is transmissible to monkeys, rabbits, guinea pigs, newborn mice, and man. Herpes B virus can be grown on the chorioallantoic membrane of chick embryonated eggs or tissue culture cells derived from rabbits, monkeys, or man. Infected tissue culture cells exhibit intranuclear inclusions and multinucleated giant cells.

E.   Rhabdovirus Group

1. Rabies Virus

Structure and Antigenic Composition. The virion is characteristically "bullet-shaped," with one flattened end (Fig. 13-3) and consists of a helical nucleocapsid enclosed in an envelope containing peplomeres. The genome of the virus is single-stranded RNA. Virus particles mature

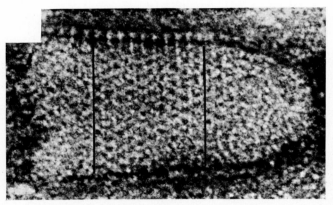

Figure 13—3. Negative-stained preparation of a typical rabies virus particle. Note the "bullet-shaped" morphology and knob-like peplomeres arranged on the surface. ×400,000. (Reprinted with permission from Hummelar, K., Kaprowski, H., and Wiktor, T.: Structure and development of rabies virus in tissue culture. J. Virol. *1:* 152, 1967.)

by budding through the plasma membrane. There is one major serotype of rabies virus. Recent evidence shows that "classical" rabies viruses and several virus isolates from the African continent contain a common nucleoprotein antigen that can be detected by immunofluorescence, CF, and precipitin tests. These viruses differ in cross-neutralization tests, indicating that membrane proteins are different. Recently, these criteria have been used to classify rabies viruses into 4 serotypes.

The term *street virus* is used to describe rabies virus isolated in nature from domestic or wild animals, as opposed to *fixed virus,* which is considered to be an "attenuated" variant of a street virus. These terms were coined by Louis Pasteur, who chose the term fixed viruses to describe viruses obtained by serial passage of street viruses in the brains of rabbits. Fixed viruses were used in Pasteur's first human rabies vaccine.

Host Range and Culture. Rabies virus has a wide host range that includes man and all other warm-blooded animals. In infected animals, the virus is distributed in the nervous system, saliva, urine, lymph, milk, and blood. In bats the virus is present in the salivary glands. Infected bats can transmit rabies virus in aerosolized saliva for extended periods without having apparent disease. Latent rabies viruses are known to be reactivated in infected animals (e.g., skunks, foxes, dogs). The virus can be grown in chick embryos and newborn mice as well as hamster kidney cell or human diploid cell cultures.

References

ANDREWS, C., and PEREIRA, H. G.: *Viruses of Vertebrates.* 3rd ed. Baltimore: Williams & Wilkins Co., 1972.

BORDEN, E. C. SHUPE, R.E., and MURPHY, F. A.: Physiochemical and morphological relationships of some arthropod-borne viruses to bluetongue virus: A new taxonomic group. Physiochemical and serological studies. J. Gen. Virol. *13:* 261, 1971.

FENNER, F., McAUSLAN, B., MIMS, C. A., SAMBROOK, J., and WHITE, D. O.: *The Biology of Animal Viruses.* 2nd ed. New York: Academic Press, 1974.

HENDERSON, B. E., and COLEMAN, P. H.: The growing importance of the California arboviruses in the etiology of human disease. Progr. Med. Virol. *13:* 404, 1971.

HORZINEK, M. C.: Comparative aspects of togaviruses. J. Gen. Virol. *20:* 87, 1973.

McLERRAN, C. J., and ARLINGHAUS, R. B.: Structural components of a virus of the California encephalitis complex: La Crosse virus. Virology *53:* 247, 1973.

MUSSGAY, M.: Growth cycle of arboviruses in vertebrate and arthropod cells. Progr. Med. Virol. *6:* 193, 1964.

WHO Expert Committee on Rabies. 6th Report. World Health Organization Technical Report Series No .523. Geneva, 1973.

Viral Neurotropic Diseases

Viruses are responsible for most cases of meningitis and essentially all cases of encephalitis in man. *Viral encephalitis* by definition is an inflammatory disease of the cerebrospinal axis produced by the direct effect of virus on neurologic tissues. The inflammation may spread to the meningeal spaces, resulting in *meningoencephalitis,* or to the spinal cord, resulting in *meningomyeloencephalitis.* In some cases of encephalitis, disease is not due to direct action of virus. For example, *postinfectious encephalitis* following smallpox vaccination is considered to be invoked by an allergic reaction. The etiology and pertinent characteristics of viral diseases involving the central nervous system (CNS) will be discussed in this chapter.

A.   Poliomyelitis

Until the present century, poliomyelitis was primarily a disease of infants, hence the name *infantile paralysis*. However, as a   result of improved sanitation over the past 50 years, the age distribution of the disease has changed to include young adults. During a peak incidence of poliomyelitis in the USA in 1953, about 1,500 deaths and 7,000 cases with residual paralysis occurred. The unfortunate crippling of many survivors of polio, including Franklin D. Roosevelt, caused great concern about the disease. Although it was one of the most feared diseases only some 2 decades ago, some medical students of today may never have occasion to diagnose and treat a clinical case of poliomyelitis. This remarkable change in the incidence of poliomyelitis was due to research, supported in large part by the March of Dimes Fund. Enders, Weller, and Robbins (1949) were the first to report the successful growth of poliovirus in tissue cultures of nonneural cells. This work, which earned for them the Nobel Prize in Medicine, provided great impetus to modern research in virology and led to the subsequent production of the Salk and Sabin vaccines. Widespread use of these vaccines has almost completely eradicated poliomyelitis from developed countries. This is dramatically documented in Table 14–1,

TABLE 14—1

Poliomyelitis in the United States

Average Annual Number of Cases			
1951-1955	1961-1965	1966-1970[a]	1972[b]
37,864	573	52	20

[a] Number of cases: 1966, 113; 1967, 41; 1968, 53; 1969, 20; 1970, 33.
[b] Includes 11 cases reported in a polio outbreak in Connecticut.
  Data from Weekly Epidemiological Record 47 (No. 31): 294-295, 1972. (Geneva: World Health Organization).

which summarizes the average annual number of cases in the USA before, at the time of, and after mass immunization with poliomyelitis vaccines. Although the consensus among the lay public in developed countries is that poliomyelitis no longer poses a health threat, serious outbreaks of paralytic poliomyelitis still occur in some parts of the world, such as Trinidad and Tobago (Table 14–2).

The history of the research that led to a successful poliomyelitis

TABLE 14—2

Poliomyelitis in Trinidad and Tobago[a]

Number of Cases					
1966	1967	1968	1969	1970	1971[b]
1	3	1	9	3	153

[a] Total population of Trinidad and Tobago is 1,040,000.
[b] Through February 1, 1972.
  Data from Weekly Epidemiological Record 47 (No. 31): 24-95, 1972. (Geneva: World Health Organization).

vaccine is especially deserving of comment because, like many other important areas in science and medicine, it illustrates admirably how formidable a problem can be before needed concepts and techniques are developed and how simple the solution always seems in retrospect. The first breakthrough in poliomyelitis came in 1947 when strong arguments and data were presented by Evans and Green to support the concept that the virus grows in nonneural as well as neural tissue, a view that opposed the long-held dogma that the organism was obligatorily neurotropic. The second breakthrough, the cultivation of the virus in cultures of nonneural cells, followed rapidly (1949); the development of the first vaccine (Salk) was finally accomplished in 1953. Thus, within the short span of a few years after the acceptance of a new concept, an effective method for controlling this important disease, so terrifying to parents, was at hand.

Because of the great historical importance of poliomyelitis and the knowledge that has accumulated about the virus and the disease, together with the contributions that poliomyelitis research has made to the study and development of other important virus vaccines, a discussion of poliomyelitis and poliovirus is instructive and important to students of medicine and related sciences.

Etiologic Agents.   Three antigenic types of poliovirus exist that are distinguishable by neutralization tests using specific antisera. *Poliovirus type 1 is the most common cause of paralytic polio.* Avirulent mutants of poliovirus have become widely distributed in nature because of the widespread use of attenuated virus vaccines (Sabin).

Clinical Symptoms.   When a nonimmune individual is infected with poliovirus, one or more of the following responses may occur: (1) inapparent infection (occurs most often); (2) mild infection characterized by fever, malaise, and sore throat with or without nausea and headache; (3) aseptic meningitis; or (4) paralytic poliomyelitis. *Only about 1% of persons with apparent poliovirus infection develop paralysis.* After an incubation period of 5 to 20 days, the disease may follow a *diphasic course*: The initial mild infection may be followed by a few symptom-free days prior to the development of muscle stiffness and pain commencing 1 to 3 days later. Paralysis develops rapidly after infection of the motor cortex of the brain. Infection of the anterior horn cells or brain stem results in bulbar polio, which may be fatal because of cardiac and respiratory failure. Some degree of recovery of motor function may occur during the first few months, but paralysis remaining at the end of this period is permanent.

Pathogenesis.   Virus enters the alimentary tract following ingestion of contaminated food or drink. The virus first multiplies in the tonsils, lymph nodes of the neck, Peyer's patches, and the mucosa of the small intestine. It appears in the throat and feces before symptoms develop. One week after the onset of symptoms, virus is found in the blood; virus is excreted in the feces for several weeks despite the development of high levels of circulating Abs. Occasionally, the CNS is invaded during the viremic phase of the disease. Virus can spread from the blood or along axons of peripheral nerves to the anterior horn cells of the spinal cord. In severe cases, the intermediate gray ganglia as well as the posterior horn and dorsal root ganglia are involved (Chapter 6). Intracellular multiplication of the virus in neurons leads to complete destruction of nerve cells. Inflammation occurs secondary to infection of neurons, with infiltration of lymphocytes, sometimes neutrophils, plasma cells, and microglial cells. Cells injured as the direct result of virus infection or by the inflammatory response of the host may recover completely during convalescence. The probability of CNS involvement with residual paralysis is enhanced in adults and in circumstances such as pregnancy, tonsillectomy, trauma, and fatigue. In particular, tonsillectomy increases the incidence of bulbar poliomyelitis. Irritation resulting from injection of various materials or trauma predisposes to paralysis in the affected limb. Nerves in areas of irritation or trauma are highly susceptible to invasion by virus. Virus spreads from these areas along peripheral nerves to reach the corresponding segment of the spinal cord or brain stem.

In contrast to the thousands of cases of paralysis caused by polioviruses in the past, there have been relatively few cases of pseudopoliomyelitis caused by other viruses (echoviruses and coxsackieviruses A and B). These enteroviruses were discovered by accident in the course of investigations on poliomyelitis. The differential diagnosis of enterovirus infections is very difficult clinically, and virologic diagnosis is imperative. Polioviruses have a high affinity for the nervous system, whereas other enteroviruses have a weak affinity for this organ system. Although rare, a poliovirus infection can coexist with infection due to either echovirus or coxsackievirus.

Immunity. Passive immunity against polioviruses is transferred from mother to offspring during pregnancy. It results from maternally derived Abs and gradually decreases during the first 6 to 9 months of life. In contrast, passive immunity conveyed by the administration of hyperimmune serum lasts only 3 to 5 weeks. Naturally acquired active immunity is permanent and is usually *type-specific* (*homotypic*), which explains why second attacks of poliomyelitis can occur. Occasionally, a low degree of *cross-resistance* (*heterotypic immunity*) between types 1 and 2 polioviruses can develop.

Diagnosis. During the early stages of disease, virus can be cultured from pharyngeal secretions by inoculating monkey kidney cells. After paralysis has become apparent, virus is readily isolated from the intestinal tract but is not easily recovered from the cerebrospinal fluid (CSF). Virus multiplies rapidly (1 to 3 days), and the isolate can be identified by tissue culture neutralization tests using hyperimmune serum. The immune status of patients can be established by determining their serum titers of neutralizing Ab against the 3 poliovirus serotypes.

Epidemiology. The only known reservoir of poliovirus is man. The virus is maintained in the population by carriers and is usually spread by direct contact. Poliovirus can be recovered from the pharynx and feces of patients for several weeks after the acute phase of the disease, as well as from healthy carriers, and is moderately stable in the external environment. These facts explain how, under crowded conditions and poor sanitation, the virus can easily spread from infected to noninfected individuals.

When conditions of hygiene and sanitation are poor, almost all infants are heavily exposed to the virus while they are still under the protection of maternally-derived Ab and thus acquire active immunity early in life without appreciable danger of developing paralytic disease.

Poliovirus infections are endemic throughout the world. *In isolated populations,* such as the Eskimos, poliomyelitis occurs in all age groups. *In crowded primitive areas with poor sanitation,* clinical poliomyelitis is infrequent because essentially all children and older individuals have developed active immunity from heavy exposure to the virus. In these areas, the susceptible individuals are primarily those few infants who do not receive sufficient maternal Ab to protect them. *Epidemics in temperate zones* are most likely to occur during the summer and fall. Spread of infection takes place most readily among nonimmunized schoolchildren and family contacts. Poliovirus type 1 is the most common serotype in Western countries. *In many developed countries,* the greatest age incidence of the disease has shifted to older unvaccinated individuals. This change has been brought about by strong "herd immunity" induced in the younger age groups by the widespread use of poliovirus vaccine. The practices of immunization and improved hygiene have essentially eliminated the wild-type virus from many communities and, in consequence, have reduced the booster value of frequent exposure to poliovirus for maintaining immunity in later years. Although waning immunity in an individual residing in a virus-free population does not ordinarily pose appreciable risk to him, he may be at high risk if he travels to an area where virulent virus is abundant in the population.

Compared with most diseases, paralytic poliomyelitis in unvaccinated populations is a paradox, the lowest incidence of paralytic disease being favored when crowding is greatest and sanitation is the poorest.

Treatment and Prevention. Both live (Sabin) and killed (Salk) vaccines are available for general use (Chapter 7). *Immunization with the Salk or Sabin vaccine is of prophylactic but not therapeutic value.* The Sabin vaccine is administered orally; it contains live attenuated virus grown in cultured monkey kidney cells. Viral contaminants may be present in some cultured monkey kidney cells; hence the human diploid cell strain (WI-38), free of detectable microbial contamination, has recently been licensed for vaccine production. The poliovirus contained in the oral vaccine invades the intestinal epithelium and multiplies; as a consequence, it immunizes the recipient by inducing the production of both humoral Abs and "coproantibodies," (mainly IgA Abs) in the wall of the small intestine. Recipients are protected not only against spread of natural polioviruses through the bloodstream to the spinal cord but also against initial multiplication of such viruses in the small intestine. Repeated vaccinations are recommended to establish permanent immunity (Chapter 7). During the initial period of use of the oral poliovirus vaccine (1961–1965), the average annual number of cases was about 573. During the period 1966–1970, the average annual number of cases dropped to about 52 (Table 14–1). The protection induced by the Sabin vaccine is 80 to 90% effective; however, due to the high "herd immunity" and reduction in carriage rate that results from vaccination, the overall effectiveness of vaccination approaches 100%.

The killed (Salk) poliovirus vaccine induces humoral Abs and protects the CNS from invasion by wild-type virus. *In contrast to the Sabin vaccine, the Salk vaccine does not prevent intestinal infection by poliovirus.*

Hyperimmune gamma globulin affords limited (3 to 5 weeks) prophylactic protection against the paralytic disease; it has no value after symptoms appear.

During an epidemic, which is defined as 2 or more local cases caused by the same serotype of poliovirus in any 4-week period, bed rest is recommended for children with fever. Nose and throat operations should be avoided. Quarantine of patients or household contacts is ineffective for controlling spread of the disease. Food and human excreta should be protected from flies. All pharyngeal discharges are considered to be infectious and should be disposed of properly. Once the serotype of poliovirus responsible for the epidemic has been determined, type-specific monovalent Sabin vaccine should be administered to all susceptible individuals in the population.

B. Aseptic Meningitis

Most cases of viral meningitis are secondary to infection elsewhere in the body; most are of the aseptic type. The term "aseptic" refers to the type of meningitis in which the spinal fluid is clear, in contrast to the purulent spinal fluid often seen in bacterial meningitis. Before the advent of antibiotic therapy, bacteria, rather than viruses, were the most frequent cause of meningitis. Mumps virus, certain coxsackieviruses, and echoviruses are among the common causative agents. Less common etiologic agents of aseptic meningitis include other enteroviruses (e.g., polioviruses), herpes simplex, mengo, and lymphocytic choriomeningitis (LCM) viruses (Table 14–3).

Untreated cases of viral meningitis carry an excellent prognosis; this is in sharp contrast to bacterial meningitis. Even though viral meningitis occurs in epidemic proportions, mortality generally is low. Lumbar puncture is necessary in order to distinguish between viral and bacterial meningitis.

TABLE 14–3

Etiology of Aseptic Meningitis Due to Viruses

Etiologic Viruses	
Common	Less Common
Mumps	Other Coxsackie and ECHO Serotypes
Coxsackie A 7, 9, 23	Polio types 1, 2, 3
ECHO 4, 6, 9, 16, 30	Herpes simplex
Coxsackie B 1-6	Mengo
	Lymphocytic choriomeningitis
	Hepatitis

1. Mumps Virus Meningitis

Meningitis may appear before, during, or after mumps parotitis. In some cases, meningitis may be the only apparent manifestation of mumps virus infection. It often occurs in a crowded environment (e.g., schools and military camps). *In comparison to other viral meningitides, mumps meningitis is the most common, the most prolonged, and often the most violent.*

Etiologic Agent.   A single serotype of mumps virus is responsible for disease in man; structurally it resembles other paramyxoviruses (Chapter 9).

Clinical Symptoms.   The incubation period ranges from 16 to 20 days. One out of every 3 cases of mumps virus infection is inapparent. A prodromal period of malaise and anorexia may or may not be followed by enlargement of the parotid glands before invasion of the CNS. Mumps virus is responsible for about 10-15% of the cases of aseptic meningitis in the USA and is more common in males than females. The disease usually develops 5 to 7 days after the prodromal period. The CSF contains an average of 200 to 600 leukocytes per cm^3, most of which are lymphocytes. Other rare complications of mumps include polyarthritis, pancreatitis, nephritis, and thyroiditis.

Pathogenesis.   Virus enters through the respiratory tract. Primary replication of virus is thought to occur in the parotid gland or epithelium of the respiratory tract. Virus is then carried by the blood to the CNS and other organs of the body (Chapter 18).

Immunity. Acquired immunity as a result of apparent or inapparent infection is considered to be lifelong.

Diagnosis. In cases of mumps aseptic meningitis without parotitis, laboratory studies are necessary to establish the etiologic diagnosis. Virus is generally recovered from saliva, blood, and CSF for the first few days of illness and later from urine. The specimen is inoculated directly into primary human or monkey kidney tissue cultures or chick embryos. After 3 to 5 days' incubation, the cell cultures are monitored by hemadsorption (HAd), or the amniotic fluid from inoculated chick embryos is assayed for viral hemagglutinin.

Complement-fixation (CF) or hemagglutination-inhibition (HI) tests using acute and convalescent sera may be used to diagnose mumps virus meningitis. The CF test is recommended for sensitivity, specificity, and accuracy. A 4-fold increase in Ab titer in convalescent serum is considered to be diagnostic of a preceding mumps virus infection.

Skin test Ag for detecting susceptible persons who have escaped mumps virus infection is available commercially; however, the test is of no value in diagnosis. Delayed hypersensitivity to mumps virus Ag develops during convalescence; sensitivity usually appears within 3 to 4 weeks after the onset of symptoms. A positive skin test indicates previous exposure to mumps virus; about 80% of the adult population is skin-test-positive.

Differential diagnosis should include meningitis caused by *Mycobacterium tuberculosis, Leptospira* sp., *Cryptococcus neoformans,* and some common bacteria (e.g., *Haemophilus* sp., staphylococci, and pneumococci).

Epidemiology. Mumps virus is endemic throughout the year, with peak periods during the winter and spring. Aseptic mumps virus meningitis, which carries a low mortality, reaches its highest incidence in children 5 to 15 years of age; however, epidemics also occur in army camps.

Mumps virus is spread by direct contact, droplets, and fomites, and is excreted in the urine of infected individuals. The disease is communicable from about 4 days before to about 7 days after symptoms develop. More intimate contact is needed for transmission of mumps than for measles or varicella-zoster viruses. In about 30 to 40% of cases, invasion by mumps virus causes inapparent infections; these individuals can carry and transmit the virus to susceptible individuals. Protective maternal Abs specific for mumps virus cross the placenta and gradually diminish during the first 6 to 9 months of life.

Treatment and Prevention. Prevention of mumps virus infection does not carry the same priority as prevention of measles, polio, diphtheria, or tetanus. However, vaccination with live attenuated mumps virus vaccine is recommended at puberty if there is no clinical history of mumps. Adults who show a negative skin test or who lack humoral Abs to mumps virus should also receive the vaccine. A single dose of vaccine induces detectable Abs in 95% of vaccinees; however, the duration of immunity following vaccination is not known. There is no specific treatment for mumps virus meningitis.

2. Echovirus Meningitis

The echoviruses form the most important and best-defined group of viruses causing aseptic meningitis; they cause many summer epidemics of the disease.

Etiologic Agents.   Echovirus meningitis is most commonly due to virus types 4, 6, 9, 16, and 30.

Clinical Symptoms.   The incubation period is short (3 to 6 days), followed by a rapid onset with headache, vomiting, sore throat, muscle pains, and fever. In 35 to 60% of cases, the first symptoms disappear briefly before a second phase of clinical disease, characterized by fever and meningeal signs, begins. A maculopapular rash, which may appear at the onset of the second phase, usually persists during the febrile period and greatly facilitates diagnosis during epidemics. The nonitching maculopapular rash, which is found on the face, neck, thorax, trunk, and extremities, presents a pale red lesion, about 2 to 4 mm in diameter. Occasionally, discrete grayish-white lesions 1 to 2 mm in diameter are present on the tonsils, buccal mucosa, and sometimes the tongue.

Pathogenesis.   The pathogenesis of echovirus meningitis is very similar to that of meningitis caused by other enteroviruses. Virus multiplication occurs in the alimentary tract (throat and small intestine) before viremia and invasion of the CNS occurs. Infection with two or more enteroviruses may occur simultaneously.

Immunity.   Both neutralizing and CF Abs are detectable following recovery.

Diagnosis.   The procedure of choice is to isolate the virus from feces, a throat swab, or the CSF by propagation in human or monkey kidney cell cultures. If possible, the isolate should be identified by the virus neutralization test or the HI test.

Epidemiology.   The epidemiology of echovirus infections is similar to the epidemiology of other enterovirus infections. The echoviruses are distributed worldwide; they produce only transitory infections, primarily in young individuals. Infections occur chiefly during the summer and autumn and are most prevalent in children from lower socioeconomic levels. Most infections are inapparent or subclinical. Echoviruses are rapidly disseminated among household contacts.

Treatment and Prevention.   No specific measures for controlling echovirus meningitis are available. Very young infants should be separated from young children exhibiting an acute febrile illness with a maculopapular rash. Medical housestaff should be screened for possible carriage of echoviruses, particularly during outbreaks of aseptic meningitis.

3. Coxsackievirus Meningitis

This syndrome occurs in large epidemics, usually in late summer or early fall, and may involve individuals of every age group, including young infants.

Etiologic Agents. Coxsackievirus meningitis is caused by all types of group B and 3 types of group A viruses (7, 9, and 23).

Clinical Symptoms. The incubation period ranges from 2 to 9 days. In cases of meningitis caused by coxsackie A serotypes, characteristic discrete vesicular lesions of "herpangina" may be seen on the anterior pillars of the fauces and sometimes on the palate, uvula, tonsils, and tongue. Coxsackievirus B meningitis is generally accompanied by painful myalgia. Late meningitis may occur 5 to 9 days after the onset of headache, vomiting, fever, neck or back stiffness, and sometimes convulsions, herpangina, or pleurodynia. A maculopapular rash may accompany coxsackievirus meningitis. Family contacts may not suffer from meningitis but instead from an inapparent infection, a mild undifferentiated upper respiratory tract infection, or perhaps from epidemic myalgia, myocarditis (coxsackievirus B), herpangina (coxsackievirus A), or exanthem (coxsackievirus A or B). Some paralysis may occur, but it is reversible.

Pathogenesis. The pathogenesis of coxsackievirus is similar to that of other enterovirus infections (e.g., poliomyelitis). Mortality is highest in infants; it is attributable to acute interstitial myocarditis and lesions that may be present in the CNS and liver as a result of a generalized systemic disease.

Immunity. Immunity against coxsackieviruses is type-specific. Passive transfer of neutralizing and CF Abs from mother to offspring occurs. In contrast to children, who often lack Abs, most adults possess Abs against several types of coxsackieviruses, suggesting that multiple exposure to these viruses occurs with increasing age.

Diagnosis. Virus can be recovered from throat swabs or blood early during infection and from rectal swabs during the first few weeks following apparent infection. Virus can also be isolated from the CSF. The laboratory procedures for the isolation and identification of coxsackieviruses are similar to those used for enteroviruses in general (e.g., poliovirus) and should include inoculation into suckling mice. The virus is identified by immunologic tests and by the characteristic lesions it produces in mice (Chapter 9).

Epidemiology. Coxsackieviruses are widely distributed in the human population. Once the virus is introduced into a household, all nonimmune persons usually become infected; however, not all develop apparent disease. The coxsackieviruses share many epidemiologic characteristics with other enteroviruses. Consequently, enteroviruses often occur together in nature (e.g., in sewage or on flies) and in the same human host.

Treatment and Prevention. No specific measures for controlling coxsackieviruses are known. Infants and young children should be separated from persons exhibiting acute febrile illness, especially those with a rash.

C. Encephalitis

Encephalitis is the most serious viral disease in man; fortunately it is rare. It is usually a complication of an inapparent infection. When apparent disease occurs, residual effects such as mental retardation, epilepsy, paralysis, deafness, or blindness are common in those who recover. Most cases of viral encephalitis are caused by togaviruses (arboviruses) that cause outbreaks or epidemics in restricted areas of the world; this is in sharp contrast to rabies virus, which is endemic and essentially worldwide. In special cases, encephalitis due to delayed hypersensitivity may follow natural recovery from measles, varicella-zoster, mumps, and more rarely rubella (Table 14–4). Viral encephalitis may also follow active immunization with vaccinia or rabies viruses. Less common causes of viral encepha-

TABLE 14—4

Etiology of Viral Encephalitides in the United States

Viruses	
Common	Less Common
Togaviruses (EEE, WEE, SLE, California groups)[a]	Herpes simplex
	Vaccinia[b]
Measles[b]	Rubella[b]
Varicelle-zoster[b]	Rabies
Mumps[b]	Polio
	Measles (SSPE)[c]
	Mengo[b]
	Lymphocytic choriomeningitis (LCM)[d]

[a] EEE, eastern equine encephalitis; WEE, western equine encephalitis; SLE, St. Louis encephalitis.

[b] Postinfectious encephalitis is not common, but when it occurs the pathogenesis is probably due to a hypersensitivity reaction. Virus has not been recovered from the brain.

[c] Subacute sclerosing panencephalitis. Virus recovery from the infected cerebral tissue has been reported.

[d] Virus of rodents which may be transmitted to man.

litis include herpes simplex virus, B virus, and mengo viruses and the unusual condition called subacute sclerosing panencephalitis, which sometimes follows recovery from measles.

The following discussion will encompass viral encephalitis associated with togaviruses and rabies virus and the subject of postinfectious encephalitis. Subacute sclerosing panencephalitis will be included in a discussion (Chapter 22) of the chronic progressive neurologic diseases of probable viral etiology that affect the CNS (e.g., kuru and progressive multifocal leukoencephalopathy).

1. Togavirus Encephalitis

Most cases of viral encephalitis, especially among children, are caused by viruses grouped as togaviruses (arboviruses). This group includes over 250 different viruses, of which about 65 have been isolated from man.

Etiologic Agents. The principal togaviruses of importance in the USA include Eastern equine encephalitis (EEE) virus, Western equine encephalitis (WEE) virus, St. Louis encephalitis (SLE) virus, and the California encephalitis virus (CEV) complex.

Clinical Symptoms. Clinical disease caused by togaviruses may vary from an inapparent infection to an acute febrile syndrome with hemorrhagic fever and involvement of the CNS. Acute encephalitis begins with a rapid onset of convulsions and abnormalities in consciousness. Headache and fever may precede neurologic symptoms. After a few days, death or extensions of abnormalities in consciousness may occur, including coma, and neurologic and psychologic signs (delirium, confusion, and excitement). In the early stages of disease, the CSF is usually abnormal, with moderate lymphocytosis and elevation of protein. The level of sugar remains normal. Prognosis in encephalitis caused by togaviruses is variable. Although recovery is common and usually takes place after about 10 days of severe illness, death may occur after a few days of illness (Table 14–5).

The disease caused by EEE virus is always severe in horses and in human beings, particularly children. It tends to run a more acute course and presents more severe symptoms than are seen in cases of encephalitis due to other togaviruses. The case mortality rate is high (80%), and surviving children are left with permanent physical and mental sequelae.

Most persons infected with WEE have inapparent illness or at least no involvement of the CNS. The severity is inversely proportional to age. The incidence of infection is highest among children, who experience the most severe illness and the highest death rate (5 to 15%). In children, the disease is associated with convulsions, vomiting, and excitement. Children who recover from the disease usually are left with serious physical and mental handicaps. Symptoms in adults include lethargy, neck and back stiffness, and often mental confusion and temporary coma.

TABLE 14—5

Summary of Four Viral Encephalitides Encountered in the Americas

Togavirus Group	Viral Species	Clinical Disease	Pathology	Vector(s)	Distribution of Disease
A	EEE	Encephalitis; severe; high mortality; residual neurologic damage; mortality 80%	Lesions in white and gray matter; prominent in brain stem and basal ganglia; spinal cord shows milder changes	*Culex* and *Aedes* species	Eastern and SE USA, Canada, Cuba, Central and South America
A	WEE	Encephalitis; recovery usually complete; incidence of disease and permanent neurologic damage highest in children; can have inapparent disease or fever and headache; mortality 5-15%	Chiefly affects brain; produces lymphocyte infiltration of meninges and parenchyma; lesions consist of necrosis of neurons; glial infiltration and perivascular cuffing	*Culex tarsalis*	Western USA, Canada, Mexico, Argentina
B	SLE	Encephalitis; mild lesions; little neurologic damage; mortality 20%	Same as for Group A but always less severe	*Culex tarsalis; Culex pipiens*	Texas, New Jersey, St. Louis, Mo.; major Group B infection in USA; most important in USA
California	CEV	Mild, undifferentiated illness, ranging from influenza-like syndrome to acute CNS disease; major sequelae uncommon; mortality low	Brain edema; neuronal degeneration; inflammation and perivascular edema	*Aedes* and *Culex* species; *Dermacentor andersoni*	California, North Carolina, Minnesota, Indiana, New York, Florida

Viral encephalitis caused by SLE virus is the most important Group B togavirus disease in the USA. In 1966, the worst epidemics of SLE occurred in Texas; they involved more than 700 cases and 32 deaths. It is likely that many cases of SLE virus infection escape diagnosis. *As with most togaviruses, the majority of infections are inapparent.* Estimates during large epidemics suggest that, whereas 60 to 70% of the population become infected, only a few individuals develop encephalitis. Benign forms of the disease are limited to a short febrile influenza-like illness of a few days' duration, with headache and aching stiffness of muscles. Severe clinical disease has an abrupt onset, with headache, fever, and vomiting followed rapidly by clinical evidence of encephalitis or meningoencephalitis. Neurologic symptoms are usually more severe in aged persons. The mortality rate is usually between 10 and 20%, and most deaths occur in persons over 50 years of age. Death may result from the primary encephalitis or from complications, including bacterial infection, pulmonary embolism, or hemorrhage in various organs of the body. Recovery may be followed by the late development of neurologic abnormalities (defects in sensory perception) or psychologic changes (irritability and instability).

Encephalitis caused by CEV has a good prognosis, and complete recovery occurs in 7 to 14 days (Table 14–5). An incubation period of 4 to 6 days is followed by an acute nonexanthematous febrile stage, with headache and severe pain in muscles of the back and legs.

Pathogenesis. Man is infected by the bite of an infected mosquito. The infected arthropod introduces its proboscis into the capillary bed beneath the skin and injects its virus-laden saliva; virus multiplication takes place in the vascular endothelium and RE cells in lymph nodes, liver, spleen, and other organs. Virus released from these cells sets up a viremia that initiates the "systemic phase" of the disease characterized by chills, fever, and aches. Progress of the disease depends on the presence of neutralizing Abs in the blood and on the amount of virus present. Other organs and systems may become infected, such as joints and muscles (arthritis and myositis), skin (rash), liver and kidneys (hepatitis and nephritis), or the brain (encephalitis that may be fatal). The skin rash, if present, is characterized by swelling of the capillary endothelium, perivascular edema, and infiltration of mononuclear cells. Lesions in the skin possess eosinophilic intranuclear inclusions, *"Torres bodies,"* and larger eosinophilic masses of hyaline material resulting from fusion of necrotic cells, *"Councilman bodies."* Fatty degeneration is prominent in kidney tubules and is seen to a lesser extent in spleen, heart, lymph nodes, and brain. In cases of encephalitis, inflammatory foci in the brain show necrosis of neurons and glial cells, perivascular cuffing, capillary thrombosis, infiltration of lymphocytes, and a variable degree of meningitis.

Immunity. Type-specific acquired immunity to the virus is believed to be permanent. This may be due to the strong stimulus provided by intimate contact of virus Ag(s) with the spleen and lymph nodes during the viremic stage of the disease and the booster effect of repeated exposure to or subclinical infections with related viruses of the same serologic group. For example, repeated infection with one or more group B togaviruses (e.g., SLE) broadens immunity against other group B togaviruses (e.g., yellow fever) (Chapter 16).

Diagnosis. Virus can be isolated (with difficulty) from the blood during the incubation period and before symptoms appear. The virus can usually be recovered from the brain in fatal cases, provided the specimen is taken soon after death and inoculated intracranially, subcutaneously, or intraperitoneally into suckling mice. Tentative identification of the virus isolate can be made by the HI or the CF test and confirmed by neutralization of virus infectivity using known reference antisera. More commonly, a laboratory diagnosis is made by detecting a rise in titer of specific Abs by tests on acute and convalescent sera.

Epidemiology. Persistence of togaviruses in nature rests upon a suitable bloodsucking vector (invertebrate host) and a vertebrate host (Figure 14–1). Only the female mosquito feeds on blood, and only she can transmit the virus. The growth cycle of several togaviruses in the infected mosquito has been determined. The primary site for virus multiplication involves the cells of the midgut, followed by viremia and subsequent infection of the salivary glands and nerve tissue, where secondary virus multipli-

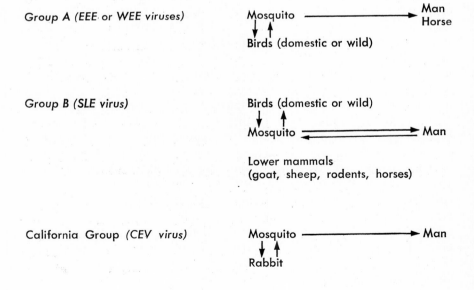

cation occurs. Infected mosquitoes do not become ill; they carry the virus for their lifetime. However, their lifespan is short (several weeks to months). Infected vertebrates (e.g., rodents) rapidly recover, eliminate the virus, and develop long-lasting immunity. Man, an unnatural and terminal host for most togaviruses, becomes infected accidentally when he is bitten by an infected bloodsucking arthropod carrying one of the togaviruses (e.g., EEE or WEE). Togaviruses persist in nature where arthropods coexist with birds and mammals. The events concerned with survival of togaviruses in temperate zones are similar to those that take place in tropical zones during the summer months, but "overwintering" is not completely understood. There is evidence that suggests that some arthropod-borne viruses (e.g., EEE and WEE) produce latent infections in hibernating animals (e.g., snakes and other reptiles). Following hibernation, a viremia occurs, and the virus is transmitted to a new host by mosquitoes that bite the awakened animal. Another possibility is that the virus survives the winter in mosquito vectors that can hibernate *(Culex tarsalis)*. Some togaviruses (group B) can be maintained in ticks by transoviral transmission through successive generations of hosts.

Treatment and Prevention. There are no effective vaccines and no specific treatments for encephalitis caused by togaviruses. Prevention of infection is accomplished by (1) avoidance of exposure in arthropod-infested areas and (2) eradication of vectors.

2. Rabies Virus Encephalitis

Rabies is the most lethal of all infectious diseases. Man has lived in fear of the rabid (*rabidus* = mad) dog throughout the centuries. In 1884, Louis Pasteur developed the first man-made viral vaccine. His demonstration of its efficacy in saving the life of a peasant boy bitten by a rabid dog was a milestone in microbiology.

Etiologic Agents. Rabies virus is classified as a rhabdovirus. Only one major serotype exists in nature. However, 4 distinct serotypes of rabies virus have recently been isolated from infected animals in remote areas of the world.

Clinical Symptoms. The incubation period depends on the distance of the nerve path from the point of virus entry to the brain. Accordingly, the shortest incubation periods (2 to 4 weeks) occurs following bites about the face, neck, and arms.

In man, two prodromal signs are pathognomonic: (1) the earliest but most inconsistent sign is a tingling sensation at the site of the bite, and (2) the most consistent but later sign is a state of anxiety and laryngopharyngeal spasm during the act of swallowing (nervous hydrophobia). This phase is generally followed by convulsive seizures and usually death within 3 to 5 days after onset.

In dogs, the incubation period for rabies is variable (3 to 8 weeks), but it may be as short as 10 days. Three phases of disease have been noted: (1) prodromal (fever, change in temperament, slow corneal reflexes), (2) excitative (irritability, nervousness, exaggerated response to light and sound stimuli), and (3) paralytic (convulsive seizures, coma, and death due to asphyxia). Unlike man, hydrophobia does not occur in dogs. During the terminal stages of the disease, the dog's saliva contains a high titer of infectious virus, which makes the animal dangerous, particularly if rabies is not suspected.

Pathogenesis.   Rabies virus multiplies in muscle and connective tissue and passes along sensory nerves to the CNS. The virus multiplies in the CNS and may spread through peripheral nerve trunks to the salivary glands. The pathology involves extensive nerve cell damage in the cerebrum, cerebellum, cortex, midbrain, basal ganglia, pons, and medulla. Demyelination occurs in the white matter, and there is extensive degeneration of axons and of the myelin sheath. If the bite wound is in the arm or leg, the corresponding posterior horns in the spinal cord will be destroyed by the virus. Cellular infiltrates are usually richer in mononuclear leukocytes and tend to be extensive when the disease is prolonged.

Immunity.   In the past, rabies was considered to be uniformly fatal in nonimmunized persons; however, in 1970, a case of the disease was treated and the patient recovered. Animals immunized before exposure to rabies virus are in general resistant to the infection if virus-neutralizing Abs are present in their serum. The same is probably true for man.

Diagnosis.   Any dead or dying animal suspected of having rabies should be subjected to laboratory diagnostic tests. The technique involves sending the head of the suspected animal to the laboratory in an ice-filled container or submerged in a container filled with glycerin. The diagnosis of rabies is based on finding intracytoplasmic inclusions (Negri bodies) in nerve cells (Fig. 14–2). Negri bodies consist of an acidophilic matrix containing basophilic granules. If Negri bodies are not detectable by direct examination of fluorescent-Ab stained impression-smears of brain, a suspension of the brain (hippocampus) or submaxillary salivary gland should be inoculated intracranially into suckling animals (mice, hamsters, rabbits).

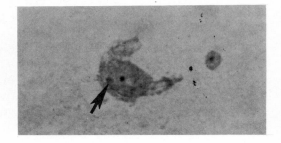

Figure 14–2.   Infected nerve cells showing intracytoplasmic inclusion bodies (Negri bodies). Presence of Negri bodies is diagnostic for rabies virus infection.

Positive diagnosis in the inoculated animals is made on the basis of clinical symptoms (e.g., convulsions) and demonstration of Negri bodies in brain sections. Laboratory diagnosis in man is of only retrospective interest but is necessary in order to establish the clinical diagnosis with certainty.

Dogs suspected of rabies are routinely quarantined for 14 days. If the dog remains asymptomatic for this period, the animal is presumed to be healthy. However, if symptoms of rabies develop, the dog should be held in isolation for several more days before tests are made in order to permit Negri bodies to develop in the brain cells.

Epidemiology. Rabies is found worldwide, except in Australia and the United Kingdom. Man is an unnatural host of the rabies virus and does not serve as a reservoir for natural transmission of the disease. The natural hosts responsible for perpetuating the virus in nature have not been defined; they may be members of the family Mustelidae (weasel and skunk) and the family Viverridae (civet and ferret). Recent evidence indicates that insectivorous and vampire bats are important natural hosts of rabies virus. Although the virus tends to remain latent in the bat, it multiplies in the olfactory mucosa and is shed by aerosols that can transmit the disease to other bats and probably to other animals and man by the respiratory route. It should be noted that vampires roost in wells in some areas and contamination of well water could easily occur. Bat bites may also serve to transmit the disease. In consequence of these circumstances, speleologists run a high risk of contracting rabies. Dogs and cats serve as the most important sources of human infection because of their close association with man. However, many wild animals (e.g., skunks, raccoons, and foxes) are common carriers of the virus and sometimes serve as sources of human infection. Spread of rabies depends on growth of the virus in salivary glands of infected animals. About 50% of rabid dogs shed virus in their saliva.

Treatment and Prevention. Treatment of confirmed rabies in man should include the use of sedatives to relieve anxiety and pain and appropriate drugs to control spastic muscular contractions. Hydration and diuresis should be ensured by intravenous perfusions and the administration of diuretics. Personnel attending rabid patients should be warned of possible contamination and should wear goggles, masks, and gloves.

Prophylaxis against rabies includes destruction of wild animal reservoirs, quarantine of animals suspected of being rabid, and routine vaccination of domestic dogs and cats. For their own protection, most dogs and cats are immunized with a live attenuated rabies virus adapted to grow in chick embryos (Flury vaccine). This vaccine is not suitable for man because of the small antigenic mass of the vaccine. Two types of vaccines are available for man in the USA, a duck embryo vaccine (DEV) and a rabbit nerve tissue vaccine (Semple vaccine). The DEV vaccine is prepared in duck

244   FUNDAMENTALS OF VIROLOGY

embryos infected with the Flury strain of rabies virus; it is subsequently inactivated with beta-propiolactone before human use. The Semple vaccine is made from rabbit brains infected with Pasteur rabbit brain "fixed virus" and inactivated by phenol. Several tissue-culture-grown rabies vaccines have recently been licensed for use in domestic animals. A new tissue-culture-grown vaccine (inactivated) for use in human beings is currently being tested for efficacy in the USA. The vaccine is administered in a single injection, rather than a series of 14 injections.

In the USA, the number of rabies cases reported annually in man is low (1 to 3); however, 30,000 persons receive postexposure prophylaxis. A guide for postexposure antirabies vaccination is given in Table 14–6. *It should be emphasized that all persons bitten by bats should receive immediate antirabies vaccine, since 50% of infected bats have no detectable Negri bodies in brain smears even though they shed virus in their salivary glands and nasal secretions.* Prophylactic rabies vaccination with DEV is recommended for persons exposed to high risk (e.g., veterinarians and speleologists).

3. Postinfectious Encephalitis

Postinfectious encephalitis is an acute or subacute disease of the CNS characterized by focal demyelinative lesions that are prominent in white matter and meninges. The disease occurs as a "postinfectious" complication of many common viral diseases that do not usually affect the CNS. It may also occur as a result of viral vaccination and sometimes without an apparent cause. The disease may present as acute aseptic meningitis, disseminated encephalomyelitis, optic neuritis, or polyneuritis.

Etiologic Agents. Postinfectious encephalitis has been observed following recovery from smallpox, measles, varicella-zoster, herpes simplex, rubella, poliomyelitis, lymphocytic choriomeningitis, mumps, Epstein-Barr and mengo virus infection. Postinfectious encephalitis may develop following vaccination for smallpox or rabies.

Clinical Symptoms. The latent period is usually 2 to 6 days after measles, rubella, or varicella-zoster exanthems. After smallpox vaccination, neurologic symptoms appear on the 10th to the 12th day. About 14 to 21 days after rabies vaccination, the disease may start abruptly, with convulsions, fever, headache, vomiting, and behavioral disturbances. Occasionally, the onset is more gradual. Postinfectious encephalitis following smallpox or rabies vaccination carries a case mortality of about 50%. Following measles, varicella-zoster, rubella, infectious mononucleosis, and mumps, the case mortality ranges from 10 to 20%. Recovery may be complete in 2 to 3 weeks after onset or may take several months. Permanent neurologic sequelae may follow recovery from measles encephalitis.

Pathogenesis. The consensus is that the lesions of postinfectious en-

TABLE 14—6 Treatment of Rabies

Local Treatment of Wounds Involving Possible Exposure to Rabies

(1) Recommended in all exposures

(a) *First-aid treatment*

Since elimination of rabies virus at the site of infection by chemical or physical means . . . is the most effective mechanism of protection, immediate washing and flushing with soap and water, detergent, or water alone is imperative (recommended procedure in all bite wounds including those unrelated to possible exposure to rabies). Then apply either 40-70% alcohol, tincture or aqueous solutions of iodine, or 0.1% quaternary ammonium compounds.[1]

(b) *Treatment by or under direction of a physician*

(1) Treat as above (a) and then:

(2) apply antirabies serum by careful instillation in the depth of the wound and by infiltration around the wound;

(3) postpone suturing of wound; if suturing is necessary use antiserum locally as stated above;

(4) where indicated, institute antitetanus procedures and administer antibiotics and drugs to control infections other than rabies.

[1] Where soap has been used to clean wounds, all traces of it should be removed before application of quaternary ammonium compounds because soap neutralizes the activity of such compounds.

Specific Systemic Treatment

| Nature of exposure | Status of biting animal irrespective of previous examination | | Recommended treatment |
	At time of exposure	During 10 days[a]	
I. Contact, but no lesions; indirect contact; no contact	Rabid	—	None
II. Licks of the skin; scratches or abrasions; minor bites (covered areas of arms, trunk, and legs)	(a) Suspected as rabid [b]	Healthy	Start vaccine. Stop treatment if animal remains healthy for 5 days [a, c]
		Rabid	Start vaccine; administer serum upon positive diagnosis and complete the course of vaccine
	(b) Rabid; wild animal[d] or animal unavailable for observation		Serum + vaccine
III. Licks of mucosa; major bites (multiple or on face, head, finger, or neck)	Suspect [b] or rabid domestic or wild [d] animal, or animal unavailable for observation		Serum + vaccine. Stop treatment if animal remains healthy for 5 days [a, c]

[a] Observation period in this chart applies only to dogs and cats.

[b] All unprovoked bites in endemic areas should be considered suspect unless proved negative by laboratory examination (brain fluorescent Ab test).

[c] Or if its brain is found negative by fluorescent Ab test.

[d] In general, exposure to rodents and rabbits seldom, if ever, requires specific antirabies treatment.

cephalitis result from an allergic reaction, due in most instances to an antigenic component of virus persisting in the nervous system. Evidence supporting this view is provided by the following example: In postvaccinial encephalitis, vaccinia virus can be isolated from the brain and CSF during the first 5 days of illness. Encephalitis following rabies vaccination (i.e., Semple vaccine), in which repeated doses of nervous tissue containing rabies is administered, is an exception that probably represents an auto-allergic (autoimmune) disease.

Immunity. Techniques are being developed to detect and measure the responses leading to allergic lesions in the CNS. These investigations should lead to a better understanding of the causative Ag(s) and the allergic mechanism(s) involved in postinfectious encephalitis.

Diagnosis. Diagnosis of postinfectious encephalitis depends on either direct virus isolation from CSF or postmortem examination. In cases of diseases caused by smallpox, vaccinia, or measles viruses, the agent can be isolated from the brain or CSF during the first few days of illness. In the case of mumps virus, diagnosis may be established by isolating the virus from saliva of patients with accompanying parotitis as well as by isolating the virus from the CSF, by detecting a rise in Ab titer, or by noting the appearance of specific skin reactivity (delayed hypersensitivity) to mumps virus skin test antigen (Chapter 18).

Epidemiology. Patients with exanthems and accompanying encephalitis should be separated from young children and nonimmune persons. In the case of mumps virus encephalitis, the agent is shed in the urine, which may serve as a source of infection for others.

Treatment and Prevention. Smallpox vaccine should be given only to persons traveling to a country reporting smallpox within the preceding 14 days (Chapter 7). In the case of rabies prophylaxis, the newer vaccine made in eggs should be used if possible. Immunization against measles and rubella is recommended for children and nonimmune adults to induce active immunity to these diseases; mumps virus vaccination is recommended at puberty in cases where there is no clinical history of mumps.

In one study, corticosteroid therapy started within 48 hr of onset of postinfectious encephalitis was successful in up to 50% of the patients treated. Gamma globulin is without therapeutic effect.

D. Encephalitides of Probable Viral Origin

1. Von Economo's Disease

The recorded history of von Economo's disease began in 1915, when a worldwide outbreak occurred. The pandemic lasted for 10 years and then mysteriously disappeared. Small epidemics (60 to 70 cases) are still reported occasionally, particularly in the United Kingdom and West Germany. During the pandemic, von Economo, a physician, reported that essentially every practitioner in most of Europe, America, and Australia observed at least several patients in whom they identified the disease with certainty. The disease is characterized by progressive onset of weariness, headache, weight loss, bouts of hiccups, and fever, followed by a number of nervous disorders (e.g., mental, ocular, paralytic), including parkinsonian syndrome. The acute phase of the disease is dominated by drowsiness. The prognosis of the disease is unfavorable, the mortality being 30 to 60%. Sequelae may consist of attacks of headache, sleep disturbances, oculomotor and mental disorders, and complete parkinsonian syndrome. Drugs that are useful for treating parkinsonism (Atropine, Artane, Isomadrin) may be indicated for the treatment of von Economo's disease.

2. Acute Necrotizing Encephalitis

This condition develops rapidly and ends in death 1 to 2 weeks after symptoms develop. In all cases, the disease begins with an "influenza-like" fever, followed by severe disturbances in consciousness, psychiatric changes, abnormal movements, temporal epilepsy, and meningoencephalitis. Although some reports suggest that acute necrotizing encephalitis may be due to herpesviruses, other etiologic agents may be involved.

References

CONSTANTINE, O. G., EMMONS, R. W., and WOODIE, J. D.: Rabies virus in nasal mucosa of naturally infected bats. Science *175*: 1255, 1972.

EMMONS, R. W., LEONARD, L. L., DeGENARO, F., JR., PROTAS, E. S., BAZELEY, P. L., GIAMMONA, S. T., and STURCKOW, R.: A case of human rabies with prolonged survival. Intervirology *1*: 60, 1973.

ENDERS, J. F., WELLER, T. H., and ROBBINS, F. C.: Cultivation of the Lansing strain of poliomyelitis virus in cultures of various human embryonic tissues. Science *109*: 85, 1947.

EVANS, C. A., and GREEN, R. G.: Extraneural growth of poliomyelitis virus. J.A.M.A. *134*: 1154, 1947.

HENDERSON, B. E., and COLEMAN, P. H.: The growing importance of California arboviruses in the etiology of human disease. Progr. Med. Virol. *13*: 404, 1971.

KIBRICK, S.: Current status of coxsackie and ECHO viruses in human disease. Progr. Med. Virol. *6*: 27, 1964.

LONGSON, M. (ed.): Acute necrotizing encephalitis and other herpes simplex virus infections. A symposium held at the University of South Manchester. Postgrad. Med. J. *49*: 373, 1973.

LOOFBOUROW, J. D., CABASSO, V. J., ROBY, R. E., and ANUSKIEWIG, W.: Rabies immune globulin (human). Clinical trials and dose determination. J.A.M.A. *217*: 1825, 1971.

TABER, L. H., MIRKOUIC, R. R., ADAM, V., ELLIS, S. S., YOW, M. D., and MELNICK, J. L.: Rapid diagnosis of enterovirus meningitis by immunofluorescent staining of CSF leukocytes. Intervirology *1*: 127, 1973.

THIEFFRY, S., and FARKAS, E.: Acute anterior poliomyelitis, p. 49. In R. Debré and J. Celers (ed.), *Clinical Virology: The Evaluation and Management of Human Viral Infections*. Philadelphia: W. B. Saunders Co., 1970.

WHO Expert Committee on Rabies. 6th Report. World Health Organization Technical Report Series No. 523. Geneva, 1973.

Chapter 15

Properties of Viruses
Associated with Hepatitis

Acute liver injury and jaundice may result from a variety of physical, chemical, viral, and bacterial agents. Acute viral hepatitis is commonly caused by one or the other of two specific viruses: hepatitis A virus, the causative agent of infectious hepatitis (IH) or hepatitis type A; and hepatitis B virus, the causative agent of serum hepatitis (SH) or hepatitis type B. Yellow fever virus is responsible for an acute, febrile, arthropod-borne illness (yellow fever) that is characterized by jaundice. Other viruses (e.g., Epstein-Barr virus) may cause hepatic enlargement with jaundice as part of a more generalized viral infection (Chapter 16).

A.   Hepatitis Viruses (Unclassified)

1. Hepatitis A (Infections Hepatitis) and Hepatitis B (Serum Hepatitis)

There is sufficient historical, epidemiologic, and experimental evidence to show that infectious hepatitis (IH) and serum hepatitis (SH) are caused by antigenically distinct viruses. Investigations on the properties of these viruses are fragmentary; consequently, hepatitis viruses have not yet been grouped into one of the major virus groups.

In 1964, Blumberg, a human geneticist, discovered an Ag referred to as Australia Antigen (Au Ag) in the serum of an Australian aborigine. Subsequently, Au Ag was recognized as a specific marker of SH virus infection in patients who had received multiple blood transfusions; in addition, this Ag has been detected in the sera of patients with Down's syndrome, lepromatous leprosy, or chronic renal failure as well as in patients on immunosuppressive therapy. These findings have greatly aided our understanding of the clinical, epidemiologic, and immunologic aspects of SH. Attempts to demonstrate a specific antigenic marker in recognizing infection of patients with IH virus have been unsuccessful thus far; however, some advances in this area of research have been made, particularly with nonhuman primates.

Structure and Antigenic Properties. Electron microscopic studies suggested that Au Ag is located in spherical or rod-shaped particles (about 20 nm in diameter) that appear to be incomplete components of SH viruses. A larger spheroid particle (about 43 nm in diameter), consisting of an outer and inner membrane and a core of "nucleic acid," probably represents the mature SH virion (Fig. 15–1). Particles with similar morphology have recently been observed in fecal material from patients with infectious hepatitis.

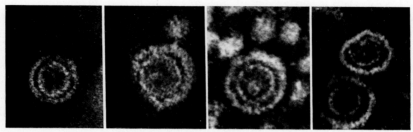

Figure 15–1. Structural variations of serum hepatitis virus particles. (Reprinted with permission from Jokelainen, P. T., Krohn, K., Prince, A. M., and Finlayson, N. D. C.: Electron microscopic observations on virus-like particles associated with SH antigen. J. Virol. *6:* 685, 1970.)

Australia Ag reacts in immunodiffusion, counter-immunoelectrophoresis, latex particle agglutination (Ab-coated) and complement-fixation (CF) tests with serum Abs of SH patients. Specific Abs to Au Ag agglutinate particles 18-21 nm in diameter that are present in the sera of patients with SH. Also, antisera against Au Ag, coupled with fluorescein isothiocyanate, stain intranuclear granules in infected liver cells. These observations indicate that Au Ag is part of the SH virus. There are no specific Ags for recognizing IH viruses.

Both SH and IH viruses are resistant to heat (60°C for 20 hr), ultraviolet light, freezing (−20°C, for more than 20 years), and many chemical disinfectants. Formalin, activated glutaraldehyde, or preparations of hypochlorite are generally used for inactivation of hepatitis viruses. The remarkable resistance of hepatitis viruses to physical agents emphasizes the need for extra precaution in dealing with hepatitis patients and their excretion products. The physical properties of SH virus are similar to those of IH virus; however, SH virus is antigenically distinct from IH virus.

Host Range and Culture. Man and perhaps nonhuman primates are the only natural hosts of both IH and SH viruses. Dogs, mice, ducks, and turkeys are susceptible to their own specific hepatitis viruses but are resistant to hepatitis viruses of human origin. Attempts to isolate IH viruses in tissue culture have resulted in a collection of "hepatitis-candidate" agents. Recent published evidence indicates that SH virus can be cultivated in human embryo liver organ cultures. Inoculation of human hepatitis materials into certain species of nonhuman primates induced viral hepatitis, and the disease was passed in series from animal to animal.

B.   Togavirus (Arbovirus) Group

1.   Yellow Fever Virus

According to the current classification of animal viruses, yellow fever (YF) virus is the prototype of the newly proposed taxonomic genus flavovirus of the group B togaviruses (arboviruses). Human isolates of YF virus exhibit viscerotropic and neurotropic characteristics. Viscerotropism is manifested by infection and injury of the liver, kidneys, and heart; neurotropism signifies infection and injury of cells of the CNS. Following successive brain passages in mice, YF virus becomes adapted and exhibits more neurotropism and less viscerotropism than the original virus. Prolonged cultivation of the virus in chick embryos has produced an attenuated strain, 17D, which is widely used as a vaccine (Chapter 7).

Structure and Antigenic Properties. Yellow fever virus is a small (30 to 40 nm) single-stranded enveloped RNA virus. The virus is stable at 4°C in 50% glycerol and withstands lyophilization. It is rapidly inactivated by boiling water (100°C) or by 0.1% formalin. The YF virus contains at least two distinct Ags, one a hemagglutinin and the other a CF Ag. Only one antigenic type of YF virus exists in nature.

Host Range and Culture. Yellow fever virus multiplies in nonhuman primates, mice, chick embryos, and mosquitoes. All strains (viscerotropic and neurotropic) of YF virus produce encephalitis in adult mice following intracranial inoculation. Infant mice develop encephalitis following subcutaneous or intraperitoneal inoculation. The virus is readily grown in tissue culture cells from a wide variety of vertebrate and arthropod cells.

References

ALLISON, B., and BLUMBERG, B.: An isoprecipitation reaction distinguishing human serum protein types. Lancet *1*: 634, 1961.

ANDREWS, C., and PEREIRA, H. G.: *Viruses of Vertebrates*. 3rd ed. Baltimore: The Williams & Wilkins Co., 1972.

BLUMBERG, B.: Polymorphisms of serum proteins and the development of isoprecipitins in transfused patients. Bull. N. Y. Acad. Med. *40*: 377, 1964.

BLUMBERG, B., GERSTLEY, D., HUNGERFORD, W., LONDON, W., and SUTNICK, A.: A serum antigen (Australia antigen) in Down's syndrome, leukemia and hepatitis. Ann. Intern. Med. *66*: 924, 1967.

JOKELAINEN, P. T., KROHN, K., PRIME, A. M., and FINLAYSON, N. D. C.: Electron microscopic observations on virus-like particles associated with SH antigen. J. Virol. *6*: 685, 1970.

KRUGMAN, S., and WARD, R.: Viral hepatitis, p. 284. In Debré, R., and Celers, J. (ed.): *Clinical Virology: The Evaluation and Management of Human Viral Infections.* Philadelphia: W. B. Saunders Co., 1970.

MILLIMAN, I., LOEB, L., BAYER, M., and BLUMBERG, B.: Australia antigen (a hepatitis-associated antigen). J. Exp. Med. *131*: 1190, 1970.

MUSSGAY, M.: Growth cycle of arboviruses in vertebrate and arthropod cells. Progr. Med. Virol. *6*: 193, 1964.

WHO Expert Committee on Viral Hepatitis. World Health Organization Technical Report Series No. 512. Geneva, 1973.

WHO Expert Committee on Yellow Fever. Third Reprint. World Health Organization Technical Report Series No. 479. Geneva, 1971.

ZUCKERMAN, A. J., and BAINES, P. M.: Australia antigen as a marker of propagation of the serum hepatitis virus in cultures. Nature *263*: 78, 1972.

Chapter 16

Viral Diseases of the Liver

A. Hepatitis Type A (Infectious Hepatitis) and
   Hepatitis Type B (Serum Hepatitis)   253
B. Yellow Fever   258
C. Other Viral Hepatic Diseases   260

Acute viral hepatitis is one of the most important of the communicable diseases present in developed countries. The most common etiologic agents are hepatitis A (infectious hepatitis) virus and hepatitis B (serum hepatitis) virus. Several other viruses may infect the liver as part of a more general disseminated disease (Table 16–1). Differential diagnosis is facilitated by

TABLE 16—1
Virus Etiology of Acute Hepatic Injury

	Causative Viruses	
Common	**Uncommon**	
Infectious hepatitis	Yellow Fever	
Serum hepatitis	Epstein-Barr	
	Cytomegalovirus[a]	
	Rubella[a]	
	Herpes simplex[b]	
	Coxsackievirus[b]	

[a] Etiologic agents of prenatal hepatitis acquired *in utero*.
[b] Etiologic agents of postnatal hepatitis usually acquired during or after parturition.

characteristic features of various infections in which hepatitis may occur. For example, lymphadenopathy and pharyngitis are characteristic of infectious mononucleosis (Epstein-Barr virus etiology), together with a positive Paul-Bunnel test (heterophil Ab) and a significant titer of serum Abs specific for Epstein-Barr (EB) virus. Hepatitis caused by yellow fever virus should be considered in endemic areas. *Neonatal hepatitis caused by cytomegalovirus or other viruses presents special diagnostic problems.* In each of these cases, hepatitis is but one of the clinical signs of a generalized viral infection. Complete physical examination will always reveal other abnormalities that are useful in deciding the etiology of the hepatitis (see chapters dealing with the individual viruses concerned). *The diagnosis of viral hepatitis is considered to be a presumptive one when based on epidemiologic, clinical, biochemical, and histologic evidence.* The student of medicine must bear in mind that jaundice can also be caused by bacteria, protozoa, and noninfectious agents, such as hepatotoxic chemicals, and by physical obstruction of the biliary system.

A. Hepatitis Type A (Infectious Hepatitis) and Hepatitis Type B (Serum Hepatitis)

Viral hepatitis type A (epidemic or infectious hepatitis; IH) and viral hepatitis type B (serum hepatitis; SH) are distinct diseases. During the past decade there has been a steady rise in the incidence of SH, particularly among males in the 15- to 29-year age group. Narcotic addiction is now widespread and may account for the changing nationwide pattern of viral hepatitis in all socioeconomic levels. Serum hepatitis is a disease with a more insidious impact, longer incubation period, and higher mortality than IH. Also, the discovery of a virus-like Ag referred to as Australia antigen (Au Ag) and its persistence in the blood for prolonged periods in patients recovered from SH showed that SH virus has a worldwide distribution similar to that previously attributed only to IH virus.

It is estimated that 700,000 cases of viral hepatitis occur annually in the USA; the number of deaths associated with this disease ranges between 2,000 and 9,000 annually. With respect to hepatitis patients in the USA, it is estimated that the direct costs for hospitalization and physician's services and the indirect costs due to loss of productivity exceed one billion dollars per year.

Etiologic Agents. It is reasonably certain that SH and the virus-like Au Ag are associated with a spherical virus present in patients' sera. Studies in human volunteers demonstrated that IH is also associated with a transmissible virus-like agent. The viruses of SH and IH are epidemiologically and immunologically distinct.

Clinical Symptoms. Infectious hepatitis and SH have similar as well as distinctive clinical features (Table 16–2). Jaundice may or may not be present during the acute phase of infection. Factors that influence the severity of viral hepatitis include age and associated conditions (e.g., pregnancy, diabetes, abdominal surgery, and cancer).

Some cases of hepatitis may develop into chronic persisting or recurrent hepatitis that follows a period of recovery from typical acute hepatitis.

TABLE 16—2

Characteristics of Hepatic Viral Diseases of Man Due to IH, SH, and YF Viruses

Feature	Infectious Hepatitis (IH)	Serum Hepatitis (SH)	Yellow Fever (YF)
Transmission to human subjects	Oral, parenteral routes via nasopharyngeal secretion, fecal material in water, food, and fomites or direct contact	Oral, parenteral injection, direct contact	Bite from infected mosquito
Antigenicity	No cross-immunity to SH virus	No cross-immunity to IH virus	Cross-reacts with other group B togaviruses (arboviruses), best with HAI, intermediate with CF, least with neutralization titration
Natural communicability	Contagious	Can be transmitted nonparenterally	During viremic state
Incubation period	Short (15-40 days)	Long (50-150 days)	3-6 days
Onset	Acute, sudden rise in serum transaminases and abrupt fall 19 days later; same for IgM	Insidious prolonged rise in serum transaminases; IgM only slightly modified	Rapid with fever, headache, vomiting
Symptoms preceding jaundice	Fever, malaise, anorexia, nausea, diarrhea, abdominal discomfort	Fever, malaise, anorexia, nausea, diarrhea, abdominal discomfort	Bloodshot eyes, wine-colored face, fever, headache, vomiting
Preicteric phase duration	2-21 days	21-81 days	3-4 days, followed by remission
Icteric phase	Abrupt, high fever, jaundice	Insidious, low fever, jaundice	Jaundice, fever, vomiting, gastric hemorrhage, degeneration of myocardium, meninges, kidneys
Seasonal incidence	Autumn and winter	All year round	During mosquito season
Age incidence	Common in children and young adults	Rare in children, common in adults	All ages
Host range	Man, nonhuman primates	Man, nonhuman primates	Man, nonhuman primates

Severity	Mortality low (1%)	Mortality high (50%)	Mortality 10%; can also support inapparent infection followed by immunity
Diagnostic tests	Transaminase levels, liver biopsy	Transaminase levels, liver biopsy	Isolation of virus in newborn mice
Australia antigen in blood	Not usually present	Present during incubation period and acute phase, may persist	Not present
Virus present in:			
Feces	During incubation and acute phases	Depends on site of virus entry	Not present
Blood	During incubation and acute phases	During incubation and acute phases	During incubation and acute phases
Duration of carried virus in:			
Blood	Unknown (maybe 8 mo)	Several years	During viremic stage
Feces	Weeks to months	Not demonstrated	Not demonstrated
Prophylactic value of pooled human γ-globulin	Good	Experimentally successful if given shortly after transfusion and one month later	Not used
Preventive Measures	Good hygiene; detection of carriers; use of disposable equipment; contaminated equipment should be autoclaved, heated at 180° C for 1 hr, incinerated, or treated with formalin, hypochlorite, or activated glutaraldehyde; subjects having history of jaundice should not donate blood	Good hygiene; use of disposable needles and syringes; screening blood for Au Ag; no way to inactivate virus in blood or plasma; addition of β propiolactone shows promise experimentally; contaminated equipment should be autoclaved, heated at 180° C for 1 hr, incinerated, or treated with formalin, hypochlorite, or activated glutaraldehyde; subjects having history of jaundice should not donate blood	Vaccination, eradicate mosquito population
Carrier rate	Widespread	2-3%	Variable in nonhuman primates
Vaccine	In development	In development	17D (attenuated live vaccine)

Whether this persistence or recurrence of hepatitis is the result of a chronic viral infection or immunologic injury to the liver is not clearly understood.

Pathogenesis. Viremia during the incubation period results from multiplication of virus in the liver and gastrointestinal (GI) tract. The two types of hepatitis cause identical lesions in the liver. Lesions may extend beyond the liver to the upper GI tract and the kidney. The hepatic lesions are characterized by parenchymal cell degeneration and necrosis, proliferation of Kupffer cells, inflammation, and cell regeneration. Macrophages accumulate at sites of necrosis, as do lymphocytes, plasma cells, and neutrophils. These changes disappear with full recovery from the disease.

Immunity. There are indications that several serotypes of these etiologic agents exist. There is no cross-immunity between different serotypes, and second attacks of both diseases occur.

Diagnosis. Assessment of abnormal liver function by various means, including measurement of serum glutamic oxaloacetic acid transaminase (SGOT) and bilirubin in the urine and blood, thymol turbidity and sulfobromophthalein (SBP) tests, and histopathologic study of liver biopsy specimens, aid in the clinical diagnosis of hepatitis, particularly in cases with jaundice.

Counter immunoelectrophoresis determinations, complement-fixation (CF) tests, and radioimmunoassays are useful for detecting Au Ag in the serum or plasma of patients with SH. About 80% of patients with clinically diagnosed SH show positive tests for Au Ag. Australia Ag appears during the preicteric period; it frequently disappears during the icteric period and may reappear. Detection of virus neutralizing Ab has not proved to be of diagnostic value; however, detection of Abs against Au Ag is of diagnostic significance. Routine isolation of hepatitis virus is not feasible.

Epidemiology. There are major differences in the epidemiologic features of IH and SH (Table 16–2). Infectious hepatitis is generally transmitted by person-to-person contact or ingestion of contaminated food (e.g., shellfish). However, it is possible to transmit IH by contaminated blood products or hypodermic needles. Subclinical cases of IH are common and may serve as a possible source of spread. Small clusters of cases of viral hepatitis in human beings in close contact with nonhuman primates have been reported. In these episodes, it could not be determined whether the virus was of human or nonhuman origin. Apparently, the incidence of IH depends on opportunities for ready distribution of infected material and the susceptibility of the exposed population. Poor sanitation, overcrowding, exposure of a nonimmune population to contaminated material, and a short incubation period contribute to epidemics of IH. Explosive epidemics of IH have occurred following fecal contamination of drinking water and after consumption of shellfish from polluted water.

Serum hepatitis virus is usually transmitted by the use of contaminated needles, syringes, blood products, renal dialysis, and heart-lung machines. The incidence of SH in recipients of blood transfusions is 0.3 to 4%; the incidence is significantly increased following multiple transfusions. The present widely employed techniques for detecting Au Ag in blood are estimated to be capable of reducing the incidence of post-transfusion hepatitis by 30%. Many persons have become infected with SH virus as the result of tattooing and vaccination with improperly sterilized instruments. Serum hepatitis virus is also transmitted on occasion by direct personal contact. The estimated ratio of anicteric to icteric infections is reported to be greater than 100 to 1.

On the basis of long-term studies with SH, two definitions for the chronic carrier states have emerged: *chronic persistent hepatitis* and *chronic aggressive hepatitis*. Chronic persistent hepatitis is a mild, benign disease. It is not always preceded by recognizable acute illness. Malaise, hepatomegaly, and minor abnormalities of liver function are the clinical features. There is no progression to cirrhosis, and the prognosis is good. Only a small proportion of these patients demonstrate Au Ag. Chronic aggressive hepatitis is usually characterized by parenchymal necrosis, inflammatory cell infiltration, and varying degrees of hepatic cirrhosis. Young females are most often affected. Autoantibodies are usually present in the serum, and immunoglobulin levels are elevated. Australia Ag has been detected in about 60% of patients (usually male) with chronic aggressive hepatitis.

Fortunately, purified human gamma globulin or albumin is free of hepatitis viruses because the virus is inactivated by ethanol during the fractionation of plasma. Patients needing massive blood transfusions (e.g., patients undergoing open heart surgery and patients subjected to renal dialysis) stand the greatest risk of becoming infected. Medical personnel attending such patients are also at considerable risk.

Treatment and Prevention. The control of IH is most effectively accomplished through preventive measures, including sanitation and aseptic techniques that break the chain of transmission and through passive immunization. Pooled human gamma globulin affords some protection if given intramuscularly during the incubation period or up to 6 days before the onset of symptoms; passive immunity lasts about 3 to 6 months. Gamma globulin is especially recommended for halting epidemics in military camps or institutions. Prophylactic immunization has been practiced among military personnel entering Vietnam as well as among missionaries, Peace Corps volunteers, and travelers entering endemic areas. Every effort should be made to maintain approved sanitation procedures that prevent fecal contamination. It is recommended that food handlers be screened by determining SGOT levels. All needles, syringes, and lancets that have come in contact with blood or blood products should be autoclaved (15 psi, 120° C, 15 min) or incinerated.

The principal measure for controlling SH is to routinely screen blood plasma and other blood products for Au Ag. Persons who have a history of hepatitis should not be used as blood donors. Because the duration of carriage of SH virus is not known, estimates of the incidence of hepatitis carriers vary from 0.1 to 10%. As little as 0.004 ml of plasma can transmit the disease; therefore, the use of pooled plasma should be avoided whenever possible. If pools must be used, it is recommended that they be made from fewer than 6 donors to reduce the possibility of transmitting SH to patients. The use of disposable needles and syringes is recommended to assure sterility and to reduce the chances that a single syringe or needle will be used on more than one person. Physicians, nurses, and dentists should be made aware of the importance of decontaminating instruments that may have come in contact with blood or feces. Dry heat, autoclaving, or incineration are the most satisfactory methods for decontamination. The choice of chemical disinfectants includes formalin, activated glutaraldehyde, or preparations of hypochlorite. Disposable dialyzers should, if possible, be used for infected patients. A record of patients using dialysis monitors is desirable to trace possible cross-infections.

B.   Yellow Fever

Yellow fever (YF) is an acute viral disease characterized by sudden onset, moderately high fever, prostration, and a relatively slow pulse rate in terms of the degree of fever. Severe cases are sometimes associated with vomiting of altered blood, albuminuria, jaundice, and formation of emboli that may lead to death (Table 16–2). The disease is endemic in tropical areas of Africa and South America. The virus is transmitted from man to man by the domestic mosquito, *Aedes aegypti (urban yellow fever)*. When the virus is transmitted from monkey to man or monkey to monkey by jungle mosquitoes, the disease is called *sylvan* or *jungle yellow fever*.

Etiologic Agents.   The causative agent of YF is a small single-stranded RNA virus that is classified in the genus flavovirus (group B) of the togavirus (arbovirus) group. Fresh human isolates of YF virus exhibit viscerotropism for liver, kidneys, and heart, and neurotropism for cells of the CNS.

Clinical Symptoms.   Most attacks of YF are mild, with fever and headache of short duration. Epidemiologic features are, therefore, important in diagnosis. The incubation period is from 3 to 6 days; the onset of disease is sudden, with chills, headache, and vomiting. The acute stage of the disease lasts about 3 days and is referred to as the *period of infection*. The symptoms preceding jaundice may also include bloodshot eyes and a wine-colored face due to hemorrhages. After a short remission of about 4 days, the *period of intoxication* begins. During this period, jaundice may develop, with associated hemorrhage into the gums, nose, and gastrointestinal (GI) tract (Table 16–2). The absence of jaundice is much more frequent than its presence. Fatal cases often exhibit degenerative changes in the myocardium, meninges, and kidneys. Patients with severe disease may recover by the 7th or 8th day following onset of the period of intoxication. Convalescence progresses rapidly. Unlike IH or SH, relapses do not occur, and there are no permanent sequelae following recovery from YF; immunity following convalescence is lifelong.

Pathogenesis. Knowledge of the pathogenesis of YF has been gained largely from experiments with nonhuman primates. When the YF virus is introduced naturally into the skin of susceptible primates by an infected mosquito, the virus reaches the local lymph node and multiplies there; it then enters the bloodstream and becomes localized in the liver, spleen, kidneys, bone marrow, and lymph glands. Animals inoculated with a highly virulent strain of YF virus show the highest concentration of virus in the liver, whereas in animals inoculated with attenuated 17D strain (vaccine strain), the virus is limited to the spleen, lymph nodes, and bone marrow.

Injury due to YF results from replication of the virus in target organs. Death is due to destruction of parenchymatous cells of the liver and to hemorrhage; the most frequent site of hemorrhage is the mucosa at the pyloric end of the stomach.

Histologically, there may be irregular masses (inclusions) of hyaline material in the cell cytoplasm; these are called *Councilman bodies.* Inclusion bodies may also be present in the nucleus and are of diagnostic value. In patients who recover, the damaged hepatic cells are replaced, and liver functions are restored.

Immunity. Immunity is transmitted passively from mother to infant and is acquired actively by exposure to natural infection or by vaccination with the 17D strain of YF virus.

Diagnosis. The possibilities of isolating virus from serum are highest during the first 5 days of disease. Adult or baby mice injected intracranially with serum from a suspected case of YF develop encephalitis if virus is present. Identification of the virus is made by specific neutralization tests in mice. Neutralizing Abs may be detected in patients' sera as early as the 5th day of disease. The assay involves mixing the serum with various dilutions of YF virus and inoculating the mixtures intracranially in mice. It is imperative that samples of the original specimen be retained so that subsequent successful isolation can be confirmed by reisolation at the same laboratory and at a WHO regional reference center. Histopathologic examination of liver biopsy material for Councilman bodies from human cases is also useful for establishing a diagnosis of YF.

Epidemiology. Yellow fever occurs in 2 distinct epidemiologic cycles: (1) classic urban (epidemic), and (2) sylvan (jungle) yellow fever. *Urban YF* involves transmission of virus from man to man through the bite of infected *Aedes aegypti* mosquitoes. The mosquitoes become infected when they bite an individual during the viremic stage of disease. Infected mosquitoes remain infectious for life. When an uninfected mosquito bites an individual with viremia, the mosquito becomes infectious after an incubation period of 12 to 14 days, *the extrinsic incubation period.* During this period, the virus replicates extensively, completing its biologic cycle. Yellow fever virus cannot survive long in an urban environment unless there is a constant influx of susceptible human beings and unless the area is infested with *Aedes aegypti* mosquitoes.

Jungle YF is primarily a disease of nonhuman primates that is transmitted from monkey to monkey by jungle (arboreal) mosquitoes. Nonhuman primates are natural hosts of the virus and serve as permanent reservoirs of the virus. The disease in monkeys may be either severe or inapparent. Man, an accidental host, contracts the disease when he enters the jungle and is bitten by jungle mosquitoes carrying YF virus. The disease may also be transmitted from monkey to man by *Aedes aegypti,* which usually takes place in nonjungle environments. All age groups are susceptible, but the disease is usually milder in young infants than older persons. Inapparent infections frequently occur. The mortality rate is about 10%.

Treatment and Prevention. If a case of YF is diagnosed in an endemic area, the patient should be kept in a mosquito-proof room during the first 5 days of illness. Vaccination is essential for all persons entering an endemic area. Vaccination with live virus of the 17D attenuated strain induces effective immunity within 7 to 10 days. Booster doses of the vaccine should be given every 10 years. Urban YF has been virtually eliminated in most areas of the world by reducing or eradicating the vector mosquito *Aedes aegypti.*

C. Other Viral Hepatic Diseases

Rubella virus, cytomegalovirus, coxsackievirus, herpes simplex virus, or EB virus infection may cause hepatitis as part of a more generalized infection. The neonate is highly susceptible to hepatitis with associated jaundice and hepatosplenomegaly caused by these viral agents, with the exception of EB virus. Infection of the neonate by rubella or cytomegalovirus occurs transplacentally from mother to offspring, whereas herpes simplex or coxsackieviruses infect the infant during or after parturition. Although the liver returns to normal metabolic function following recovery from hepatitis due to the "hepatitis viruses," sequelae may include cirrhosis. Other viral diseases (e.g., measles) may be accompanied by minor, nonspecific changes in liver function.

Infectious mononucleosis in adults is caused by EB virus (Chapter 18);

it is usually accompanied by hepatic enlargement and altered liver functions (e.g., serum alkaline phosphatase) although jaundice is usually absent. In contrast to SH or IH, there is minimal cell necrosis, and chronic liver disease is not a sequela of infectious mononucleosis.

References

DEBRÉ, R., and CELERS, J. (ed.): *Clinical Virology: The Evaluation and Management of Human Viral Infections.* Philadelphia: W. B. Saunders Co., 1970.

FAULKNER, W. R., and KING, J. W. (ed.): *Australia Antigen* and *Hepatitis.* Cleveland: CRC Press, 1971.

KRUGMAN, S., GOLES, J. P., and HAMMOND, J.: Viral hepatitis, type B (MS-2 strain): 1. Studies on active immunization. 2. Prevention with specific hepatitis B immune serum globulin. JAMA *218*: 41; *218*: 1665, 1971.

LeBOUVIER, G. L., and McCOLLUM, R. W.: Australia (hepatitis-associated) antigen: Physiochemical and immunological characteristics. Adv. Virus. Res. *16*: 357, 1970.

NEILSON, J. O., DEITRICHSON, O., ELLING, P., and CHRISTOFFERSON, P.: Incidence and meaning of persistence of Australia antigen in patients with acute viral hepatitis: Development of chronic hepatitis. N. Engl. J. Med. *285*: 1157, 1971.

NEILSON, J. O., NIELSON, M. H., and ELLING, P.: Differential distribution of Australia-antigen-associated particles in patients with liver diseases and normal carriers. N. Engl. J. Med. *288*: 484, 1973

PRINCE, A. M.: An antigen detected in the blood during the incubation period of serum hepatitis. Proc. Nat. Acad. Sci. U.S. *60*: 814, 1968.

SHULMAN, N. R.: Hepatitis-associated antigen. Amer. J. Med. *49*: 669, 1970.

WHO Expert Committee on Viral Hepatitis. World Health Organization Technical Report Series No. 512. Geneva, 1973.

WHO Expert Committee on Yellow Fever, Third Reprint. World Health Organization Technical Report Series No. 479. Geneva, 1971.

Chapter 17

Properties of Viruses Associated with Glandular Infections

Virus infections of parotid glands, lymph nodes, or mesenteric glands are frequent. The etiology may involve mumps virus (parotid glands), cytomegalovirus (salivary glands), Epstein-Barr virus (lymph nodes), or echovirus (mesenteric glands). These infections sometimes are inapparent (e.g., mumps virus) or latent (e.g., cytomegalovirus). In this chapter, we shall consider properties of Epstein-Barr (EB) virus and cytomegalovirus (both are members of the herpesvirus group). For a discussion of the biological properties of echovirus, see Chapter 9, and for mumps virus, see Chapter 13.

A. Herpesvirus Group

More than 200 viruses are now classified in the herpesvirus group. The important herpesviruses of man are herpes simplex types 1 and 2 and varicella-zoster (Chapter 11), cytomegalovirus, and EB virus. Herpesviruses of monkeys include B virus (Chapter 13), which can cause disease in man.

1. Epstein-Barr Virus

Epstein-Barr virus, an antigenically distinct herpesvirus, was recently observed in cell cultures of Burkitt's lymphoma (a tumor originally described in Central African children). The virus has also been found in many lymphoid cell cultures derived from patients with Burkitt's lymphoma or infectious mononucleosis (mono) as well as from normal individuals. Epstein-Barr virus is considered to be the etiologic agent of infectious mono and is suspected of being the cause of Burkitt's lymphoma and nasopharyngeal carcinoma (Chapter 24).

Structure and Antigenic Properties. All herpesviruses, including EB virus, contain an internal core of double-stranded DNA enclosed by a capsid exhibiting icosahedral symmetry. The virion is surrounded by a lipid-containing envelope and contains 162 capsomeres. Whereas the enveloped form measures about 160 nm in diameter, the nonenveloped "naked" particle is about 90 nm in diameter. Typical herpes-like particles in infectious mononucleosis cell lines are shown in Figures 17–1 and 17–2.

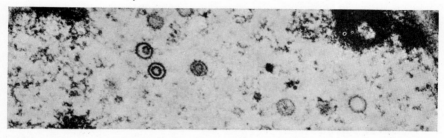

Figure 17–1. Incomplete herpes-type virus particles located within a nucleus of a peripheral blood cell in a cell culture established from a patient with heterophil-positive infectious mononucleosis. ×50,000. (Reprinted with permission from Moses, H. L., Glade, P. R., Kasel, J. A., Rosenthal, A. S., Hirshaut, Y., and Chessin, L. N.: Infectious mononucleosis: Detection of herpeslike virus and reticular aggregates of small cytoplasmic particles in continuous lymphoid cell lines derived from peripheral blood. Proc. Nat. Acad. Sci. U.S. *60:* 492, 1968.)

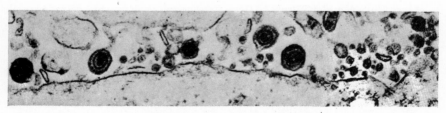

Figure 17–2. Extracellular herpes-type virus particles that have an internal core with the same dimensions as the nuclear particles (Fig. 17–1) but appear to be surrounded by an envelope giving an overall diameter of 160 nm. ×50,000. (Reprinted with permission from Moses, H. L., Glade, P. R., Kasel, J. A., Rosenthal, A. S., Hirshaut, Y., and Chessin, L.: Infectious mononucleosis: Detection of herpeslike virus and reticular aggregates of small cytoplasmic particles in continuous lymphoid cell lines derived from peripheral blood. Proc. Nat. Acad. Sci. U.S. *60:* 492, 1968.)

Epstein-Barr virus is antigenically distinct from other human herpes-viruses. However, it reportedly shares a common Ag with the herpesviruses that induce the Lucké tumor (a renal adenocarcinoma of frogs), Marek's disease of fowl (Chapter 23), infectious bovine rhinotracheitis, and cyto-megalovirus of monkeys and guinea pigs. Epstein-Barr-virus-infected lymphoblastoid cells in culture contain virus capsid Ag and a virus-specified membrane Ag. These Ags are measured by immunofluorescence or com-plement-fixation (CF) tests using hyperimmune serum.

Host Range and Culture. Infection and transformation of human em-bryo fibroblasts and human or nonhuman primate blood leukocytes with EB virus have been accomplished. The virus appears to have specific affinity for lymphoblastoid cells, in which it can exist in a vegetative or lysogenic state. In these cells, EB virus is detected by electron microscopy or with immunofluorescence using acetone-fixed cells and fluorescein-labeled EB virus antiserum. The number of cells positive for virus particles varies from 0.1 to 10%; however, the virus genome is present not only in the cells containing EB virus or EB viral Ags but also in most, if not all, cells within the culture. Cultivation of lymphoblastoid cells in media de-prived of arginine or supplemented with 5-bromodeoxyuridine increases the virus content in some cell lines. Only leukocytes that contain the EB virus genome are assumed to persist in cell culture.

2. Cytomegalovirus

Structure and Antigenic Properties. Cytomegalovirus has a structure common to all herpesviruses (Chapter 1). There are several strains of human cytomegalovirus that share many common antigenic properties, making it difficult to separate them into individual serotypes. However, cytomegaloviruses of animals are antigenically distinct. There are no firm indications that human cytomegaloviruses share common antigens with other herpesviruses.

Host Range and Culture. Since cytomegaloviruses are species-specific with respect to host range, the human types are grown in cultured human cells. Primary or serially propagated strains of human fibroblasts (e.g., WI-38) are routinely utilized to isolate the virus, to prepare virus stocks for study, or to provide antigenic materials for serologic tests. Treatment of human fibroblast cells with 5-iododeoxyuridine enhances replication of cytomegalovirus in these cells. Infectivity is primarily cell-associated, and spread of infectious virus is from cell to cell. Infected cells become swol-len, rounded, and refractile and contain intranuclear and intracytoplasmic inclusions. Cytopathology may be recognized within 24 to 72 hours when high-virus-titer inocula are used. With low-titered inocula, lesions may not develop in the culture for several weeks. Serial passage to new cultures is best accomplished by transfer of infected cells freed by trypsinization or mechanical scraping. Cytomegalovirus loses infectivity when heated at 56° C for 30 min or when exposed to ether or to acid pH.

Recent data show that ultraviolet-inactivated cytomegalovirus can transform hamster embryo fibroblasts *in vitro* and that the transformed cells induce tumor formation when inoculated into newborn hamsters.

References

ANDREWS, C., and PEREIRA, H. G.: *Viruses of Vertebrates.* 3rd ed. Baltimore: Williams & Wilkins Co., 1972.

CARLSTROM, G.: Virologic studies on cytomegalic inclusion disease. Acta Pediat. Scand. *54*: 17, 1965.

EVANS, D. L., BARNETT, J. W., BOWEN, J. M., and DMOCHOWSKI, L.: Antigenic relationship between herpesviruses of infectious bovine rhinotracheitis, Marek's disease and Burkitt's lymphoma. J. Virol. *10*: 277, 1972.

GERBER, P.: Activation of Epstein-Barr virus by 5-bromodeoxyuridine in "virus free" human cells. Proc. Nat. Acad. Sci. U.S. *69*: 83, 1972.

MILLER, G., SHAPE, T., LISCO, H., STITT, D., and LIPMAN, M.: Epstein-Barr virus: Transformation, cytopathic changes, and viral antigens in squirrel monkeys and marmoset leukocytes. Proc. Nat. Acad. Sci. U.S. *69*: 383, 1972.

MOSES, H. L., GLADE, P. R., KASEL, J. A., ROSENTHAL, A. S., HIRSHAUT, Y., and CHESSIN, L. N.: Infectious mononucleosis. Detection of herpeslike virus and reticular aggregates of small cytoplasmic particles in continuous lymphoid cell lines derived from peripheral blood. Proc. Nat. Acad. Sci. U.S. *60:* 489, 1968.

PLUMMER, G.: Cytomegaloviruses of man and animals. Progr. Med. Virol. *15*: 92, 1973.

PROBERT, M., and EPSTEIN, M. A.: Morphological transformation in vitro of human fibroblasts by Epstein-Barr virus: Preliminary observations. Science *175*: 202, 1972.

ST. JEOR, S., and RAPP, F.: Cytomegalovirus: Conversion of nonpermissive cells to a permissive state for virus replication. Science *181*: 1060, 1973.

WELLER, T. H.: The cytomegaloviruses: Ubiquitous agents with protean clinical manifestations. N. Eng. J. Med. *285*: 203, 1971.

ZUR HAUSEN, H., DIEHL, V., WOLF, H., SCHULTE-HOLTHAUSEN, H., and SCHNEIDER, U.: Occurrence of Epstein-Barr virus genomes in human lymphoblastoid cell lines. Nature New Biol. *237*: 189, 1972.

Glandular Viral Diseases

A. Mumps

Mumps was one of the earliest diseases recognized as a clinical entity. Hippocrates described its characteristic features (nonsuppurative swelling of the parotid glands) as early as the 5th century B.C. About 1790, Hamilton stressed the importance of orchitis as a complication of mumps and noted that CNS disorders sometimes accompany parotitis (Chapter 13). In 1940, physicians began to recognize pancreatitis and involvement of other organs and tissues as additional expressions of infection with mumps virus.

In 1934, Goodpasture and Johnson proved the viral etiology of mumps by reproducing the disease in nonhuman primates inoculated with filtrates of human saliva. The subsequent development of a skin test Ag for determining hypersensitivity to mumps virus revealed that mumps virus frequently causes inapparent infections that are followed by immunity.

Etiologic Agents. Mumps is caused by an RNA virus belonging to the paramyxovirus group (Chapter 9). The virus agglutinates chicken or human erythrocytes and induces parotitis and fatal meningoencephalitis in suckling mice or hamsters.

Clinical Symptoms. In most cases, the incubation period is 16 to 20 days. Swelling of one or both parotid glands is the first sign of disease. However, in adult males, pain in the testes may be the first symptom. Rarely, aseptic meningitis appears first, followed by parotitis (Chapter 14); the incidence of aseptic meningitis is variable but may be as high as 25%.

In severe cases of mumps, the prodromal period with fever, malaise, headache, chills, sore throat, earache, and tenderness along the region of the parotid ducts lasts as long as 2 or 3 days. Parotid swelling is usually

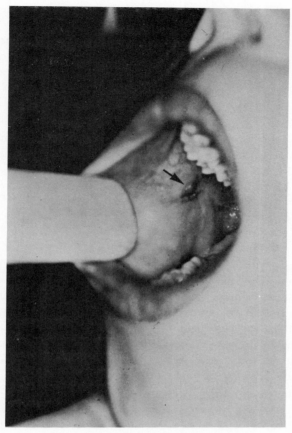

Figure 18–1. Swollen Stensen's duct opening in mumps. Note papillae at the opening of the duct. Involvement of Stensen's duct may be diagnostically helpful. (Reprinted with permission from *Physician's Bulletin,* 1959. Eli Lilly Co., p. 92.)

observed below the ear. There is sharp pain if Stensen's duct becomes partially occluded as the gland swells (Fig. 18–1). The papillae at the opening of Stensen's duct may be reddened, but this feature is inconsistent. Symptoms tend to be mild in children and more severe in adults. The duration of swelling and fever depends on the extent and severity of the infection.

Orchitis is rare before puberty but may occur in 25% of adult patients. The onset is variable but usually occurs between the 5th and the 10th day of illness as the parotid swelling subsides. Inflammation of the testes is usually unilateral. Even if both testes are involved, the necrosis is commonly spotty and seldom results in complete sterility. Pancreatitis occurs in about 10% of all cases. More rarely, other organs (e.g., prostate, mastoid, ovaries, thyroid, thymus, spleen, liver) are involved, particularly in adults.

Pathogenesis. Mumps virus enters and multiplies first in the respiratory tract. Viremia with invasion of other organs, including CNS, occurs later. The parotid glands are highly susceptible to virus infection and become markedly inflamed. Degenerative changes can occur in the testes and ovaries; lesions found in the CNS are those of postinfectious encephalitis (Chapter 14).

Immunity. Only one antigenic type of the virus exists, and immunity is permanent after the first infection. There is no basis for the old wives' tale that individuals who develop and recover from unilateral mumps parotitis can later develop the same disease involving the other side. Mumps is rare in infants because of passively acquired maternal Ab. Skin test Ag is available commercially for determining the immune status of an individual.

Diagnosis. It is impossible to diagnose mumps clinically if the salivary glands are not involved. Laboratory specimens should include saliva, spinal fluid, or urine; the urine specimen should be collected 4 or 5 days after the onset of illness. The specimen is inoculated into the amniotic cavity of chick embryos. Demonstration of mumps virus is then made by hemagglutination and hemagglutination-inhibition (HI) tests using known antisera. Inoculation of monkey kidney cells and identification of mumps virus by hemadsorption and hemadsorption-inhibition tests can also be done. The skin test is of no value for diagnosis.

Epidemiology. Mumps infections occur worldwide, and man is the only natural host and reservoir. Children are particularly susceptible to the virus. Spread of mumps virus occurs by direct contact and droplet infection. Saliva of patients during the 6 days preceding parotitis and of persons harboring inapparent infections is highly infectious. Virus is also excreted in the urine until the 15th day of the disease. The length of the virus excretion period contributes to the highly contagious nature of the disease. The fact that man is the only natural reservoir of the virus and that virus transmission is by direct contact and by droplet nuclei explains the regional variation in the epidemiology of the disease.

Treatment and Prevention. The administration of hyperimmune gamma globulin prior to the development of clinical symptoms will prevent or attenuate the disease in persons exposed to mumps virus. A vaccine comprised of live virus attenuated by culture in chick embryos is available commercially. A single dose of vaccine produces an inapparent infection that is not transmissible to other individuals. The vaccine has been shown to be 95% effective (Chapter 7).

B. Infectious Mononucleosis (Glandular Fever)

Infectious mononucleosis (mono) is characterized by irregular fever, pharyngitis, lymph node enlargement, splenomegaly, lymphocytosis (due to morphologically atypical lymphocytes), high titers of heterophil Abs that react with sheep erythrocytes, and the development of Abs to Epstein-Barr (EB) virus capsid Ags.

Etiologic Agent. In 1968, Gertrude and Werner Henle concluded that EB virus is the cause of infectious mono; their conclusion was based on seroepidemiologic data. Originally, this conclusion was not widely accepted, since EB virus is also associated with other diseases, namely, Burkitt's lymphoma, nasopharyngeal carcinoma, and possibly Hodgkin's disease (Chapter 24). Evidence supporting an EB virus etiology of infectious mono is based on the following data: (1) it occurs only in individuals lacking Abs that react with EB virus; (2) all individuals with a documented history of infectious mono have anti-EB virus capsid Abs; (3) infectious mono is a lymphoproliferative disease, and EB virus stimulates growth of cultured lymphocytes *in vitro;* and (4) EB virus can occasionally cause an infectious-mono-like syndrome and Ab conversion in patients following heart surgery supported by blood transfusions. Epstein-Barr virus is often present in circulating leukocytes of healthy blood donors. The infrequency of EB-virus-induced infectious mono following blood transfusions may be due to the fact that the transfused blood also contains EB virus Abs that might abort or prevent the disease. Recent evidence has shown that EB virus can be isolated from the nasopharynx during the acute stages of infectious mono, which strongly supports the EB virus etiology of this disease.

Clinical Symptoms. The "incubation period" of infectious mono can vary from 3 days to several weeks. Initial symptoms include malaise, fever, sore throat, headache, and severe pharyngitis. Between the 5th and 12th day, a palatal exanthem consisting of sharply circumscribed red spots can be observed. Cervical lymph node and splenic enlargement is almost always noted. Jaundice with or without hepatomegaly may occur between the 4th and 14th day of illness. A skin rash consisting of maculopapular, faintly erythematous eruptions has been described. Involvement of the CNS and peripheral nerves, heart, or lung rarely occurs. The disease course lasts about 1 to 2 weeks, but convalescence may be prolonged. Relapses or death are very rare. Death is generally attributable to traumatic rupture of the spleen.

Pathogenesis. The highly varied and numerous clinical features of infectious mono reflect the wide distribution of lesions in the body. Little information is available concerning the pathogenetic mechanisms responsible for diseases due to the EB virus. *In vitro* experiments suggest that EB virus can produce a latent infection and perhaps persist for the life of the individual. Epstein-Barr virus can be detected in peripheral or bone marrow leukocytes derived from a wide diversity of healthy donors. The virus has the *in vitro* capacity to transform normal leukocytes into established cell lines.

Immunity. Antibodies engendered against EB virus persist for many years, in contrast to "heterophil" Abs against sheep erythrocytes. Up to 85% of the adult population have EB virus Abs despite the lack of any documented history of apparent disease. These data indicate that EB virus is ubiquitous in nature and commonly causes inapparent infections.

Diagnosis. Epstein-Barr virus may be isolated from nasopharyngeal swabs of patients with infectious mono, although routine isolation of the virus for diagnosis is not done. Diagnosis is usually made by examining blood samples taken during the acute stages of disease for (1) lymphocytosis characterized by the presence of atypical lymphocytes (Fig. 18–2) involving 20% or more of the cells and (2) heterophil Abs measured by the Paul-Bunnell test. Heterophil Ab titers of over 1:100 are significant. From 60 to 80% of clinically and hematologically diagnosed cases of infectious mono show a positive Paul-Bunnell test. This test will no doubt soon be replaced by CF, gel diffusion, immunofluorescence, or other specialized serologic tests for Abs specific for EB virus Ags (e.g., early Ag, virus capsid Ag, membrane Ag). The SGOT (serum glutamic oxalacetic transaminase) and cephalin-cholesterol flocculation tests for liver damage are usually positive.

Epidemiology. Infectious mononucleosis is principally a disease of young persons between the ages of 15 to 40 years. The disease is not highly contagious and occurs sporadically. Transmission of the disease occurs principally by direct contact, especially through saliva and especially as the result of kissing. Some reports indicate that it is possible to contract the disease indirectly from fomites contaminated by persons with apparent or inapparent infections or following massive transfusions of blood.

Treatment and Prevention. No effective infectious mono vaccine has been developed. The course of infectious mono is generally benign, and no effective therapy is available. Palliative treatment with aspirin may be used to alleviate the symptoms of the fever and pharyngitis. Rest and inactivity are recommended to prevent possible splenic rupture during the acute and convalescent phases of the disease.

C. Cytomegalic Inclusion Disease (Salivary Gland Virus Disease)

Cytomegalovirus infection is manifested in a variety of ways, depending on age and physical condition of the patient and whether the disease is

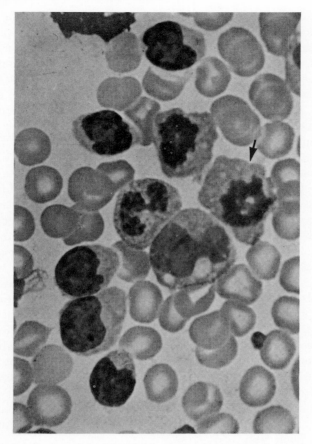

Figure 18–2. Smear of peripheral blood showing "atypical lymphocytes" associated with infectious mononucleosis. Apart from the central monocyte (with vacuoles) and a segmented neutrophil, the nucleated cells are all lymphocytes. The mitotic figure (in telophase) shows the increased cytoplasmic basophilia often seen in the abnormal lymphocytes (↑) of this disease. Mitoses in lymphocytes are very uncommon in normal peripheral blood but are frequently seen in infectious mononucleosis. (Reprinted with permission from Hayhoe, F. G. J., and Flemans, R. J.: *An Atlas of Haematological Cytology.* New York: Wiley-Interscience, 1970.)

associated with primary or latent infection. Originally, the disease was recognized only retrospectively by the postmortem finding of enlarged epithelial cells bearing intranuclear and cytoplasmic inclusions in salivary glands, liver, spleen, lungs, kidneys, and occasionally the brain, and by seroepidemiologic surveys. Recently, however, the disease is being recognized more often during life and has emerged to prominence because of its association with extensive blood transfusions (e.g., for open-heart surgery), immunosuppressive therapy, congenital infections, and renal transplantation. Whereas inapparent infection is common during childhood and adolescence, most fatalities occur among children under 2 years of age.

Etiologic Agent. The causative agent of cytomegalic inclusion disease is a typical herpesvirus (cytomegalovirus). It replicates best in human cells and is relatively unstable at 37°C (the half-life is 1 hour at 37°C). Cytomegalovirus grows slowly and produces a low yield of virus in tissue culture.

Clinical Symptoms. Cytomegalovirus infections are most often inapparent. Infections become apparent more commonly in congenitally infected infants than in infants infected postnatally. Most often, the disease in infants is associated with hepatosplenomegaly with hepatitis (Chapter 16). A maculopapular erythematous rash is sometimes seen in childhood infections. Primary infection in young adults resembles the febrile type of infection associated with infectious mono but without the pharyngitis or lymphadenopathy. Damage to the liver often accompanies cytomegalic inclusion disease. The atypical lymphocytes seen in patients with infectious mono are also seen in cytomegalic disease; however, the patient does not exhibit an elevated titer of heterophil Abs.

Cytomegalovirus mononucleosis (postperfusion mononucleosis) sometimes occurs in recipients of recent blood transfusions. The disease may be the result of either a primary infection or of reactivation of a latent infection. The febrile symptoms of the disease are particularly severe in debilitated or immunosuppressed patients (leukemic children) who require massive blood or plasma transfusions. It is now the consensus that cytomegalovirus, along with EB virus, accounts for most of the cases of postperfusion febrile syndromes.

Observations on kidney transplant patients also suggest that immunosuppression activates latent cytomegalovirus or renders the patients susceptible to reinfection.

Pathogenesis. The prolonged incubation period (months) of disease caused by cytomegalovirus is paralleled by the slow replication cycle of cytomegalovirus in tissue culture. Intrauterine infection of the neonate may lead to hepatosplenomegaly with jaundice, microcephaly, mental retardation, and death (Chapter 6). Infection of the newborn presents generalized visceral involvement with viremia and viruria.

The characteristic cytopathology of infected cells includes cell enlargement and eosinophilic inclusion bodies in the nucleus and/or basophilic inclusion bodies in the cytoplasm (Fig. 18–3). A mononuclear cell infiltrate may be associated with the infected cells in many organs, including salivary glands, lymph nodes, liver, spleen, lungs, and kidneys.

Immunity. Complement-fixing (CF) and neutralizing Abs are present in a high proportion of the sera of healthy human beings. Young healthy children may excrete virus in the urine or saliva despite circulating Abs in the blood. This suggests that cytomegalovirus commonly produces chronic

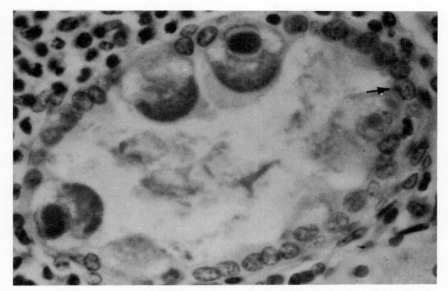

Figure 18—3. Microscopic section of cytomegalic inclusion disease virus-infected kidney. Note the swollen "cytomegalic" cells with intranuclear inclusions (↑) and the characteristic enlargement of the affected cells in the renal tubule. (Reprinted with permission from *Physician's Bulletin* No. 1, 1959, Eli Lilly Co., p. 83.)

or inapparent infections. The frequency with which cytomegalovirus can be isolated from individuals decreases after the first few years of life. Evidence for reinfection is provided by a rise in serum Abs above the previous level which can be detected at the time of virus isolation from apparent disease. Furthermore, infants infected during intrauterine life are born with IgM Abs synthesized during the fetal period; titers of IgM Abs continue to rise after birth, and there is continued excretion of virus in the urine. This condition is similar to that observed in congenital rubella infection (Chapters 6 and 12).

Diagnosis. The presence of "cytomegalic cells" containing characteristic inclusion bodies in urinary sediments or in autopsy material from the kidney and other viscera assures the diagnosis of cytomegalovirus infection. Virus isolation in human fibroblast cultures can be accomplished using specimens obtained from the nasopharynx or the urine. The presence of serum IgM neutralizing Abs to cytomegalovirus in newborns is suggestive of congenital infection. An increase in the titer of IgM Abs against cytomegalovirus during the first year of life also can be of diagnostic value.

Epidemiology. Cytomegalovirus infections are widespread and, except for infants under one year of age, are usually subclinical. Approximately 60 to 70% of adults have circulating Abs to the virus. Infants with cyto-

megalic inclusion disease discharge virus through the nasopharynx and
urine for many months after birth. In this respect, the disease resembles
congenital rubella. Cytomegalovirus may also be spread in a similar manner by asymptomatic carriers.

Treatment and Prevention. There is no effective treatment for cytomegalovirus infections, and no vaccine is currently available.

D.   Mesenteric Adenitis

This disease, which involves mesenteric lymph nodes and appendix, results from infection by echoviruses or adenoviruses. Clinically, the disease
resembles an appendicitis attack. However, at the time of surgery, the
signs noted are enlarged lymph nodes in the ileocecal region and an apparently normal appendix. The etiologic agent can be isolated from stools or,
in case surgery is carried out, from mesenteric lymph nodes. For further
details on the biological properties of adenoviruses and echoviruses, see
Chapter 9 on Respiratory Viruses and Chapter 13 on Neurotropic Viruses.

References

BIGGS, P. M., DE-THÉ, G., and PAYNE, L. N. (ed.): *Oncogenesis and Herpesviruses.*
   Lyon, France: International Agency for Research on Cancer, 1972.
HANSHAW, J. B.: Congenital cytomegalovirus infection: A fifteen year perspective.
   J. Infect. Dis. *123:* 555, 1971.
HENLE, G., HENLE, W., AND DIEHL, V.: Relation of Burkitt's tumor-associated
   herpes-type virus to infectious mononucleosis. Proc. Nat. Acad. Sci. U.S. *59:*
   94, 1968.
PEREIRA, M. S., FIELD, A. M., AND BLAKE, J. M.: Evidence for oral excretion of EB
   virus in infectious mononucleosis. Lancet *1:* 710, 1972.
PLUMMER, G.: Cytomegaloviruses of man and animals. Progr. Med. Virol. *15:* 92,
   1973.
WANER, J. L., AND WELLER, T. H.: Serological and cultural studies bearing on the
   persistent nature of cytomegaloviral infections in man. Perspect. Virol. *8:* 211,
   1973.
WELLER, T. H.: The cytomegaloviruses: Ubiquitous agents with protean clinical
   manifestations. N. Eng. J. Med. Part I:*285:* 203. Part II:*285:* 267, 1971.

Chapter 19

Viral Diseases of the Eye

The eye and associated tissues may be affected during the course of many cutaneous and systemic viral diseases. Infections of the eyelid and conjunctiva that accompany pharyngoconjunctival fever, varicella, and other benign illnesses usually lead only to minor and transient clinical symptoms. However, ocular infections with viruses such as herpes simplex, vaccinia, varicella-zoster, or variola can involve the cornea and cause serious and permanent damage to the eye. In addition, congenital rubella may cause cataracts and glaucoma, and cytomegalic inclusion disease may involve the retina. Epidemic keratoconjunctivitis, Newcastle disease conjunctivitis, and occasionally herpetic keratoconjunctivitis may occur in the absence of generalized infection and characteristically produce localized eye lesions.

A. Epidemic Keratoconjunctivitis (Shipyard Eye)

Epidemic keratoconjunctivitis is an acute infectious inflammation of the conjunctiva at the border of the cornea.

Etiologic Agent. This disease is caused by adenovirus type 8, which produces more serious ocular disease than those adenoviruses that cause pharyngoconjunctival fever and conjunctivitis (Chapter 10).

Clinical Symptoms. The incubation period of this disease ranges from 5 to 10 days. The onset is usually abrupt and is characterized by a unilateral follicular conjunctivitis or an intense catarrhal conjunctivitis without perceptible corneal involvement. The other eye frequently becomes infected within a few days, but the involvement usually is less severe. A pseudomembrane sometimes forms, and subconjunctival hemorrhages and an iritis may develop. The preauricular lymph node on the affected side is almost always enlarged. A moderate fever, headache, and malaise are usually the only systemic manifestations. Within a few days, the cornea becomes inflamed; the corneal lesions consist of small foci of subepithelial infiltration in the form of thin corneal opacities. There is intense lacrimation, photophobia, blurred vision, and pain. The disease may last from 2 weeks to several months; repeated relapses may take place. The corneal lesions may persist for weeks, months, or years after clinical recovery. However, healing usually occurs with few sequelae and with complete return of visual acuity.

Pathogenesis. Epidemic keratoconjunctivitis is characterized by marked edema and hyperplasia of the ocular mucosa and by numerous follicles. The pseudomembrane that may cover the conjunctivae (Fig. 19–1) contains many mononuclear cells and degenerating epithelial cells; in severe cases, there may be conjunctival scarring. The corneal subepithelial foci are composed mainly of mononuclear cells and do not ulcerate. One of the characteristics of epidemic keratoconjunctivitis is the absence of corneal neovascularization either during the development of lesions or later. It has been suggested that the stromal opacities are caused by an immune response to viral Ags that are elaborated in the corneal epithelium and diffuse to the stroma. However, the possibility that continuing viral infection is responsible for the opacities cannot be excluded. The intranuclear inclusion bodies characteristic of adenovirus infection are seldom seen in corneal cells from human patients. However, electron microscopic examination of corneal epithelium from severe infections has occasionally revealed intranuclear virus particles, indicating that the virus replicates in the cornea.

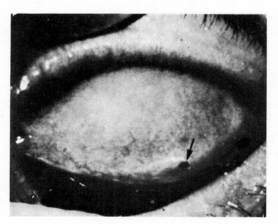

Figure 19–1. Upper tarsal conjunctivae of patient eight days after onset of epidemic keratoconjunctivitis. Entire tarsus is covered with inflammatory membrane. Hole (arrow) indicates membrane's thickness. (Reprinted with permission from Dawson, C. R., Hanna, L., and Togni, B.: Adenovirus type 8 infections in the United States. IV. Observations on the pathogenesis of lesions in severe eye disease. Arch. Ophthal. *87:* 258, 1972.)

Immunity. Serum neutralizing Abs to adenovirus 8 develop during the course of the disease; however, there is a relatively rapid fall in titer following recovery, and immunity may be short-lived.

Diagnosis. During an epidemic, adenovirus keratoconjunctivitis may be diagnosed by the clinical features of the disease. However, the first cases that appear during an outbreak may be difficult to distinguish from keratoconjunctivitis or keratitis caused by other viruses or by chlamydiae. Since the latter infections can be effectively treated with antibiotics or chemotherapeutic agents, it is of utmost importance to establish an etiologic diagnosis.

The virus may be isolated by inoculating susceptible cells with conjunctival scrapings. The presence of virus is recognized by the characteristic cytopathic changes that occur; the virus is identified by serologic procedures (Chapter 10). The diagnosis also can be established or confirmed by demonstrating a significant increase in serum neutralizing Ab to adenovirus type 8.

Epidemiology. Epidemic keratoconjunctivitis is endemic in the Near and Far East, where there are yearly outbreaks. It was introduced into the USA during World War II and caused large epidemics among shipyard employees. For this reason, the disease was called "shipyard eye." In the USA the disease now occurs mainly as localized outbreaks that can usually be traced to eye clinics or eye specialists. Adenovirus is not inactivated by some of the routine procedures used to clean ophthalmic instruments. Accordingly, a patient with the disease can serve as a source of contamination of such instruments, which then spread the disease to other individuals.

Treatment and Prevention. There is no specific treatment. Topically applied steroids are effective in treating persistent corneal opacities that may cause reduction of vision. However, steroid therapy should be reserved for severe corneal involvement, since it does not appear to reduce the intensity of conjunctival inflammation.

No vaccines for epidemic keratoconjunctivitis are available.

B. Newcastle Disease Conjunctivitis

Newcastle disease is a natural disease of fowl; the disease manifestations include a pneumoencephalitis in young chickens and an influenza-like illness in adult birds. Infections in man, who is an unnatural host, cause an inflammation of the conjunctivae.

Etiologic Agent. The etiologic agent of this disease is Newcastle disease virus (NDV), a member of the paramyxovirus group.

Clinical Symptoms. The incubation period in man is 1 to 2 days. The onset of disease is abrupt, and the principal symptoms are an acute follicular-type inflammation of the conjunctivae, edema of the lids, profuse lacrimation, and preauricular adenopathy. The infection is usually unilateral. The cornea is not involved, and photophobia is unusual. Pulmonary involvement may occur, but it is usually inconspicuous and may not be recognized. In most cases, the temperature remains normal. The conjunctivitis lasts only 3 or 4 days, and recovery is complete within 1 to 2 weeks.

Pathogenesis.   The pathogenesis of NDV infections in chickens has been studied extensively because of the economic importance of the disease. In man, the virus causes only a self-limiting conjunctivitis with no residual effects. The ocular mucosa is hyperemic and may be dark red; edema is marked, and there may be an inflammatory pseudoptosis.

Immunity.   The limited involvement of the eye in man probably accounts for the low level of neutralizing Ab in serum.

Diagnosis.   Diagnosis can usually be made on the basis of clinical symptoms coupled with a history of laboratory exposure to the virus or contact with infected fowl.

An etiologic diagnosis can be made by culturing the virus in embryonated chicken eggs or in tissue cultures, followed by identification using neutralization or hemagglutination-inhibition tests. Serologic confirmation using patients' sera may be difficult because the infection does not elicit a good Ab response.

Epidemiology.   Birds are the natural hosts of NDV. Infection in man is an occupational disease, limited almost exclusively to poultry workers or meat processors and laboratory personnel associated with NDV research. The virus becomes airborne and is spread by droplet nuclei. Although the virus is somewhat more resistant to environmental conditions than most of the paramyxoviruses, close association with contaminated materials is required for infection.

Treatment and Prevention.   No effective treatment of Newcastle disease conjunctivitis is available.

Prevention of human infections involves control of the disease in poultry and extreme caution when working with the virus in the laboratory. Live attenuated virus vaccines as well as inactivated virus vaccines are useful for preventing generalized systemic disease in fowl but are less effective for preventing infection of the avian respiratory tract. Slaughter of infected flocks and quarantine of infected premises can eliminate or control the disease.

C.   Herpetic Keratoconjunctivitis

Herpes simplex virus type 1 is the etiologic agent of herpetic keratoconjunctivitis. This potentially serious ocular disease is discussed in Chapter 12.

References

DAWSON, C. R., HANNA, L., WOOD, T. R., and DESPAIN, R.: Adenovirus type 8 keratoconjunctivitis. Amer. J. Ophthal. *69:* 473, 1970.

FENNER, F., McAUSLAN, B. R., MIMS, C. A., SAMBROOK, J., and WHITE, D. O.: *The
Biology of Animal Viruses.* New York: Academic Press, 1974.

FENNER, F., and WHITE, D. O.: *Medical Virology.* New York: Academic Press, 1970.

GRAYSTON, J. T.: Viral infections of the eye. In: M. M. Wintrobe, G. W. Thorn, R. D.
Adams, I. L. Bennet, Jr., E. Braunwald, K. J. Isselbacher, and R. G. Petersdorf
(eds.), *Principles of Internal Medicine.* New York: McGraw-Hill Book Co., 1970.

GRIST, N. R., BELL, E. J., and GARDNER, C. A.: Epidemic keratoconjunctivitis. A continuing study. Health Bull. (Edinb.) *28:* 47, 1970.

HANNA, L., and TOGNI, B.: Adenovirus type 8 infections in the United States, IV.
Observations on the pathogenesis of lesions in severe eye diseases. Arch. Ophthal.
87: 258, 1972.

NATAF, R., and COSCAS, G.: Involvement of the eyelid, conjunctiva, cornea, sclera,
and anterior segment. In R. Debré and J. Celers (eds.), *Clinical Virology.* Philadelphia: W. B. Saunders Co., 1970.

Viral Gastroenteritis

Diarrhea and vomiting are symptoms frequently observed in many systemic virus infections. Although there is little doubt that virus infections can cause diseases in which digestive tract symptoms predominate, the etiologic agents in most cases have not been isolated. Certain types of echoviruses are the only known viruses that have been associated with gastrointestinal disorders with statistically significant frequency. Adenoviruses, coxsackieviruses, and reoviruses also have been isolated from patients with gastroenteritis, but the etiologic significance of these agents has not been clearly established. However, gastrointestinal symptoms may accompany respiratory infections caused by the adenoviruses.

A. Epidemic Nonbacterial Gastroenteritis

Epidemic nonbacterial gastroenteritis is an acute, self-limiting infection characterized by symptoms of profuse watery diarrhea, abdominal cramps, nausea, and vomiting that may occur singly or in combination. The incubation period varies from 1 to 5 days; the onset of symptoms is often abrupt. Systemic signs are relatively mild and include headache, dizziness, and malaise. Fever, when present, is low and is probably related to dehydration. The acute illness lasts only a day or two; however, loose stools may continue for a week.

The disease is worldwide in distribution and affects all age groups. It is highly communicable and occurs in large epidemics as well as sporadically. The disease is transmitted by the fecal-oral route and has been passed serially in volunteers fed bacteria-free fecal filtrates. At least two unidentified viruses have been implicated.

Immunity lasts for a year or longer, and there is no cross-protection among the causative viruses. It appears likely that there is more than one antigenic type of each virus, since cases may recur in families and communities at yearly intervals. Although the causative viruses have not been cultured routinely, one has been serially passed in organ cultures of human intestinal epithelium. One agent has been observed in the electron microscope; it appears to be a small, naked icosahedral virus.

Diagnosis is based on clinical symptoms and negative bacteriologic findings. Treatment is nonspecific and consists only of fluid replacement.

B. Infantile Diarrhea

Infantile diarrhea appears to be distinct from adult viral gastroenteritis; it is a more severe disease, is of longer duration, and may be caused in part by a simultaneous bacterial infection. The disease usually occurs in the summer in the form of explosive epidemics in nurseries, orphanages, and in large families living under crowded conditions with poor sanitation.

The incubation period is 3 to 4 days. The disease is characterized by an abrupt onset with fever; a profuse watery diarrhea may cause rapid dehydration and death, particularly in newborn and premature infants. Certain types of echoviruses have been isolated more often from infants with infantile diarrhea than from matched controls; infected infants also develop significant increases in serum neutralizing Ab to the isolates.

Treatment involves prompt intravenous administration of fluids to combat dehydration and salt imbalances, which can be fatal.

C. Epidemic Vomiting (Winter Vomiting Disease)

Epidemic vomiting is a benign illness of short duration characterized by abrupt onset of nausea and vomiting. Headache, diarrhea, and abdominal pain may be present; some patients develop a rubella-like rash. There is little or no fever. The disease frequently is observed in association with upper respiratory tract infections and may last only a few hours or up to 1 to 2 days. Recovery is rapid and uncomplicated.

The disease occurs most frequently in the winter months and is probably spread by droplet transmission. All age groups are affected. Because of its benign nature, there have been few laboratory investigations of the disease. Echoviruses have been isolated, but their etiologic significance has not been established with certainty.

References

BERROVICH, S., and KIBRICK, S.: Echo 11 outbreak in newborn infants and mothers. Pediatrics *33:* 534, 1964.
DOLIN, R., BLACKLOW, N. R., DuPONT, H., FORMAL, S., BUSCHO, R. F., KASEL, J. A., CHAMES, R. P., HORNICK, R., and CHANOCK, R. M.: Transmission of acute infectious nonbacterial gastroenteritis to volunteers by oral administration of stool filtrates. J. Infect. Dis. *123:* 307, 1971.

Gastroenteritis, possible winter vomiting disease. Morbidity and Mortality Weekly Report *19:* 181, 1970.

LELONG, M. Virus infections with manifestations predominating in the digestive tract proper. In R. Debré and J. Celers (eds.), *Clinical Virology*. Philadelphia: W. B. Saunders Co., 1970.

LERNER, A. M.: Viral Gastroenteritis. In M. M. Wintrobe, G. W. Thorn, R. D. Adams, I. L. Bennett, Jr., E. Braunwald, K. J. Isselbacher, and R. G. Petersdorf (eds.), *Principles of Internal Medicine*. New York: McGraw-Hill Book Co., 1970.

RAMOS-ALVAREZ, M., and OLARTE, J.: Diarrheal diseases of children. Amer. J. Dis. Child. *107:* 218, 1964.

YOW, M. D., MELNICK, J. L., BLATTNER, R. J., STEPHENSON, W. B., ROBINSON, N. M., and BURKHARDT, M. A.: The association of viruses and bacteria with infantile diarrhea. Amer. J. Epidemiol. *92:* 33, 1970.

Chapter 21

Properties of Viruses Associated with Persistent Diseases

Viral infections of the CNS are usually associated with acute diseases characterized by inflammatory changes in the cerebrospinal fluid and brain (Chapter 14). Recently, it has been observed that some viruses cause subacute or chronic neurologic disease in which inflammatory changes are lacking and in which the pathogenesis involves a gradual degenerative or demyelinating process. Viruses that cause subacute or chronic diseases have long incubation periods lasting several weeks to years before the onset of clinical symptoms, hence the name "slow" viruses. Once initiated, such diseases follow a protracted course that usually ends in death. Slow viruses are differentiated from latent viruses (Chapter 5), such as herpes simplex or varicella-zoster, which cause recurrent acute diseases. Similarly, slow viruses are differentiated from other viruses that cause chronic infections in which the clinical course tends to be irregular and unpredictable (e.g., hepatitis virus) (Chapter 16). Tumor viruses (Chapter 23) characteristically cause cell proliferation, whereas slow viruses cause cell dysfunction. The term "slow viruses" is a misnomer because most of the slow viruses can multiply rapidly under appropriate conditions. Some slow viruses behave differently from conventional viruses in that they do not invoke a demonstrable immune response in the intact host.

This chapter presents available virologic and immunologic information about the viruses associated with slowly progressive neurologic diseases of man and animals. A summary of pertinent information pertaining to these diseases and the viruses associated with them is presented in Tables 22–1, 22–2, and 22–3.

A.   Paramyxovirus Group

1. Measles Virus

The structural, antigenic, and cultural properties of measles virus have been described in Chapter 9.

B.   Scrapie Virus

Structure and Antigenic Properties. The scrapie virus, one of the smallest known infectious agents, has a diameter of about 27 nm. The term "viroid" has recently been used to describe this subviral particle consisting of single-stranded nucleic acid without a protein capsid. It is highly resistant to heat (80°C for 45 min) and formalin. The scrapie virus is nonantigenic both in natural and experimental hosts; for example, it fails to induce Abs in the nonsusceptible rabbit. The fact that nucleic acids are poor Ags may account for its lack of antigenicity.

Host Range and Culture. The agent can be maintained *in vitro* in mouse spleen-clot cultures derived from infected animals and in primary mouse embryo cell or mouse brain cell cultures. The virus does not produce cytopathology in cultured cells. Scrapie virus is assayed by infectivity tests in mice, sheep, goats, monkeys, rats, or hamsters. The infected animals rub their bodies and bite their skin. They exhibit fatigue, weight loss, involuntary tremors, and bizarre behavior. The disease is progressive and invariably fatal. Virus is recoverable from lymph nodes, spleen, salivary glands, thymus, lungs, and brain.

C.   Visna and Maedi Viruses

Structure and Antigenic Properties. Visna virus is the cause of a slowly progressive meningoencephalitis of sheep. The agent probably represents a neurotropic variant of maedi virus, the etiologic agent of progressive pneumonia of sheep. The two viruses are similar in ultrastructure and morphogenesis; they are related serologically, and visna-like virus particles can be recovered from the brains of sheep infected with the agent that causes progressive pneumonia in sheep.

Visna virus contains a 70S single-stranded RNA genome surrounded by a lipid-containing envelope. Extracellular virus possesses an RNA-directed DNA polymerase, "reverse transcriptase," (Chapter 24) as an integral component of the virion. The virus is pleomorphic (diameter 60 to 100

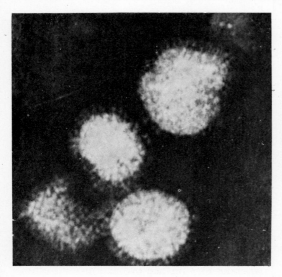

Figure 21–1. Structure of visna virus as observed by electron microscopy. Note outer envelope covered with numerous spikes. ×250,000. (Reprinted with permission from Thorman, H.: The structure of visna virus studied by negative staining. Virology 25:145, 1965.)

nm). The virion surface is covered with spikes (Fig. 21–1); a central core of 35 nm is evident in sectioned particles.

Visna and maedi viruses resemble the oncornaviruses in several ways: (1) sensitivity to physical and chemical agents, (2) ultrastructural appearance of the virions, (3) possession of a 70S RNA genome, and (4) presence of reverse transcriptase activity in virions. Visna and maedi viruses can cause transformation of embryonic mouse cells in culture and interfere with subsequent replication of murine leukemia-sarcoma viruses. However, based on molecular hybridization tests, visna and maedi viruses are genetically unrelated to oncornaviruses. Antibody made against visna virus partially neutralizes the closely related maedi virus, but not oncornaviruses.

Host Range and Culture. Visna virus can infect all organs of sheep; however, pathologic changes are confined primarily to the brain, lungs, and the RES. There is a long incubation period, with virus release lasting up to 4 years after infection. Visna and maedi virus can be grown *in vitro* in sheep choroid plexus and bovine tracheal cells. Maximum yields of virus are obtained in cell cultures 40 to 72 hours after infection. Virus-induced cytopathic effects include polykaryon formation followed by cell degeneration.

D. Arenavirus Group

1. Lymphocytic Choriomeningitis Virus

Structure and Antigenic Properties. Lymphocytic choriomeningitis (LCM) virus has an RNA genome. Particles observed by electron microscopy are quite pleomorphic and range in size from 60 to over 300 nm in

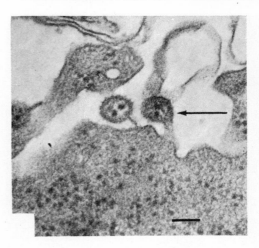

Figure 21–2. LCM virus particle budding (arrow) from an infected mouse 3T3 cell. Peplomeres (spikes) are apparent on the surface of the other particle. ×70,000. (Reprinted with permission from Dalton, A. J., Rowe, W. P., Smith, G. H., Wilsnack, R. E., and Pugh, W. E.: Morphological and cytochemical studies on lymphocytic choriomeningitis virus. J. Virol. 2:1465, 1968.)

diameter. Sectioned particles show spike-like surface projections and often have one or more dense granules (22 nm) in the virus core, hence the group name arenavirus (from *arenasus*, L. sandy). The types of symmetry in the virion and the strandedness of the RNA are not completely known. Arenaviruses differ from other viruses in that they contain unique intravirionic granules (Fig. 21–2).

Host Range and Culture. Many mammals, including man, mice, dogs, monkeys, and guinea pigs, can be infected with LCM virus. Chronically infected animals shed virus in the urine and feces and represent a hazard to animal handlers. Female mice can transmit LCM virus to their offspring *in utero;* the offspring in turn can become healthy carriers. Later in life, these animals may develop a fatal debilitating disease of the CNS or chronic glomerulonephritis due to immune complexes. The virus can be propagated in African green monkey kidney cells and mouse embryo fibroblasts.

E. Aleutian Mink Disease Virus

Structure and Antigenic Properties. The causative agent of Aleutian mink disease is considered to be a virus on the basis of disease transmission in susceptible animals with cell-free filtrates and passage through a 50-nm nitrocellulose membrane filter. No information is available concerning its antigenic properties or growth in tissue culture.

F. Mink Encephalopathy Virus

Structure and Antigenic Properties. Infectious particles from cell-free homogenates pass through membranes of 100-nm pore size. Infectivity is not destroyed by exposure to formalin or ether. Like scrapie virus, the mink encephalopathy virus is heat resistant.

Host Range and Culture. Infected mink or ferrets develop progressive CNS disease. If convulsions occur, the disease may progress to coma and death 3 to 8 weeks after initial symptoms appear. No successful *in vitro* system has been developed for virus propagation.

G. Papovavirus Group

1. Viruses Closely Related to Simian Virus 40 (SV_{40})

Particles resembling papovaviruses have been consistently found in brain tissue from patients with progressive multifocal leukoencephalopathy (PML), a subacute demyelinating disease (Fig. 21–3).

Structure and Antigenic Properties. The virus associated with PML exhibits icosahedral symmetry, a naked capsid, and a diameter of about 45 nm. Structurally and antigenically, it is related to SV_{40} of primates, but it appears to be antigenically distinct from polyoma and human wart viruses as judged by immunofluorescent staining.

Host Range and Culture. Original isolation of the virus was achieved by inoculating a homogenate of brain tissue from a patient with PML onto monolayers of human fetal brain cells. Virus has also been grown in tissue culture by fusing infected brain cells to African green monkey kidney cells *in vitro*.

H. Picornavirus Group

1. Enterovirus

Cases of the Guillain-Barré syndrome have been shown to be associated with certain types of echoviruses that can be isolated from patients' CSF.

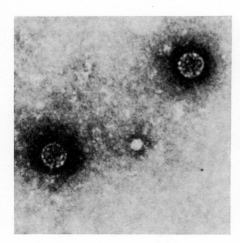

Figure 21–3. Papovavirus (SV_{40})-like particles isolated from the brain of a patient with PML. $\times 150,000$. (Reprinted with permission from Penney, J. B., Weiner, L. P., Herndon, R. M., Narayan, O., and Johnson, R. I.: Virions from progressive multifocal leukoencephalopathy: Rapid serological identification by electron microscopy. Science *178*:60, 1972. Copyright © 1972 by the American Association for the Advancement of Science.)

The patients studied also showed a rise in neutralizing Abs to echoviruses. The physical and biological properties of echoviruses have been described in Chapter 13.

References

CASPARY, E. A., and BELL, T. M.: Growth potential of scrapie mouse brain *in vitro*. Nature *229*:269, 1971.

DIENER, T. O.: Is the scrapie agent a viroid? Nature New Biol. *235*:218, 1972.

FENNER, F., and WHITE, D.: *Medical Virology*. New York: Academic Press, 1970.

HARTER, D. H., AXEL, R., BURNY, A., GULATI, S., SCHLOM, J., and SPIEGELMAN, S.: The relationship of visna, maedi and RNA tumor viruses as studied by molecular hybridization. Virology *52*:287, 1973.

HORTA-BARBOSA, L., FUCILLO, D., and SEVER, J. L.: Chronic viral infections of the central nervous system. JAMA *218*:1185, 1971.

OUTRAM, G. W., DICKINSON, A. G., and FRASER, H.: Developmental maturation of susceptibility to scrapie in mice. Nature *241*:536, 1973.

PAYNE, F., and BAUBLIS, J. V.: Measles virus and subacute sclerosing panencephalitis, p. 279. *In* M. Pollard (ed.): *Persistent Virus Infections: Perspectives in Virology VIII*. New York, Academic Press, 1973.

PENNEY, J. B., WEINER, L. P., HERNDON, R. M., NARAYAN, O., and JOHNSON, R. T.: Virions from progressive multifocal leukoencephalopathy: Rapid serological identification by electron microscopy. Science *198*:60, 1972.

PORTER, D.: A quantitative view of the slow virus landscape. Progr. Med. Virol. *13*: 339, 1971.

WEINER, L. P., JOHNSON, R. T., and HERNDON, R. M.: Direct serological identification of virions from progressive multifocal leukoencephalopathy by electron microscopy. N. Eng. J. Med. *288*:1103, 1973.

Persistent Viral Diseases

The phrase "persistent viral diseases" or "slow virus infections" refers to the long incubation period and the chronic nature of the disease; these diseases tend to progress gradually. There may be remissions and relapses, which ultimately lead to irreversible deterioration and demise of the host. "Slow virus" is actually a misnomer because under optimal conditions several of these viruses replicate rapidly *in vitro.* Slow virus diseases are a group of persistent, degenerative, usually fatal diseases that are associated with intermittent or continuous infection throughout life. At any given time, the presence of virus may or may not result in apparent infection and disease. If infection with slow viruses results in disease, symptoms appear after an incubation period of weeks to years, and the pathogenesis of the disease may be mediated by the immunologic responses of the host to the infection (Chapter 6). Several subacute and chronic neurologic diseases of man having a virus etiology are listed in Table 22–1. Other slowly progressive neurologic diseases of man of possible viral etiology include Guillain-Barré syndrome, multiple sclerosis (MS), and Parkinsonian dementia (Table 22–2). In addition, there are several diseases in animals that also appear to be caused by slow viruses (Table 22–3). This chapter includes information on slow virus–host interactions and the pathogenesis of selected diseases in man and animals in which neurologic manifestations predominate.

TABLE 22—1

Slowly Progressive Neurologic Diseases in Man of Probable Viral Etiology

Probable Etiologic Agent	Disease	Host Range	Incubation Period	Major Findings
Measles virus	Subacute sclerosing panencephalitis	Man	2 to 20 years	Ataxia; mental and motor deterioration; coma; measles virus in CNS
Kuru virus	Kuru	Man, chimpanzee	Months to years	Cerebellar ataxia; incoordination; status spongiosus
Papova-virus (SV$_{40}$-like)	Progressive multifocal leukoencephalopathy (PML)	Man	Months to years	Patchy foci of demyelination; gliosis; loss of memory; dysarthria; incoordination
C-J Virus	Creutzfeld-Jakob (C-J)	Man, chimpanzee	Months to years	Progressive dementia; ataxia; spasticity; cell loss; astrocytic proliferation

TABLE 22—2

Slowly Progressive Neurologic Diseases in Man of Possible Viral Etiology

Possible Etiologic Agent	Disease	Major Findings
Echovirus	Guillain-Barré syndrome	Petechial hemorrhages in spinal cord; demyelination; perivascular infiltration; polyneuritis; paralysis
Measles virus	Multiple sclerosis	Sclerotic plaque; demyelination; gliosis; incoordination; dysarthria; nystagmus; paraplegia
Paramyxovirus	Parkinsonian dementia	Ganglion cell degeneration; gliosis; neurofibrillary degeneration; bradykinesia; rigidity; dementia

Modified from Horta-Barbosa, L., Fucillo, D., and Sever, J.: Chronic viral infections of the central nervous system. JAMA *218*:1185, 1971.

TABLE 22—3

Probable Viral Etiology of Slowly Progressive Neurologic Diseases of Animals

Probable Etiologic Agent	Disease	Animal Host(s)	Incubation period	Major Findings
15-30-nm viroid?	Scrapie	Sheep, goat, mouse	Months to years	Noninflammatory degeneration of CNS; incoordination; no detectable antibodies in host
70-100-nm enveloped particle	Visna (maedi)	Sheep	Months to years	Demyelination of CNS; virus in brain, lungs, and blood; *in vitro* growth in sheep choroid plexus cells
LCM virus	Lymphocytic choriomeningitis (LCM)	Mouse	Days to months	Rapid death or persistent tolerant infection; may be immune-complex disease
50-nm particle?	Aleutian disease of mink (AD)	Mink	Months	Diseases of the liver and kidney; hypergammaglobulinemia; persistent viremia; glial scarring; polyarteritis
50-nm particle?	Mink encephalopathy (ME)	Mink, other mammals	Weeks to months	Extraneuronal vacuolation of gray matter; neuronal degeneration; astrocytic proliferation

A. Subacute Sclerosing Panencephalitis (SSPE)

This disease is relatively uncommon in the USA, the estimated frequency being 1 per million. Almost all cases involve children.

Etiologic Agent. Measles virus (Chapter 11) has been observed and isolated in tissue culture from brain tissue and lymph nodes of patients with SSPE.

Clinical Symptoms. Early symptoms of disease are gradual deterioration followed by motor neuron dysfunction (e.g., jerks, convulsions, and incoordination). Visual difficulties and ultimate blindness follow (Table 22–2). Finally, coma and death occur 1 to 3 years after the onset of clinical symptoms. This disease should not be confused with postinfectious encephalitis (Chapter 14), another neurologic complication of measles that begins within a few days after the primary infection.

Pathogenesis. Brain sections show round cell infiltration, perivascular round cell cuffing, and occasionally Cowdry type A intranuclear inclusions in neuronal and glial cells.

Immunity. High titers of humoral Ab to measles virus are detectable in the patient's serum.

Diagnosis. There is a marked increase in IgG in the CSF. Measles virus has been isolated from cell cultures of SSPE human brain tissue and lymph nodes at postmortem. A disease resembling SSPE can be produced in the laboratory by inoculating SSPE-infected brain material into ferrets.

Epidemiology. Although rare, SSPE may develop years after recovery from apparent measles. Viruses isolated from infected brain tissue have biologic and morphologic characteristics similar to those of measles virus (Chapter 11). These data suggest that, in SSPE, the measles virus becomes cell-associated following initial *in vivo* infection of human brain cells and persists in the brain in latent form for the life of the individual. A specific defect in the cellular immune system may be responsible for the persistence of the SSPE infection.

Treatment and Prevention. There is no specific treatment for SSPE.

B.   Kuru

Kuru is an endemic disease of Melanesian tribal people inhabiting a remote area in the highlands of New Guinea. Until recently, kuru had been the most common cause of death in this limited area, predominantly affecting children and adult women.

Etiologic Agent. The putative virus etiology of kuru is based on a kuru-like syndrome produced in chimpanzees inoculated with brain material from a patient who died from kuru.

Clinical Symptoms and Pathogenesis. The incubation period in man is months to years. The symptoms and laboratory findings of kuru (Table 22–1) are similar to those of scrapie (Table 22–3). Symptoms of the disease include slowly progressive ataxia with tremors of the head, trunk, and extremities. There is no febrile phase, no changes in CSF, biochemical values, or peripheral blood cells, and no inflammation. Late in the course of disease, abnormalities of extraocular movements and mental changes develop. The disease leads to death in 3 to 6 months.

Epidemiology. The first hypothesis regarding the etiology of kuru was that it was a sex-linked genetic disease in which a mutant gene had become widely disseminated throughout the isolated Melanesian tribe by centuries of inbreeding. Recent investigators have discredited the genetic hypothesis, since the disease has become less common. Close interrogation of tribal members revealed that women of the tribe practiced cannibalism, beginning about 1910. Deceased relatives were eaten following a "nonsterilizing" cooking ritual; children were given an occasional morsel. The men played a minor role in these rituals and rarely ate any of the brain, which was considered a gourmet's delight by the women. This interesting, but unresolved, disease is considered to have a virus etiology; however, unanswered questions are: (1) what is the natural source of the virus and (2) what are its biologic properties?

C. Progressive Multifocal Leukoencephalopathy (PML)

This is a rare demyelinating syndrome of the CNS that generally occurs in elderly persons with a debilitating disease (e.g., leukemia, Hodgkin's disease, tuberculosis).

Etiologic Agent. Large numbers of papovavirus-like particles have been observed repeatedly in infected brain tissue. A virus like SV_{40} or wart virus has been isolated in monolayers of human fetal brain cells inoculated with homogenates of infected brain tissue.

Clinical Symptoms. Gross abnormalities of motor function, vision, and speech occur. The CSF is unchanged, and the electroencephalogram shows only diffuse slowing. The time from first observation of clinical symptoms to death is about 3 to 4 months.

Pathogenesis. Pathologic changes include areas of demyelination that are numerous in the cerebral hemispheres, cerebellum, and brain stem. Eosinophilic intranuclear inclusions are observed in oligodendrocytes; however, there is no detectable inflammatory response to the infected cells (Table 22–1).

Epidemiology. It is not known whether the infection represents endogenous reactivation of a latent or noninvasive virus, such as the human wart virus, or recent infection by an exogenous virus.

D. Creutzfeld-Jakob (C-J) Disease

This uncommon disease of the CNS is a complex subacute presenile encephalopathy in which the patient becomes progressively incoordinated and demented as a result of a "spongy deterioration" of the brain. These findings resemble kuru and scrapie; however, the clinical symptoms are clearly distinguishable, in that there is severe dementia, myoclonic fasciculation, and somnolence with C-J disease (Table 22–1). Death usually follows in less than a year after symptoms appear. A similar disease has been produced in chimpanzees inoculated with brain homogenates obtained from patients who died of C-J disease; the experimental disease had an incubation period of about one year. The causative agent of this disease does not evoke a demonstrable immune reaction.

E. Slowly Progressive Neurologic Diseases in Man of Possible Viral Etiology

1. Guillain-Barré Syndrome

In several cases of Guillain-Barré syndrome (Table 22–2), echoviruses have been isolated from the CSF. Concomitant increases in specific Ab titers suggest that the syndrome and echovirus infection were concurrent.

2. Multiple Sclerosis (MS)

Multiple sclerosis is the most common demyelinating disease of man; about 100,000 persons in the USA are afflicted. There is suggestive evidence, based on recent epidemiologic, immunologic, and pathologic data, that measles virus may be the causative agent of MS. In this regard, isolation of measles virus from the brain tissue of MS patients has recently been reported. These studies indicate that from 3 to 23 years may elapse between virus exposure and the onset of clinical disease. Patients with MS have high IgG levels in the CSF. Also, inclusion bodies and small multinucleated giant cells have been found in demyelinating scarred areas of the brains of MS patients. Recent reports indicate that intranuclear paramyxovirus-like particles are present in mononuclear cells infiltrating perivascular areas of active myelin deterioration. These observations suggest that MS may involve activation of latent viruses in lymphocytes that interact with cells of the CNS. Ultimately, the virus induces cell injury and death. Similarly, in Marek's disease of chickens (Chapter 24), circulating lymphoid cells bearing Marek's disease herpesvirus in a latent state can incite destruction of myelin.

3. Parkinsonian Dementia

The possibility that parkinsonian dementia is a slow virus infection has been entertained. The major clinical findings include ganglia cell destruction, gliosis, neurofibrillary degeneration, bradykinesia, rigidity, and dementia (Table 22–2).

F. Slowly Progressive Neurologic Diseases in Animals of Probable Viral Etiology

The term slow virus infection was originally used in veterinary literature to describe several transmissible diseases of sheep (Table 22–3). Two of these slow virus infections (scrapie and visna) are of particular interest because they cause persistent, progressive neurologic diseases similar to those found in man.

1. Scrapie

The best-known slow virus infection in animals is scrapie, a natural disease of sheep (Table 22–3). The disease was first recognized in Scotland by sheep farmers and was thought to be a hereditary condition. However, in 1936, it was transmitted to healthy sheep with brain suspensions from diseased animals. The animals rub their bodies (hence the name scrapie) and nibble their skin on the lower extremities. They exhibit fatigue, weight loss, disturbed gait, tremors, and abnormal behavior. Later they develop ataxia and blindness. The disease is invariably fatal 6 weeks to 6 months after the onset of symptoms.

Scrapie is characterized by a noninflammatory, focal degeneration of gray matter that is distributed symmetrically in various parts of the brain. Perineuronal gray matter becomes spongy, astrocytes hypertrophy, and there is sporadic degeneration of myelin. Neurons become necrotic and vacuolated. Status spongiosus and edema, associated with hypertrophy of astrocytes, are the most common lesions of scrapie. The disease can be transmitted to mice and hamsters, which show similar lesions.

The virus can be isolated from lymph nodes and spleen about one week after infection. Several weeks later, it is present in the salivary glands, thymus, and lungs, and by 16 weeks it is recoverable from the brain. Although eosinophilic bodies are often seen in vacuoles, no virus particles have been observed in tissue sections of infected brain by employing electron microscopy.

2. Visna and Maedi Viruses

It is now well established that visna, a progressive neurologic disease of sheep, is caused by an RNA-containing virus structurally similar to measles virus (Chapter 11). The virus can be grown in sheep choroid plexus tissue cultures; infected tissue culture fluids can transmit the disease. These criteria fulfill Koch's postulates for assigning a virus etiology to visna. A related virus, maedi, causes progressive hemorrhagic pneumonia in sheep. The agent of maedi has properties very similar to those of visna and can be grown in the same tissue culture system.

In infected sheep, the incubation period of visna varies from 8 months to 4 years. During the incubation period, virus can be recovered from the CSF, blood, saliva, RES, brain, and lungs by culture in cells derived from the choroid plexus of sheep. The disease in sheep has an insidious onset. The animal first develops paresis of the hind limbs, which progresses to total paralysis and death. The primary lesions are in the CNS. The histopathology is characterized by meningeal and subependymal infiltration and proliferation of RES cells. There is demyelination of white matter, but gray matter is unaffected. Virus-neutralizing Abs are produced in high titer by infected sheep (Table 22–3).

3. Lymphocytic Choriomeningitis

Adult mice inoculated with LCM virus usually develop a fatal generalized infection. In contrast, infant mice inoculated with the same virus a few hours after birth or infected *in utero* develop a chronic infection that resembles slow virus infections. After 10 months of age, many of these mice develop a progressive disease involving the CNS. During development of disease, there is a gradual Ab response resulting in accumulation of Ag-Ab complexes in the kidneys that causes chronic immune-complex glomerulonephritis, which is lethal (Table 22–3).

4. Aleutian Disease (AD) of Mink

Aleutian disease is contagious in mink, but the mode of spread (i.e., vertically from mother to offspring or horizontally from animal to animal) is not completely understood. The pathology in diseased animals is characterized by proliferation of plasma cells and high levels of IgG. Although the Abs incited can interact with the AD virus, they do not neutralize virus infectivity. In addition, anti-IgM Abs develop in AD-infected mink, suggesting that an autoimmune response involving autologous Ag-Ab complexes may be involved in this disease.

The incubation period of AD is 8 to 12 months. Death is sudden, often by exsanguination as the result of rupture of major blood vessels. At autopsy the liver and kidneys are most severely affected. Capillary membrane thickening in the glomeruli of the kidney has been described. Both organs show fibrin thrombosis and plasma cell infiltration of perivascular areas that ultimately involves all organs. Lymph nodes and spleen show plasmacytosis.

5. Mink Encephalopathy (ME)

Transmissible mink encephalopathy was first recognized in Wisconsin some 20 years ago and later at Idaho mink farms. The pathologic changes in ME (Table 22–3) are quite similar to the changes in scrapie and slow virus diseases of man (e.g., kuru and C-J disease). The major pathologic lesions in ME are found in the CNS and consist of vacuolization of the gray matter and a reactive astrocytosis. In contrast to AD, there is a general lack of humoral and cellular immune responses in ME. Clinical symptoms are characterized by locomotor incoordination, convulsions, and ultimately a state of semicoma. Death follows 3 to 8 weeks after the development of the initial symptoms.

References

BEESON, P. B., and McDERMOTT, W. A., (ed.): *Textbook of Medicine.* 13th ed. Philadelphia: W. B. Saunders Co., 1971.

DIENER, T. O.: Is the scrapie agent a viroid? Nature New Biol. *235*:218, 1972.

GAJDUSEK, D. C., and GIBBS, C. J.: Subacute and chronic diseases caused by atypical infections and unconventional viruses in aberrant hosts, p. 279. *In* M. Pollard (ed.): *Persistent Virus Infections: Perspectives in Virology VIII.* New York: Academic Press, 1973.

HORTA-BARBOSA, L., FUCILLO, D. A., and SEVER, J. L.: Chronic viral infections of the central nervous system. JAMA *218*:1185, 1971.

KOPROWSKI, H., and KATZ, M.: Disease caused by slow viruses, p. 235. *In* R. Debré and J. Celers (ed.): *Clinical Virology—The Evolution and Management of Human Viral Infections.* Philadelphia: W. B. Saunders Co., 1970.

NATKINS, A. L., and KOPROWSKI, H.: How the immune response to a virus can cause disease. Sci. Amer. *228*:22, 1973.

PORTER, D.: A quantitative view of the slow virus landscape. Progr. Med. Virol. *13*: 339, 1971.

PRINEAS, J.: Paramyxovirus-like particles associated with acute demyelination in chronic relapsing multiple sclerosis. Science *178*:760, 1972.

Chapter 23

Properties of Viruses
Associated with Oncogenesis

The purpose of this chapter is to present an overview of the comparative structure and biology of cancer-inducing (oncogenic) viruses. Biologically, the oncogenic viruses differ from other mammalian viruses specifically in their capacity to induce cell transformation. Over 100 known oncogenic viruses comprising oncogenic RNA viruses and oncogenic DNA viruses are listed in Table 23–1. Oncogenic RNA viruses show greater variation in their chemical and physical properties and in the mechanisms by which they replicate and induce cell transformation than oncogenic DNA viruses.

TABLE 23—1

Classification of the Major Oncogenic Viruses

A. Oncogenic RNA viruses (about 100)

   1. Leukovirus (oncornavirus) group

     a. Avian leukosis viruses (>20)

     b. Murine leukosis viruses (several isolates reported, but the number of different types is not well established)

     c. Murine mammary tumor virus (3 types) (Bittner virus)

     d. Leukosis-sarcoma viruses of the cat, hamster, rat, guinea pig, and monkey

B. Oncogenic DNA viruses (about 50 different types)

   1. Papillomavirus subgroup

     a. Papillomaviruses of man, rabbits, dogs, cows, and other animals

   2. Polyomavirus subgroup

     a. Polyomavirus (murine)

     b. SV_{40} virus (simian)

   3. Adenovirus group

     a. Adenoviruses of man, nonhuman primates, birds, and cows

   4. Poxvirus group

     a. Molluscum contagiosum (man)

     b. Yaba virus (nonhuman primates)

   5. Herpesvirus group

     a. Herpesviruses of

        Burkitt's lymphoma, nasopharyngeal carcinoma[1] (man)
        Hodgkin's disease[1] (man)
        Cervical carcinoma[2] (man)
        Lucké's adenocarcinoma[1] (*Rana pipiens*)
        Marek's disease[1] (birds)
        Monkey lymphoma[1] (owl monkey)
        Guinea pig leukemia[1]

[1] Evidence associates these diseases with new members of the herpesvirus group.
[2] Epidemiologic evidence associates this disease with herpes simplex virus type 2.

I. ONCOGENIC RNA VIRUSES

A. Leukovirus (Oncornavirus) Group

The oncogenic RNA viruses listed in Table 23–1 share several common properties: (1) they are oncogenic in their natural host; (2) they acquire an envelope by budding from the cell surface and measure 90 to 120 nm in diameter; (3) the nucleoprotein in the budding virion is a helix, supercoiled as a hollow sphere; (4) their RNA genome is single-stranded with a sedimentation value of 70S; (5) their replication involves a DNA intermediate that requires the enzymatic machinery for reverse transcription. Morphologically, two distinct forms of the oncornaviruses have been described: (1) C-type viruses associated with leukemias and sarcomas of a variety of animals and (2) the B-type viruses associated with mammary tumors of mice; an A-type particle, devoid of a nucleoprotein core, that is observed in some infected cells represents an immature form of B-type particles. Virus infectivity is associated with either C-type (avian, murine, or feline leukosis-sarcoma viruses) or B-type (mammary tumor virus) particles.

The virus genome can be disrupted with heat or dimethylsulfoxide, resulting in a breakdown of 70S RNA into 20S and 35S RNA subunits. Oncornavirus particles contain at least two polymerase activities: an *RNA-directed DNA polymerase* or "reverse transcriptase" and a *DNA-directed DNA polymerase*. These polymerases function during oncornavirus replication to transcribe the 70S RNA into an RNA-DNA hybrid form and then a double-stranded DNA "provirus" form. Several other enzyme activities have been detected in oncornaviruses (i.e., endonuclease, ligase, protein kinase, nucleotide kinase). The genetic origin (host or viral) and function of these enzyme activities in oncornavirus replication and cell transformation are not completely understood.

Two types of Ags are found in oncornavirus particles: (1) glycoproteins with the type-specific or virion envelope (V) Ags and (2) the nonglycoproteins with the group-specific (gs) internal Ags. The type-specific Ags associated with the virus envelope are measured by virus neutralization, CF, and immunofluorescence tests with sera from animals bearing the virus-induced tumor or immunized with purified virions. Group-specific Ags are associated with the nucleoprotein core of C-type and B-type particles; they are assayed by CF, immunofluorescence, and immunodiffusion tests using sera from animals bearing the virus-induced tumor. The gs Ags are of two classes: (1) those that are restricted to oncornaviruses of a single animal species and (2) those that are shared by oncornaviruses of more than one animal species (interspecies Ags). All oncornaviruses possess species-specific Ags, whereas the leukosis-sarcoma viruses of mammalian origin possess interspecies Ags (e.g., murine, feline, hamster). The gs Ags are used as specific markers of oncornavirus gene expression under conditions where infectious virus production is not detectable in infected cells.

Aside from their oncogenic capacity, the most striking biological characteristic of oncogenic RNA viruses is that they can establish an endosymbiotic association with the host cell that allows simultaneous production of virus and multiplication of the host cell. Furthermore, this relationship can vary (e.g., the virus can enter a latent or provirus state and be passed on to daughter cells). Association of oncornaviruses with cells is not necessarily

TABLE 23–2

Classification of Avian Leukosis-Sarcoma Viruses Based on Their Antigenicity and Ability to Replicate in Genetically Defined Avian Cells

Antigenic Subgroup	Viruses[1]		Ability of Viruses to Grow in Genetically Defined Chick Embryo Cells				
	Leukosis Strains	Rous Sarcoma (RSV) Strains	C/O	C/A	C/B	C/AB	C/BC
A	RAV-1 RAV-3 RAV-4 RAV-5 RIF-1 AMV-1 FAV-1	Bryan Standard (BS-RSV) Schmidt-Ruppin-A (SR-RSV-A) Fuginami (FSV) Mill-Hill (MH-RSV) Prague-A (PR-RSV-A) Carr-Zilber-A (CZ-RSV-A)	Yes	No	Yes	No	Yes
B	RAV-2 RIF-2 AMV-2	Harris (HA-RSV) Schmidt-Ruppin-B (SR-RSV-B) Prague-B (PR-RSV-B)	Yes	Yes	No	No	No
C	RAV-7 RAV-49	Carr-Zilber-C (CZ-RSV-C) Prague-C (PR-RSV-C) B-77	Yes	Yes	Yes	Yes	No
D	RAV-50 CZAV	Schmidt-Ruppin-D (SR-RSV-D) Carr-Zilber-D (CZ-RSV-D)	Yes	Yes	Yes	Yes	Yes

Reprinted with permission from Jawetz, E., Melnick, J., and Adelberg, E.: *Review of Medical Microbiology*. 10th ed. Los Altos, Calif., Lange Medical Publishers, 1972.

[1] Abbreviations: RAV (Rous-associated virus) = leukosis viruses used as "helper"viruses for the defective Bryan "high titer" (BH-RSV) strain of RSV; RIF (resistance-inducing factor) = field strains of avian leukosis viruses that interfere with the focus-forming capacity of RSV; AMV = avian myeloblastosis virus; FAV = leukosis virus associated with the Fuginami sarcoma virus; CZAV = leukosis virus associated with the Carr-Zilber sarcoma virus; B-77 = a recent sarcoma virus isolate.

accompanied by cell transformation; the virus can multiply for long periods in nontransformed cells without cell destruction. For example, the murine mammary tumor virus can multiply in the mammary gland cells long before the cells become neoplastic; the virus can also propagate in other tissues of mice without giving rise to visible tumors. Unlike oncogenic DNA viruses, infectious oncogenic RNA viruses can be recovered from most of the tumors they induce as well as from nontransformed target cells of infected animals.

1. Avian Leukosis-Sarcoma Viruses

This virus group consists of related avian viruses that induce leukoses (lymphomatosis virus, myeloblastosis virus, erythroblastosis virus) or sarcomas in chickens (e.g., Rous sarcoma virus).

Structure and Antigenic Properties. The virions of this group have a mean diameter of about 100 nm and are similar in structure. They are enveloped and contain a single-stranded RNA (70S) genome as well as reverse transcriptase activity. Avian leukosis-sarcoma viruses share a common gs Ag that can be detected by using the complement-fixation avian leukosis (COFAL) test employing sera from rodents bearing Rous sarcoma virus (RSV) tumors. These viruses have been classified into 4 subgroups (A to D) based on type-specific envelope Ags and their ability to replicate in genetically defined avian cells (Table 23–2). Certain oncogenic viruses can promote their own replication, whereas other "defective viruses" require the help of another virus (helper virus) to replicate. The helper activity results from complementation and phenotypic mixing of the two viruses within the same cell (Chapter 4).

Host Range and Culture. Most of the avian leukosis viruses replicate in chick embryo fibroblast cultures without causing any CPE or cell transformation. Virus replication is detected by immunofluorescence assay or by failure of the infected cells to transform when superinfected with RSV (interference test).

Unlike avian leukosis viruses, avian sarcoma viruses (e.g., RSV) are unique in that they can induce almost 100% malignant transformation of infected chick embryo cells. Infection with RSV results in production of foci of transformed cells (Fig. 23–1); virus infectivity is assayed by determining the number of focus-forming units (FFU) in a given volume of inoculum (one infectious unit of virus gives rise to one focus of transformed cells). Some strains of RSV will induce transformation of mammalian (mouse, rat, hamster, primate, human) fibroblast cells. However, assay for infectious RSV in mammalian transformed cells is accomplished by cocultivating the transformed cells with chick embryo cells and assaying for FFU.

Some stocks of RSV contain a second virus, Rous-associated virus (RAV). The RSV is "defective" in that it can cause cell transformation

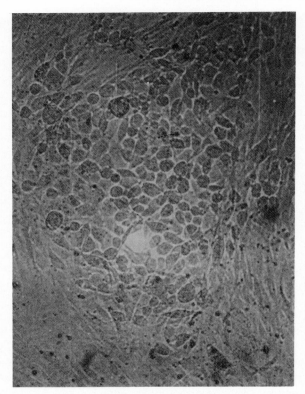

Figure 23–1.   Focus of chick embryo cells transformed by Rous sarcoma virus.
×80 (Reprinted with permission from Temin, H., and Rubin, H.: Characteristics of
an assay for Rous sarcoma virus and Rous sarcoma cells in tissue culture. Virology 6:
669, 1958.)

but cannot replicate to form new infectious virus in the absence of RAV
"helper" virus, which is not oncogenic for fibroblasts. Since cells transformed by RSV alone do not produce virus, they are called nonproducer
(NP) cells. Nonproducer cells contain the gs avian leukosis-sarcoma Ags,
reverse transcriptase, and the RSV-70S genome. When NP cells are superinfected with RAV "helper" virus, the cells yield new infectious RSV.
Since the "helper" virus codes for RSV envelope proteins (type-specific
Ags), RSV possesses the envelope Ags and exhibits the host range of its
"helper" virus.

2. Murine Leukosis-Sarcoma Viruses

Many different strains of murine leukemia and sarcoma viruses, named
for the investigators who first described them (e.g., Gross, Friend, Maloney,
Harvey, Rauscher), are associated with leukemias and sarcomas in mice.

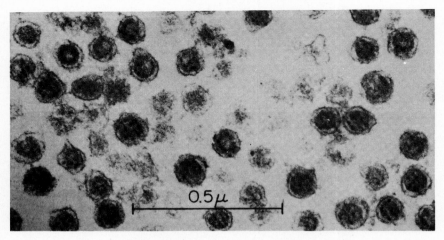

0.5μ

Figure 23–2. Electron micrograph of negatively stained Friend leukemia virus. Most of the particles are of the C-type with central electron-dense cores; some are of the A-type and share an electron-lucent center. ×80,000 (Reprinted with permission from Friend C.: Structure of virus particles partially purified from the blood of leukemic mice. Virology *23*:119, 1964.)

Structure and Antigenic Properties. Purified murine leukemia viruses possess an envelope, which is essentially smooth, and a condensed central nucleoid (core) (Fig. 23–2). The viral core is surrounded by a shell containing subunits that are regularly arranged to form icosahedral symmetry (Chapter 1).

Murine leukemia viruses possess gs and type-specific Ags. Neutralization tests have revealed at least two distinct gs Ags, one common to Friend, Maloney, and Rauscher viruses and the other common to Gross and Harvey viruses. These gs Ags are detectable in both transformed and non-transformed infected cells by the CF test employing sera from rats carrying a transplantable Rauscher leukemia virus-induced lymphosarcoma. Murine sarcoma viruses are antigenically related to the murine leukemia viruses.

Host Range and Culture. Murine leukemia viruses can be grown in mouse embryo fibroblast cells or in mice. Virus replication occurs without observable cytopathic effects (CPE); however, infected cells contain gs Ags and continue to release virus particles. Virions produced in tissue culture systems are 10,000 times less infectious than particles generated in leukemic mice. Cells infected with murine leukemia virus are resistant to subsequent transformation by murine sarcoma virus (viral interference test), similar to the phenomenon observed with avian leukemia viruses and RSV.

A plaque assay for murine leukemia viruses has recently been developed. Rat cells (XC cells) transformed by the Schmidt-Ruppin strain of RSV are NP cells. However, for some unknown reason, XC cells fuse with murine leukemia virus-infected mouse cells to form giant syncytia (Chapter 2), which are detected as virus plaques.

Some murine leukemia viruses (e.g., Friend, Gross, Rauscher) can cause *in vitro* transformation of mouse, rat, and hamster embryo cells. The transformed cells contain the viral-specific gs Ags, reverse transcriptase, and 70S RNA; they release infectious viruses that are oncogenic *in vivo*.

Newborn mice or rats (immunologically immature) are more susceptible to leukemogenic viruses than older animals; genetic factors also play an important role in the susceptibility of mice to the virus. Thymectomy reduces the incidence of acute lymphocytic leukemia (T-cell malignancy) but not of myeloid leukemia; however, it has no effect on the multiplication of murine leukosis virus in other organs of the host. Large amounts of infectious viruses are released into the blood of infected animals and can be transmitted congenitally.

Murine sarcoma virus (MSV) is a "defective" virus that requires a murine leukemia "helper" virus to form infectious MSV in tissue culture cells (derived from rat, mouse, or hamster embryos). Infection with MSV and "helper" virus results in foci of transformed cells as well as virus production that can be measured by FFU. Murine sarcoma viruses cause rhabdomyosarcomas in newborn mice, rats, and hamsters.

3. Murine Mammary Tumor Virus (MMTV)

This virus, also known as *milk factor* or *Bittner virus,* induces mammary tumors in mice. It is transmissible from mother to offspring through the milk.

Structure and Antigenic Properties. The MMTV resembles the murine leukemia viruses. It has an envelope with peplomeres (Fig. 23–3) and

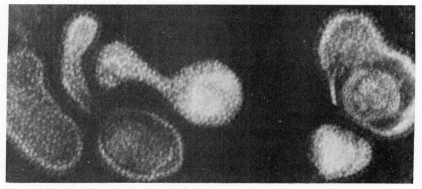

Figure 23–3. Structure of purified murine mammary tumor viruses as observed by negative staining in the electron microscope. Note knobs (peplomeres) on the surface of the virus envelope. ×200,000. (Reprinted with permission from Lyons, M. J., and Moore, D. H.: Isolation of mouse mammary tumor virus: Chemical and morphological studies. J. Nat. Cancer Inst. *35*:549, 1965.)

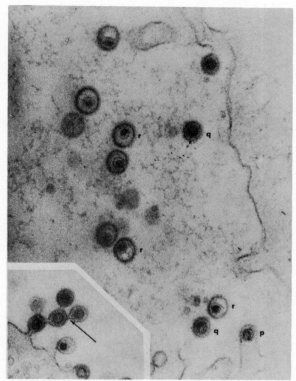

Figure 23—4. Electron micrograph of a thin section of a mouse mammary tumor virus infected cell. q = immature type-A particles; r = mature type-B particles; p = virus particle budding through the plasma membrane. Arrow in insert indicates viruses sharing a common envelope ×100,000. (Reprinted with permission from Lyons, M. J., and Moore, D. H.: Isolation of the mouse mammary tumor virus: Chemical and morphological studies. J. Nat. Cancer Inst. 35:549, 1965.)

contains reverse transcriptase and a 70S RNA genome. The virus presents two morphologic types (Fig. 23–4); a small immature particle (called type A) and a larger mature particle (called type B). Particles morphologically similar to MMTV have been observed in human milk and human mammary carcinoma cells; the particles possess a 70S RNA genome and reverse transcriptase activity.

The MMTV possesses type-specific envelope Ags and internal gs Ags; the latter are antigenically related to gs Ags of murine oncornaviruses.

Host Range and Culture. Murine mammary tumor viruses are found naturally in certain genetically susceptible "high cancer" strains of mice. Virus multiplies in the mammary gland and is released into the milk. Newborn or adult mice are susceptible to virus given by the oral, sc, or ip routes. Females can develop inapparent infections and transmit the virus to both male and female offspring.

4. Feline Leukosis-Sarcoma Viruses

This is a newly discovered group of viruses that have the capacity to induce leukoses and sarcomas in cats, dogs, rabbits, and monkeys. They resemble C-type particles associated with murine leukemias and sarcomas. Feline leukosis viruses possess unique type-specific Ags and gs Ags.

5. Hamster Leukosis-Sarcoma Viruses

Hamster sarcoma viruses resemble, but are antigenically distinct from, murine sarcoma viruses; they are oncogenic for hamsters but not for mice. The hamster leukosis viruses have some properties in common with known murine leukosis viruses; however, they possess unrelated type-specific Ags.

6. Other Leukosis-Sarcoma Viruses

Particles with the morphology of oncornaviruses have been detected in malignant tumors of reptiles, guinea pigs, swine, nonhuman primates, and man. Information on the biological properties of these viruses is incomplete.

II. ONCOGENIC DNA VIRUSES

A. Papillomavirus Subgroup

Papillomaviruses cause tumors (papillomas or warts) in their natural hosts (e.g., man, rabbits, cows, dogs). They are antigenically distinct by CF tests.

1. Human Papillomavirus

The human papillomavirus is the causative agent of warts; the genital wart (condyloma acuminatum) may become malignant. For a description of the virus, see Chapter 11.

2. Rabbit Papillomavirus

This virus causes large papillomas when inoculated sc into wild cottontail rabbits or domestic rabbits. Deoxyribonucleic acid isolated from rabbit papillomavirus is also infectious for both wild and domestic rabbits. Unlike most oncogenic DNA viruses, infectious papillomavirus can be recovered from papillomas of wild cottontail rabbits.

B. Polyomavirus Subgroup

1. Polyomavirus

Polyomavirus causes latent infections in laboratory and wild mice. Infection may occur within the first two weeks of life due to contaminated urine or saliva shed by infected adult mice. These viruses are highly tumorigenic when inoculated into newborn mice or hamsters; the tumors produced are of various histologic types, hence the name polyoma.

Structure and Antigenic Properties. Polyomaviruses are morphologically indistinguishable from papillomaviruses; however, they are antigenically distinct and have the capacity to agglutinate red blood cells.

Host Range and Culture. Whereas polyomaviruses grow and induce CPE in mouse embryo fibroblast cells, inoculation of hamsters results in tumor formation. The tumor cells can be cultivated *in vitro* and retain malignancy. The 3T3 cell line of mouse fibroblasts and BHK21 (baby hamster kidney) cells can be readily transformed *in vitro* with these viruses (Fig. 23–5).

2. Simian Virus 40 (SV_{40})

The properties of SV_{40} have been described elsewhere (Chapter 21).

C.   Adenovirus Group

1. Adenovirus

Several simian, bovine, avian, and human adenoviruses are tumorigenic when inoculated into newborn hamsters, mice, and rats. Although these

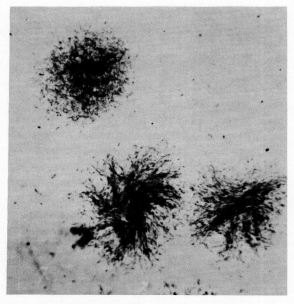

Figure 23–5. Transformation of BHK21 cells by polyomavirus. Two colonies of nontransformed BHK21 cells in the center of the figure showing the regular parallel arrangement of the fibroblastic cells. In the upper left-hand corner, note the BHK21 cells transformed by polyomavirus showing the criss-cross random orientation of the more rounded cells. ×15. (Reprinted with permission from Stoker, M., and Abel, P.: Conditions affecting transformation by polyoma virus. Cold Spring Harbor Symposium on Quantitative Biology 27:375, 1962.)

viruses can also transform hamster embryo or mouse embryo cells *in vitro,* they are not known to be associated with cancer in man. Rodents infected with adenoviruses have been used as experimental models for studying the mechanisms of tumor induction by viruses. For a description of the structure, antigenic properties, and host range of human adenoviruses, see Chapter 9.

D. Poxvirus Group

Several members of the poxvirus group produce only slight epithelial proliferation in infections of their natural hosts. Two poxviruses, Yaba virus and molluscum contagiosum virus, produce localized skin tumors in nonhuman primates and man, respectively.

1. Yaba Virus

Structure and Antigenic Properties.   Structurally and antigenically, the Yaba virus is morphologically similar to vaccinia and molluscum contagiosum (Chapter 11); however, there is no cross-neutralization between the Yaba virus and other poxviruses.

Host Range and Culture.   The Yaba virus is tumorigenic for several species of nonhuman primates and man, whereas animals of other species are refractive to the tumorigenic effects of the virus. It can be grown in monkey cells and human cells with stimulation of cell growth followed by cytopathology. Under natural conditions, the virus appears to be transmitted by insect vectors.

2. Molluscum Contagiosum Virus

The properties of molluscum contagiosum virus have been described elsewhere (Chapter 11).

E. Herpesvirus Group

1. Herpes Simplex Virus

There is strong evidence that herpesviruses cause certain tumors in chickens, nonhuman primates, guinea pigs, and frogs (Table 23–3). In man, a high degree of association has recently been observed between Epstein-Barr (EB) virus, a new member of the herpesvirus group (Chapter 17), and Burkitt's lymphoma (a tumor found in African children), nasopharyngeal carcinoma (most common in Chinese), and infectious mononucleosis (a benign lymphoproliferative disorder) (Chapter 18).

Seroepidemiologic surveys have shown that a significant association exists between herpes simplex virus type 2 (HSV-2) and malignant cervical carcinoma in women. Recent evidence suggests that HSV-1 may be

TABLE 23—3

Properties of Herpesviruses Associated with Malignant Disease

Virus	Disease	Antigens	Host Range	
			Transformation	Productive Infection
Herpes simplex type 2 (HSV-2)	Cervical carcinoma	Type-specific capsid Ags; shares group-specific Ags with HSV-1	Hamster embryo cells; human fetal cells	Rabbit kidney or human kidney cells; chick embryo cells
Epstein-Barr (EB)	Burkitt's lymphoma; nasopharyngeal carcinoma	Shares group-specific Ags with MDHV and Lucké herpesvirus	Leukocytes from man, marmosets, squirrel monkey; human embryo fibroblasts	Human lymphoblastic cells
Marek's disease herpesvirus (MDHV)	Lymphoproliferative	Shares group-specific Ags with herpes simplex, cytomegalovirus and Lucké herpesvirus; neutralized by Abs made against turkey herpesvirus	Chick leukocytes	Chick, duck, or quail embryo cells
Herpesvirus saimiri (HVS)	Lymphoma	Type-specific capsid Ags	Leukocytes from marmosets	Squirrel monkey or marmoset kidney cells
Lucké herpesvirus	Renal adenocarcinoma	Shares group-specific Ags with MDHV and EB virus	Frog (Rana pipiens)	Explants of kidney tumor tissue
Guinea pig herpesvirus	Lymphoblastic leukemia	Distinct from guinea pig cytomegalovirus	Guinea pig leukocytes	Guinea pig embryo cells or kidney cells
Herpesvirus sylvilagus	Lymphoma	Viral Ags demonstrated by immunofluorescence in transformed lymphoblastic cells	Leukocytes and viscera of wild rabbits (genus Sylvilagus)	Rabbit or mammalian kidney cells

causally related to lip and prostatic carcinoma in humans. Further support for the oncogenic potential of HSV-1 and HSV-2 has been provided in reports showing that these viruses have the capacity to transform hamster embryo cells and human embryo lung cells *in vitro*. For a discussion of the properties of herpes simplex viruses, see Chapter 11.

2. Epstein-Barr Virus

The properties of Epstein-Barr virus are described in Chapter 17. The virus can transform human fetal cells and nonhuman primate (marmoset) lymphocytes *in vitro*. The transformed lymphoctyes induce tumors in marmosets.

3. Cytomegalovirus

The properties of cytomegalovirus are described in Chapter 17. Recent evidence shows that this virus can transform hamster embryo fibroblasts and that the transformed cells induce tumors in newborn hamsters.

References

BIGGS, P. M., DE-THÉ, G., PAYNE, L. N. (eds.): *Oncogenesis and Herpesviruses.* Lyon, France: International Agency for Research on Cancer, 1971.

DARAI, G., and MUNK, K.: Human embryonic lung cells abortively infected with herpes virus hominis type 2 show some properties of cell transformation. Nature New Biol. *241*:268, 1973.

FENNER, F., and WHITE, P. O.: *Medical Virology.* New York, Academic Press, 1970.

GROSS, L.: *Oncogenic Viruses.* New York: Pergamon Press, 1970.

HOLLINSHEAD, A., and TARRO, G.: Soluble membrane antigens of lip and cervical carcinomas: Reactivity with antibody for herpesvirus nonvirion antigens. Science *179*:698, 1973.

KLEIN, G.: Herpesviruses and oncogenesis. Proc. Nat. Acad. Sci. U.S., *69*:1056, 1972.

NAWINSKI, R. C., FLEISSNER, E., and SARKAR, N. H.: Structural and serological aspects of the oncornaviruses, p. 31–60. In Pollard, M. (ed.): *Perspectives in Virology Vol. VIII.* New York: Academic Press, 1973.

NAYAK, D. P.: Isolation and characterization of a herpesvirus from leukemic guinea pigs. J. Virol. *8*:579, 1971.

RAPP, F., and DUFF, R.: In vitro cell transformation by herpesviruses. Fed. Proc. *31*: 1660, 1972.

TEMIN, H.: The RNA tumor viruses—background and foreground. Proc. Nat. Acad. Sci. U.S. *69*:1015, 1972.

TEMIN, H.: Mechanism of cell transformation by RNA tumor viruses. Ann. Rev. Microbiol. *25*:610, 1971.

TODARO, G., and HUEBNER, A.: NAS Symposium: New evidence as the basis for increased efforts in cancer research. The viral oncogene hypothesis: New evidence. Proc. Nat. Acad. Sci. U.S. *69*:1009, 1972.

VIGIER, P.: RNA oncogenic viruses: Structure, replication and oncogenicity. Progr. Med. Virol. *12*:240, 1970.

Chapter 24

Viruses and Oncogenesis

The aim of this chapter is to present an overview of some of the processes involved in the virus causation of cancer and particularly to indicate
how the tools and models of basic research have aided in exploring the
virus etiology of human malignancies.

Oncogenic viruses have the capacity to induce either *benign* or *malig-*

nant neoplasms in susceptible animals. The oncogenic potential of most oncogenic viruses can be demonstrated also in tissue cultures, where they induce characteristic cell alterations designated as *cell transformation*. When a virus induces cell transformation in a tissue culture, small foci of cells resembling microtumors (Fig. 23–5) often appear; the number of foci is proportional to the number of infectious virus particles present in the virus inoculum.

Viral oncology has advanced rapidly as the result of studies with 3 major groups of viruses:

1. The oncornaviruses include leukosis and sarcoma viruses of various animal species and the murine mammary tumor virus (Bittner agent). A recent observation of singular interest is that particles resembling murine mammary tumor virus were detected in human mammary carcinomas and the milk of American women with a familial history of breast carcinoma.

2. The small oncogenic DNA viruses, which include the polyomavirus of mice, SV_{40} of monkeys, and a number of adenovirus serotypes, have been isolated from man and other species.

3. Certain members of the herpesvirus group are associated with neoplastic or proliferative lesions in a wide variety of animal species, including man (e.g., Burkitt's lymphoma, nasopharyngeal carcinoma, lip carcinoma, and cervical carcinoma).

Both *in vitro* and *in vivo* methods for quantitative assay of the oncogenic activities of oncornaviruses, the small oncogenic DNA viruses, and herpesviruses have been devised. These achievements have resulted from the use of modern tissue culture techniques, inbred newborn animals, and the application of basic biochemical, biophysical, and immunologic research tools.

Because of the complexities involved, much of the current information on virus-induced cell transformation is still fragmentary and speculative.

A. Properties of Virus-Transformed Cells

The transformation of cells cultured *in vitro* and the induction of neoplasms in animals by oncogenic viruses are related phenomena, as exemplified by the observations that transformed cells behave like tumor cells when transplanted into suitable animals, and that tumor cells from animals behave like transformed cells when cultivated in tissue culture.

Viral-induced cell transformation *in vitro* provides a model for determining the possible mechanism(s) by which oncogenic viruses incite tumors *in vivo*. During virus-cell interactions, most oncogenic viruses do not produce cytopathologic changes that permit their recognition. However, they can be detected in infected cells by other techniques, including (1) the formation of new Ags, (2) the presence of virus-specific mRNA, (3) the presence of viral DNA or RNA genomes, and (4) virus-specific enzyme activities (e.g., reverse transcriptase).

TABLE 24—1

Properties of Cells Transformed by Oncogenic Viruses

1. Altered growth characteristics of transformed cells
   a. loss of contact inhibition
   b. increased growth rate and saturation density in culture
   c. increased capacity to persist in culture
   d. altered metabolism

2. Changes in transformed fibroblasts
   a. cells are shorter
   b. parallel orientation of cells is lost
   c. chromosomal abnormalities are present
   d. resist superinfection by the transforming virus

3. Altered immunologic properties of transformed cells
   a. new cellular antigenic components are present
   b. virus-specified antigens (T antigens, TST antigens, gs antigens, virion antigens) are produced

4. Capacity to form neoplasms

The criteria for cell transformation induced by oncogenic viruses include the following: (1) altered growth characteristics, (2) morphologic changes, (3) altered antigenic composition, and (4) the capacity to form neoplasms when inoculated into susceptible animals (Table 24–1). The most reliable criterion of true oncogenic transformation of cells is the ability of the transformed cells to produce a malignant tumor when injected into a susceptible host.

B. Viral-Induced Tumor Antigens

One of the principal properties of transformed cells is that they possess new Ags not found in uninfected cells. These new Ags are detected by CF, fluorescent Ab, and graft rejection tests and are designated by different, albeit inappropriate, terms. For example, new intranuclear Ags detected by fluorescent Ab and CF tests in polyomavirus-, papillomavirus-, and adenovirus-transformed cells are referred to simply as *T antigens* (tumor Ags). On the other hand, surface Ags responsible for tumor graft rejection are called *tumor-specific transplantation* (TST) *Ags*. The TST Ags are present in the cell plasma membrane but not in the virion. Although these TST Ags are nonvirion Ags, they are virus-specified in the sense that all tumors induced by the same virus carry the same antigenic specificity irrespective of the nature of the tissue or the species of animal in which they originated. In contrast, herpesvirus-induced tumors present a different picture. The TST Ags present in the plasma membrane of these tumors may also be present in the isolated virion. The reason for this is that herpesviruses possess an envelope that is derived from cell membranes, whereas polyoma, papilloma, and adenoviruses are nonenveloped virions.

Transplantation experiments based on the principle of graft rejection are used to demonstrate presence of TST Ags in transformed cells. Thus, inbred mice inoculated with syngeneic polyomavirus-transformed cells develop immunity to the TST Ags and reject the transformed cells. Since the TST Ags specified by this virus in different strains of animals are the same, inbred animals immunized with polyomavirus-induced tumor cells of allogeneic origin will likewise be immune to syngeneic tumors induced with the same virus. The TST Ags can also be demonstrated by the immuno-fluorescence test, the cytotoxic test, and the colony inhibition test.

Recent evidence suggests that viral-induced cell transformation results in the appearance of *"embryonic Ags"* on the plasma membrane (Fig. 24–1). The specificity of embryonic Ags is determined by the species origin of the transformed cells; their possible role in carcinogenesis is not known.

C. Oncogenic RNA Viruses

1. Leukosis-Sarcoma Viruses (Oncornaviruses)

Although an appropriate name for this group of viruses is currently being debated, the term oncornaviruses (oncogenic RNA viruses) seems most appropriate. The proposed oncornavirus group includes the avian leukosis-sarcoma viruses, the murine leukosis-sarcoma viruses, the murine mammary tumor viruses, and several recently discovered leukosis-sarcoma viruses of the cat, hamster, rat, and guinea pig. Many of these animals have indigenous oncornaviruses that may induce leukoses or sarcomas either naturally or experimentally in laboratory animals.

Oncornaviruses are remarkably similar structurally and biochemically (Chapter 23). Virions (C-type particles) consist of an internal icosahedral nucleoid (core) containing single-stranded RNA and an inner and outer membrane. The outer membrane corresponds to an envelope (host-cell-derived) formed by a budding process of the cell membrane that precedes virus liberation from the infected cells. Additionally, the virus envelope contains virus-specified Ags. Disruption of the virus envelope liberates the core components (i.e., virus 70S RNA and internal group-specific Ags). Oncornaviruses possess a unique DNA polymerase system (RNA-directed DNA polymerase or *reverse transcriptase* and a DNA-directed DNA polymerase) associated with the virus core that probably functions in virus replication and cell transformation (Fig. 24–2).

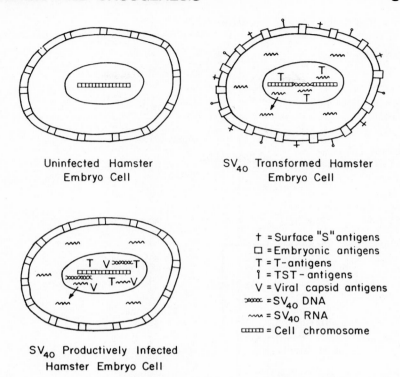

Uninfected Hamster
Embryo Cell

SV$_{40}$ Transformed Hamster
Embryo Cell

SV$_{40}$ Productively Infected
Hamster Embryo Cell

† = Surface "S" antigens
□ = Embryonic antigens
T = T-antigens
↑ = TST - antigens
V = Viral capsid antigens
xxxxx = SV$_{40}$ DNA
⌒⌒⌒ = SV$_{40}$ RNA
⊏⊐⊐⊐⊐ = Cell chromosome

Figure 24–1. Comparison of uninfected, SV$_{40}$-productively-infected, and SV$_{40}$-transformed hamster embryo cells. In transformed cells, the SV$_{40}$ genome is integrated into the cellular chromosome in the nucleus. Viral mRNA is found in the nucleus and cytoplasm. T antigens are produced and localized in the nucleus. Several changes occur at the cell surface, including the appearance of embryonic antigens, virus-specified TST antigens, and S antigens. In productively infected cells, the SV$_{40}$ genome is not integrated into the cellular chromosome, and TST antigens, S antigens, and embryonic antigens are absent or masked. However, SV$_{40}$-specified mRNA, T antigens, and viral capsid antigens are synthesized during productive infection. In comparison, all these changes are either absent or masked in uninfected cells.

Two major groups of Ags (type-specific or virion Ags and group-specific Ags) are found in oncornaviruses. The type-specific Ags are glycoproteins; they are associated with the virus envelope and are measured by virus neutralization, CF, or fluorescent Ab tests (Chapter 23). These immunologic tests utilize sera from animals immunized with virions or animals bearing the virus-induced tumor. The group-specific Ags are nonglycoproteins; they make up part of the internal virus component, and appear to consist of two distinct polypeptide Ags: (1) Ags restricted to a single viral species (species-specific Ags) and (2) Ags shared by oncornaviruses of more than one species (interspecies Ags). All oncornaviruses

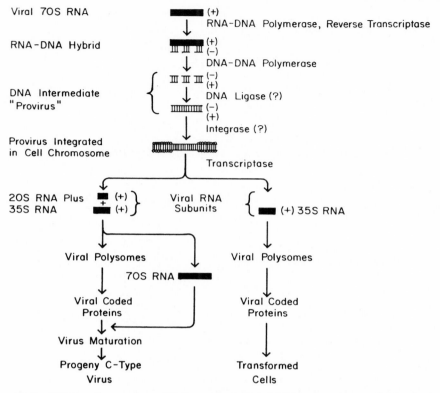

Figure 24—2. Proposed model for oncornavirus DNA polymerase activities and their possible functions in virus replication and cell transformation. Viral 70S RNA is copied into a RNA-DNA hybrid molecule by reverse transcriptase. The DNA strand of the hybrid molecule is polymerized into a double-stranded DNA intermediate "provirus." The provirus is integrated into the cell chromosome and then transcribed into viral RNA. Translation of the virus-specified RNA into proteins can lead to progeny virus production and cell transformation. The mechanism(s) that controls these events has not been elucidated. (Modified from Green, M.: Molecular basis for the attack on cancer. Proc. Nat. Acad. Sci. U.S. *69*:1036, 1972.)

possess species-specific Ags, whereas only the leukosis-sarcoma viruses of mammalian origin possess Ags of the interspecies Ags. The species-specific Ags are unrelated to the type-specific or virion Ags; they are used in serologic tests to divide the oncornaviruses into distinct classes (e.g., the avian leukosis-sarcoma viruses, the mammalian leukosis-sarcoma viruses, the reptilian leukosis-sarcoma viruses, and the mouse mammary tumor viruses).

The most striking biological characteristic of oncogenic RNA viruses, next to their oncogenic capacity, is that they establish an endosymbiotic association with their host cells that allows simultaneous production of virus and multiplication of the host cells. It is possible to recover infectious virus from most of the tumors induced by oncornaviruses as well as from noncancerous tissues of infected animals.

In cultured animal cells transformed by some strains of Rous sarcoma virus (RSV), infectious virus is not produced despite the presence of the RSV genome in the Rous cells. In this case, RSV appears to be "defective" in that it cannot code for essential RSV envelope proteins (i.e., type-specific Ags). However, the RSV genome can be "rescued" following superinfection of the Rous cells with "helper" virus (e.g., Rous-associated virus, RAV). Thus the RSV is a defective virus that retains the capacity to transform· cells while lacking the information to code for its own envelope proteins. By complementation and phenotypic mixing (Chapter 4), fully infectious RSV is formed by borrowing an RAV envelope.

Recently, it has been shown that another type of "helper" function for defective RSV multiplication exists in nature. Cells of a majority of chick embryos contain a genetic element called chick-cell-associated helper factor (chf) that is responsible for production of group-specific Ags and a viral coat protein of a certain specificity. During infection of the chf-positive cells with defective RSV, the cells provide viral coat proteins for the formation and release of new infectious RSV. The expression of chf by these chick embryo cells appears to be genetically determined, its presence being a dominant trait and its absence a recessive trait.

Infection of susceptible cells with oncornaviruses, which results in virus replication and cell transformation, involves a series of steps: (1) virus attachment and entry into the cell nucleus, (2) integration of a *"provirus"* (DNA form of oncornavirus 70S RNA) (Fig. 24–2), (3) synthesis of virus-specified RNA and proteins, (4) maturation of virions at the plasma membrane, (5) replication of the provirus, and (6) cell transformation. The replication steps in oncogenic DNA viruses are essentially the same as those for oncornaviruses except that formation of a provirus is not required. In cells transformed by most oncornaviruses, doughnut-like particles (A-type particles), believed to be immature viruses, are observed (Chapter 23). The A-type particles are converted into virions (C-type particles) by budding through the cell membrane or into cytoplasmic vacuoles. In the case of murine mammary tumor viruses, the virions are referred to as B-type particles (Chapter 23).

The requirement for DNA synthesis during oncornavirus replication and cell transformation is based on indirect evidence. Early studies demonstrated that inhibitors of DNA synthesis (5-iododeoxyuridine, cytosine arabinoside) block replication and transformation by oncornaviruses (e.g., RSV), a finding subsequently extended to other oncornaviruses. The need for DNA synthesis is transient, occurring during the first several hours after infection. If DNA synthesis is blocked or the newly synthesized early

DNA is destroyed, the oncornavirus genome is lost. A reasonable hypothesis is that the requirement for early DNA synthesis is to provide a DNA intermediate "provirus" that later serves as a template for viral RNA synthesis, e.g., 70S RNA (Fig. 24–2). This feature of oncornaviruses is unusual since the replication of all nononcogenic RNA viruses (except for orthomyxoviruses) does not require DNA synthesis or DNA transcription during their replication cycles.

A singularly interesting observation is that human cells in tissue culture can be transformed to neoplastic cells by infection with avian sarcoma viruses (e.g., RSV). The mechanism of transformation by RSV requires (1) the presence of the virion and (2) a permissive cell for transformation. The production of virions or the stable integration of "provirus" does not seem to be a requirement for the continued occurrence of cell transformation. The current opinion is that some virus-specified product(s) that is not a structural component of the virion is responsible for maintaining the transforming event.

D. Oncornaviruses and the Etiology of Human Neoplasms

Although oncornaviruses have not been shown to be clearly associated with human cancer, their role in carcinogenesis in man has been proposed because of their wide distribution among animal species and because of their demonstrated role in the genesis of certain tumors of chickens, mice, and cats. Additionally, there have been reports that C-type virus particles (Chapter 23) are present in leukemic human plasma and in human tumor cell cultures; in addition, "reverse transcriptase" and 70S RNA have been detected in human cases of leukemia and other neoplastic tissues (e.g., rhabdomyosarcoma, Hodgkin's disease, and Burkitt's lymphoma). Particles morphologically identical to the B-type particles (Chapter 23), 70S RNA, and reverse transcriptase activity found in mouse mammary tumors have also been detected in human milk and in human mammary carcinomas. A recent epidemiologic survey revealed that, whereas such B-type particles were present in the milk of 60% of American women with a familial history of breast cancer, they could be detected in only 5% of women without such familial history; moreover, fewer particles were present in the milk of subjects of the latter group. Considerable numbers of B-type particles were detected in milk from 39% of the Parsi women of Bombay, a group that has a two to three times higher incidence of breast cancer than the rest of the Bombay population. It is noteworthy that breast cancer accounts for about 50% of all cancer in Parsi women. The Parsis are descendants of Zoroastrians who emigrated from Persia some 1300 years ago and who, because of religious practices, have been inbreeding intensively ever since.

E. Theories on the Origin of Oncornaviruses

In the absence of experimental infection, oncornaviruses are thought to be transmitted vertically—that is, from parent to offspring. They are widespread among different species of vertebrates. Two hypotheses have emerged to explain the origin of oncornaviruses: the oncogene hypothesis and the protovirus hypothesis.

According to the *oncogene hypothesis,* transmission of oncogenic RNA viruses depends on viral genes carried in the provirus that are associated with genetic material of the host cell. The oncogenes may be but a portion of the virogenes, namely, the portion responsible for cell transformation. The virogenes also carry information needed for oncornavirus replication. Normally, oncogenes and virogenes are not expressed in host cells because of a cellular repressor(s) (Fig. 24–3). The repressor(s) can act coordinately to control the expression of the whole virogene or independently to allow partial expression (e.g., gs Ag production or reverse transcriptase activity).

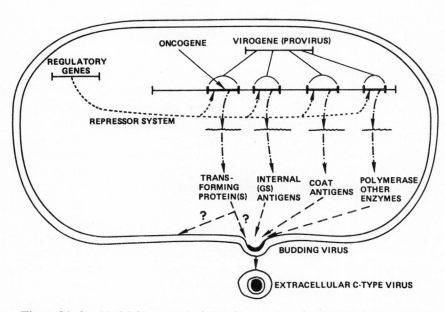

Figure 24–3. Model for control of the virogene (provirus). The virogene or provirus is depicted as having four genes, one of which is the oncogene. These genes can be repressed or derepressed individually or in any combination. When the regulatory genes are transcribed and translated into repressor molecules, the genes of the provirus are not expressed. The repressor system can act coordinately to control expression of all genes in the provirus. Partial expression could allow virus production without transformation or transformation without virus production. (Reprinted with permission from Todaro, G., and Huebner, R.: New evidence as the basis for increased efforts in cancer research. Proc. Nat. Acad. Sci. U.S. 69:1009, 1972.)

Partial expression may allow for virus replication in the absence of cell transformation. Activation of endogenous virogenes has been demonstrated in primary mouse embryo cells using 5-bromodeoxyuridine or ultraviolet irradiation. During tumorigenesis, the provirus can be entirely activated by factors such as radiation, chemical carcinogens, virus infection, aging, treatment of cells with 5-bromodeoxyuridine, and other alterations of genetic expression to make virus-specified products and virions.

In contrast, the basis of the *protovirus theory* is that the germ line of vertebrates contains regions of DNA that can evolve in various directions through DNA→RNA→DNA transfers utilizing reverse transcriptase activity of somatic cells. This type of evolution is comparable to embryonic cell differentiation; however, abnormal evolution could lead to the formation of an oncogenic RNA virus genome. Integration of the virus genome at a special chromosomal site in the host cell could then lead to the production of some specific product(s) that causes malignant transformation.

Although these hypotheses concerned with oncornaviruses are interesting and may have relevance to the etiology of some animal cancers, certain DNA viruses are also oncogenic and have the capacity to induce cell transformation without the intervention of oncornaviruses.

F. Oncogenic DNA Viruses

Of the known oncogenic DNA viruses (Chapter 23, Table 23–1), polyoma, simian virus 40, human adenoviruses, and herpesviruses have been studied in detail. The possibility that herpesviruses may have tumorigenic properties is based on seroepidemiologic studies, the identification of herpesviruses in cultured tumor cells from man and animals, and the recent demonstration that herpes simplex virus type 2 (HSV-2) can induce transformation of hamster embryo cells and possibly of human embryonic cells in tissue culture.

Infection with oncogenic DNA viruses results in either productive infection with associated virus production and cell death or abortive infection with a block in virus production. Under appropriate conditions, up to 40% of abortively infected cells may undergo malignant transformation. Unlike oncornavirus-transformed cells, cells transformed by oncogenic DNA viruses generally do not synthesize infectious virus but continuously express certain virus gene functions. Productive infection and cell tranformation by oncogenic DNA viruses are mutually exclusive. Usually, cells of the natural host are productively infected (*permissive cells*), whereas cells of the unnatural host are transformed (*nonpermissive cells*). It appears that nonpermissive cells either lack some essential component required for infectious virus replication or produce a repressor-like substance(s) that blocks the late virus gene functions required for infectious virus production.

1. Papillomaviruses

Natural tumors induced by members of the papillomavirus group are either benign (e.g., common warts—"verruca vulgaris"—in man and many animal species) or are initially benign but may become malignant (e.g., rabbit papilloma and human genital warts, condyloma acuminatum). The lesions of *condyloma acuminatum* are warts growing on moist mucous membranes of the vagina or external genitalia of the male. The cells contain intranuclear inclusions that resemble DNA-containing inclusions described in cells of common human warts caused by human papillomavirus (Chapter 11). Condyloma acuminatum presents a highly proliferative tumor and is the only type of human wart that may become malignant. Human papillomaviruses have not been successfully grown in cell culture; consequently, there is limited information on the mechanisms of virus multiplication and tumorigenesis.

2. Polyomaviruses

Considerably more information is available about the polyomavirus subgroup, which includes polyoma and simian virus 40 (SV_{40}) (Chapter 23), the smallest known oncogenic DNA viruses. Polyoma virus can spread naturally among laboratory mice or wild house mice without apparent disease or tumors. However, when high titers of infectious polyoma virus are inoculated artificially into newborn mice or hamsters, a wide variety of histologically diverse tumors are produced, hence the name "polyoma." Most tumors are spindle cell sarcomas. In polyoma-transformed cells, neither infectious virus nor infectious viral DNA can be detected; however, transformed cells contain polyoma virus-specific T Ags and TST Ags, virus-specific RNA, and multiple copies of virus DNA that are not necessarily complete but are intimately associated with host cell chromosomes. The significance of multiple polyomavirus DNA copies and their location in cell-specific chromosomes remains to be determined.

Simian virus 40 was initially discovered in apparently normal cultures of monkey kidney cells being used for the production of poliovirus vaccine. Inoculation of SV_{40} virus into newborn hamsters revealed that this virus was oncogenic. Subsequent studies showed that SV_{40} resembles polyoma virus in its physical and chemical properties. Polyoma or SV_{40} viruses induce striking biochemical alterations in transformed cells, including induction of cellular DNA synthesis, stimulation of specific enzyme activities, synthesis of virus DNA and virus-specific mRNA, and the formation of at least two nonstructural viral Ags, T Ags, and TST Ags.

Tumor Ags found in the cell nucleus can be demonstrated by CF or immunofluorescence tests using sera from animals bearing polyoma- or SV_{40}-induced tumors. The TST Ags appear in the plasma membrane of transformed cells (Fig. 24–1) and can be demonstrated by transplantation rejection tests in syngeneic animals previously vaccinated with infectious SV_{40} virus. This type of immunity occurs because the vaccine virus probably induces some TST-Ag synthesis that elicits a cellular immune response leading to subsequent rejection of the tumor.

Other Ags recently reported to be associated with SV_{40}- or polyoma-transformed hamster cells include cell surface (S) Ags (presumed to be unrelated to TST antigens) and embryonic Ags. The S Ags were detected by immunofluorescence and colony inhibition tests with sera of SV_{40}-immunized hamsters that had resisted challenge with virus-free transformed cells. The embryonic Ags (Fig. 24–1) on SV_{40}-transformed hamster cells were detected by immunofluorescence using sera from non-tumor-bearing pregnant hamsters. The mechanism of induction of detectable embryonic Ags and the relationship of these surface Ags to TST Ags, S antigens, and tumorigenesis remain to be elucidated.

The mechanism of cellular DNA induction and its role in SV_{40}-induced cell transformation is unknown. Apparently, only part of the virus genome is involved in cell transformation, since ultraviolet or gamma radiation inactivates the infectivity of SV_{40} virus 3 to 5 times more rapidly than the capacity of the virus to induce cell transformation. Viral-induced cell transformation in the SV_{40} system is a rare event, for even with inputs of 1000 PFU per cell, only about 5% of the cells eventually become transformed.

In contrast to polyomavirus- or adenovirus-transformed cells (discussed below), the complete SV_{40} genome is often present in SV_{40}-transformed cells, as evidenced by the production of infectious SV_{40} either spontaneously or as a result of artificial cell hybridization (Fig. 24–4). A notable observation is that DNA isolated from SV_{40} virions can transform human fibroblast cells in tissue culture; the transformed cells contain SV_{40} T Ags, and infectious virus is recoverable from the transformed cells.

3. Adenoviruses

The human adenoviruses are of special interest since they were the first human viruses shown to possess oncogenic properties in newborn rodents. Adenoviruses possess about 23 genes, but not all of them are expressed in adenovirus-transformed cells. Similar to polyomaviruses, adenoviruses can induce tumors in rodents, but no infectious virus has been detected in the tumor cells even after subjecting them to various physical or biological manipulations, including cell fusion techniques used to induce latent SV_{40} virus in hamster tumor cells. It is noteworthy that adenovirus-transformed cells carry the equivalent of several molecules of adenovirus DNA integrated into a number of their chromosomes; virus-specific mRNA is transcribed *in vivo* and the transformed cells always contain adenovirus-specified T and TST Ags.

Purified adenovirus virions contain at least 9 different structural poly-

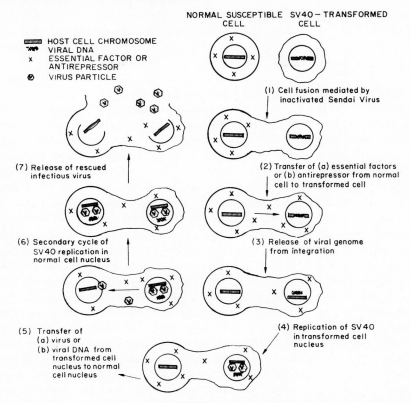

Figure 24–4.   Possible mechanism for induction of SV$_{40}$ multiplication following SV$_{40}$-transformed cell fusion mediated by inactivated Sendai virus with susceptible host cells. (Reprinted with permission from Butel, J. S., Tevethia, S. S., and Melnick, J. L.: Oncogenicity and cell transformation by papovavirus SV$_{40}$: The role of the viral genome. Adv. Cancer Res. *15*:1, 1972.).

peptides. One of the internal core polypeptides has been identified as an endonuclease that cleaves 30S viral DNA into 18S subunits. The 18S DNA species may be involved in adenovirus DNA replication and perhaps in integration of the virus genome during the process of cell transformation. Transformation by adenoviruses evidently involves an abortive infection of nonpermissive host cells and probably includes the following essential events: (1) Host cell DNA synthesis is induced, (2) T-Ag synthesis occurs, (3) virus genes are integrated into cellular DNA so that functions 1 and 2 are maintained, and (4) late virus gene functions (production of virus structural proteins and infectious virus) are blocked.

Although adenoviruses induce cancer experimentally in animals, they do not appear to induce cancer in man. A survey of more than 130 differ-

ent cancers in man for the presence of adenovirus-specific mRNA by
RNA-DNA hybridization experiments has provided no evidence that they
cause cancer.

4. Poxviruses

Several members of the poxvirus group induce slight epithelial proliferation in their natural hosts. Two poxviruses, namely, *Yaba virus* and *molluscum contagiosum virus,* which produce benign skin tumors in nonhuman
primates and in man, respectively, are of interest and merit further discussion. Yaba tumors were first described in 1957 among rhesus monkeys
kept in open-air cages in Yaba, Nigeria. The Yaba virion is morphologically similar to vaccinia virus (Chapter 9), although it may be slightly
larger. It causes large subcutaneous, nonencapsulated histiocytomas in
nonhuman primates. After intravenous inoculation into rhesus monkeys,
hundreds of small benign tumors may develop at multiple sites, including
subcutaneous tissues, heart, muscles, and lungs. Within 48 hr after inoculation, macrophages migrate into the infected area and the infected cells
undergo striking morphologic changes leading to tumor formation. The
nuclei and nucleoli of the tumor cells enlarge and multiply rapidly. The
tumor cells contain cytoplasmic inclusion bodies, infectious virus, and many
soluble viral Ags. Apparently, tumors produced in mature animals never
become malignant. Yaba virus has been transmitted to man, and *in vitro*
infection of both monkey and human cells is characterized by a prolonged
growth cycle and eventual cytopathic changes. Characteristically, Yaba
tumors in monkeys, either naturally acquired or induced, regress spontaneously within 1–2 months, probably as the result of *in vivo* cytopathic
effects of the virus. Specific Abs develop but appear to have little, if any,
effect on established tumors. Evidently, no antigenic relationship exists
between Yaba virus and other members of the poxvirus group.

Molluscum contagiosum virus produces painless, pearly white, discrete
lesions in children and young adults. Infection leads to formation of benign
tumors that can occur anywhere on the body except the soles and palms.
The "molluscum body" is a large cytoplasmic inclusion body composed of
virus particles resembling other poxviruses. The virus has been transmitted experimentally to man. Growth of the virus in tissue culture cells
has been difficult; however, the tendency to induce proliferative changes of
infected cells is more striking with molluscum contagiosum virus than with
other poxviruses.

5. Herpesviruses

In contrast to the viruses discussed above, which seldom, if ever, induce
malignant neoplasms in their natural hosts, there is convincing evidence
that viruses of the herpesvirus group are linked etiologically with certain

natural malignant neoplasms of lower animals (e.g., Lucké renal adenocarcinoma, Marek's disease, rabbit lymphoma, monkey lymphoma) and of man (e.g., cervical carcinoma, Burkitt's lymphoma, nasopharyngeal carcinoma, and Hodgkin's disease).

G. Herpesviruses and the Etiology of Animal Neoplasms

1. Lucké Renal Adenocarcinoma

Of the oncogenic herpesvirus models in animals, the Lucké tumor is the only carcinoma. The other herpesvirus-induced cancer models are lymphoproliferative diseases. The Lucké renal adenocarcinoma occurs with a low frequency in the leopard frog, *Rana pipiens*. An observation of interest is that tumor cells from hibernating frogs (4 to 9°C) contain intranuclear inclusion bodies and herpesvirus particles, whereas tumor cells of frogs held at room temperature (20 to 25°C) do not. Herpesvirus-containing extracts prepared from inclusion-containing Lucké tumor cells (4 to 9°C) induce typical Lucké renal adenocarcinomas when injected into frog embryos. When the inoculated frog embryos develop into adult frogs, up to 80% of the animals develop renal adenocarcinomas.

2. Marek's Disease

This is a highly contagious disease of chickens caused by a herpesvirus; it is characterized by lymphoid infiltration and uncontrolled cell proliferation in the nerves and visceral organs, resulting in tumor formation and paralysis. Herpesviruses multiply in the follicular epithelium of the feather from whence they can be shed into the environment. The virus is not transmitted vertically (from mother to offspring by the ovum). Prevention of the disease in flocks of chickens has been accomplished with a nonpathogenic turkey herpesvirus vaccine. This is the first instance in which a neoplastic disease caused by a virus has been controlled by vaccination.

3. Rabbit Lymphoma

This lymphoproliferative disease is caused by herpes sylvilagus, an indigenous virus of wild cottontail rabbits (genus *Sylvilagus*). The virus is unable to cross genus lines to infect the ordinary laboratory strains of rabbits of the genus *Oryctolagus*. The disease varies from benign hyperplastic tumors to malignant lymphomas. Virus can be recovered from peripheral leukocytes and from infected immature lymphoid cells that infiltrate the lymph nodes and spleen. No virus-induced cytopathic effect has been observed in parenchymal cells of any organs showing lymphocyte infiltration. It is not known whether the herpesvirus genome is present in all immature lymphoid cells.

4. Monkey Lymphoma

Two unrelated herpesviruses, herpesvirus saimiri and herpesvirus ateles, were the first oncogenic herpesviruses isolated from nonhuman primates. They differ in their host cell range in tissue culture, Ab induction in animals, antigenic structure, and oncogenic range. Herpesvirus saimiri, which was originally isolated from kidney cultures and peripheral lymphocyte cultures of squirrel monkeys, can induce leukemia and malignant lymphomas in several animal species, e.g., marmoset monkeys and rabbits. The virus remains latent in squirrel monkeys.

Herpesvirus ateles, originally isolated from kidney cultures of a spider monkey, causes leukemia and malignant lymphoma in marmoset monkeys.

H. Herpesviruses and the Etiology of Human Neoplasms

1. Cervical Carcinoma

Evidence for the herpesvirus etiology of cancer in man is mainly circumstantial. Two types of herpes simplex viruses (types 1 and 2), differing in their biologic, immunologic, and biochemical properties, infect man (Chapter 11). Herpes simplex virus type 1 (HSV-1) is usually associated with lip lesions (coldsores), whereas herpes simplex virus type 2 (HSV-2) is harbored in the genitourinary tract and is transmitted by sexual intercourse. Both viruses can be cultivated readily in tissue culture, and both types cause latent as well as active infections in man.

Exposure to HSV-1 generally occurs early in life, whereas exposure to HSV-2 does not occur until puberty. Either type of infection can develop into an apparent or inapparent disease. Apparent disease is characterized by cell destruction, which is most often self-limiting. Many herpesviruses establish latent infections following recovery from apparent disease. Latent infections often persist for the life of the individual even though circulating neutralizing Ab is constantly present.

Recent epidemiologic, serologic, and virologic evidence suggests that HSV-2 may be the causative agent of squamous cell carcinoma of the uterine cervix, the second most common cancer in women; HSV-1 is suspected of being the causative agent of lip cancer. The onset of cervical carcinoma seems to be related to the sexual exposure. For example, prostitutes, women with multiple sex partners, and those who start sexual relations early in life tend to exhibit a higher frequency of the disease and higher frequency of Abs to HSV-2 than matched control groups. In one study, HSV-2 Abs were detected in 98% of an experimental group of patients with cervical carcinoma as compared to (1) Abs in 55% of a matched control group without tumors and (2) Abs in 50% of women with malignancies at sites other than the cervix. These data suggest that there is an association between HSV-2 and carcinoma of the cervix. More recently, infectious HSV-2 has been isolated from a degenerating *in vitro* culture of cervical carcinoma cells. Also, ultraviolet-irradiated HSV-2 is oncogenic for hamster embryo fibroblasts and possibly for human embryonic fibroblasts. Similar results have been obtained with human cytomegalovirus and HSV-1, which have the capacity to transform hamster embryo fibroblasts. It has been shown that ultraviolet irradiation does not decrease the oncogenic potential of herpesviruses as rapidly as it decreases their lytic potential. Herpesvirus Ags are found in the cytoplasm and on the surface of the transformed cells. Cells transformed by HSV-1 or HSV-2 metastasize after injection into hamsters. Of interest was the observation that the number of metastases was not inhibited by previous immunization with HSV-1 or HSV-2, indicating that hamsters do not develop transplantation immunity to the HSV-transformed cells as a result of viral immunization. In spite of *in vitro* and *in vivo* studies on the potential oncogenicity of HSV-1 and HSV-2, the causal role of these viruses in human carcinogenesis remains to be established.

2. Burkitt's Lymphoma

In addition to herpes simplex viruses, a second widely distributed herpesvirus, Epstein-Barr (EB) virus, has been shown to be associated with certain human tumors, i.e., Burkitt's lymphoma in African children and nasopharyngeal carcinoma of the Chinese. The virus is also the cause of infectious mononucleosis, a common nonmalignant disease of adolescents (Chapter 18). The incidence of Burkitt's lymphoma among African children is 1 in 50,000. In most cases, the tumor starts in the region of the alveolar process of the maxilla or the mandible (Fig. 24–5); it grows rapidly and causes distortion of the face. There may be invasion of the eyelids and orbit and metastasis to the liver, kidneys, ovaries, and other visceral organs. The tumor can be successfully treated with alkylating agents such as cyclophosphamide or vincristin; recurrences are uncommon. If remission lasts more than one year, the prognosis is good. Patients with Burkitt's lymphoma, nasopharyngeal carcinoma, or infectious mononucleosis develop high Ab titers to EB virus.

The production of Burkitt's lymphoma or nasopharyngeal carcinoma occurs under unusual circumstances not as yet understood. Recent data suggest that malaria can cause immunodepression and predispose to the development of Burkitt's lymphoma.

Most cell cultures established from Burkitt's tumors synthesize EB virus particles and have been shown to synthesize IgM that is bound to the cell membrane. The maintenance of this cell marker is proof that the tumor cells are derived from lymphoid tissue. The isolation and purification of the virus have been difficult; most virus particles are structurally defective, and relatively few tumor cells in culture make EB virions. The agent appears to

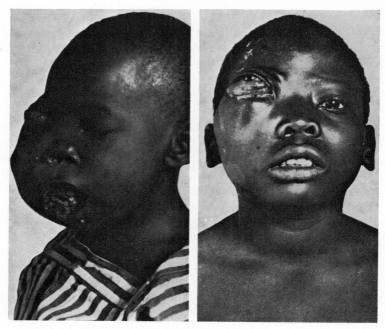

Figure 24—5. Left panel shows a Burkitt's tumor involving the right maxilla and mandible. Right panel shows a Burkitt's tumor involving the right maxilla and extending into the orbit. (Reprinted with permission from Burkitt, D.: A sarcoma involving the jaws in African children. Brit. J. Surg. *46*:218, 1958–1959.)

fulfill all the criteria of an oncogenic virus: It has been identified in peripheral blood leukocytes of patients with Burkitt's lymphoma and is capable of transforming human fetal fibroblasts and both human and non-human primate leukocytes *in vitro*. Viral genomes have also been detected in the transformed cells. More recently, DNA-DNA hybridization studies have revealed that small quantities of EB virus-DNA are present in virus-free biopsy specimens of Burkitt's lymphoma and nasopharyngeal carcinoma. Clones of somatic cell hybrids produced by fusing Burkitt lymphoblastoid cells with other human cells also carry the EB virus genome, which can be induced to replicate after exposure to 5-iododeoxyuridine. These data indicate that the entire virus genome is present in all Burkitt lymphoblastoid cells.

Virus-induced Ags detected in EB-virus-infected lymphoblastoid cells include early antigen(s) (EA) in the cell nucleus, virus capsid antigen(s) (VCA) in the cell cytoplasm, and membrane antigen(s) (MA) in the plasma membrane of the infected cells. It has been demonstrated that patients with Burkitt's lymphoma or infectious mononucleosis have serum

Continued
Clark, John.

SOCIAL AND
BEHAVIORAL
SCIENCES
Political
Science
Comparative
Politics

"collapse" duplicates work presented in many other forums during the late 1980s. It is also not clear whether the scope of the conclusions includes Poland exclusively or applies to the communist world in general. Upper-division undergraduates and above.—*J. W. Peterson, Valdosta State College*

Abs against EA that appear during the acute phase of disease and well before the appearance of Abs to VCA and MA. Detection of Abs to EA in the patient's serum by immunofluorescence or CF tests can be of diagnostic importance. The Abs to EA can no longer be detected a few months following recovery from disease, whereas Abs to VCA and MA persist for years, if not for life.

Recent data have shown that 87% of Burkitt's lymphomas tested possess detectable 70S RNA and reverse transcriptase activity. This finding is of interest because a relatively high percentage of established human leukocyte cultures contain reticular arrays of small (22 nm) virus-like particles in the cell cytoplasm. The possible relationship of these small cytoplasmic particles to EB virus particles and the etiology of Burkitt's lymphoma has not been elucidated. Whether the transformation of cells is caused by herpesviruses alone or results from interaction of herpesvirus and a second virus will require further investigation.

3. Hodgkin's Disease

Findings similar to those concerned with oncogenic herpesviruses have resulted from studies on the etiology of Hodgkin's disease. Cultured leukocytes from patients with Hodgkin's disease undergo changes that seem to be accompanied by the emergence of herpes-like virus particles (antigenically unrelated to EB virus or HSV-2) and possibly another agent containing an RNA genome. These data suggest that a dual infection (i.e., herpesvirus plus an RNA virus in the same cell) may be necessary to cause cell transformation in Hodgkin's disease.

References

BUTEL, J. S., TEVETHIA, S. S., and MELNICK, J. L.: Oncogenicity and cell transformation by papovavirus SV_{40}: The role of the viral genome. Adv. Cancer Res. *15*:1, 1972.

DUFF, R., and RAPP, F.: The induction of oncogenic potential by herpes simplex viruses, pp. 189–210. *In* M. Pollard (ed.): *Perspectives in Virology VIII*. New York: Academic Press, 1973.

GILDEN, R., and OROSZIAN, S.: Group-specific antigens of RNA tumor viruses as markers for subinfectious expression of the RNA virus genome. Proc. Nat. Acad. Sci. U.S. *69*:1021, 1972.

GREEN, M.: Molecular basis for the attack on cancer. Proc. Nat. Acad. Sci. U.S. *69*: 1036, 1972.

GREEN, M.: Oncogenic viruses. Ann. Rev. Biochem. *24*:701, 1970.

GROSS, L.: *Oncogenic Viruses*. New York: Pergamon Press, 1970.

HANAFUSA, T., HANAFUSA, H., MIYAMOTO, T., and FLEISSNER, E.: Existence and expression of tumor virus genes in chick embryo cells. Virology *47*:475, 1972.

HAUGHTON, G., and NASH, D. R.: Transplantation antigens and viral carcinogenesis. Progr. Med. Virol. *11*:248, 1969.

HELLSTROM, K. E., and HELLSTROM, I.: Cellular immunity against tumor antigens. Adv. Cancer Res. *12*:167, 1969.

HINZE, H. C., and CHIPMAN, P. J.: Role of herpesviruses in malignant lymphoma in rabbits. Fed. Proc. *31*:1639, 1972.

JONCAS, J.: Clinical significance of the EB herpesvirus infection in man. Progr. Med. Virol. *14*:200, 1972.

KUFE, D., MAGRATH, I. T., ZIEGLER, J. L., and SPIEGELMAN, S.: Burkitt's tumors contain particles encapsulating RNA-instructed DNA polymerase and high molecular weight virus-directed RNA. Proc. Nat. Acad. Sci. U.S. *70*:737, 1973.

MELENDEZ, L. V., HUNT, R. D., DANIEL, M. D., FRASER, E. O., BARAHONA, H. H., KING, N. W., and GARCIA, F. G.: Herpesvirus saimiri and ateles—their role in malignant lymphomas of monkeys. Fed. Proc. *31*:1643, 1972.

NAHMIAS, A., and ROIZMAN, B.: Infection with herpes-simplex viruses 1 and 2. N. Engl. J. Med. *289*:719, 1973.

Glossary

This Glossary includes a selected list of terms and their definitions that are commonly used for communication in basic and applied virology. The list is not intended to be inclusive of all terms.

Albumin: A protein widely distributed throughout the tissues and body fluids of animals and plants.

Alkylating agents: Chemicals or drugs that induce substitution of an alkyl radical for a hydrogen atom in a cyclic compound such as a purine or pyrimidine.

Anamnestic response (recall phenomenon, memory phenomenon): Accelerated immune response to an antigen that occurs in an animal that has previously responded to the same antigen; it may involve humoral or cellular immunity.

Antibody (Ab): A substance (commonly, if not always, a gamma globulin) that can be incited in an animal by an antigen or by hapten combined with a carrier and that reacts specifically with the antigen or hapten. Some antibodies occur naturally without known antigen stimulation.

Antigen (Ag): A substance that can react specifically with antibodies and, under appropriate conditions, can incite an animal to form specific antibodies.

Aseptic meningitis: An infection of the meninges caused primarily by viruses; occasionally other microorganisms may be etiologic agents of this disease but they are not detectable in spinal fluid.

Asthenia: A syndrome characterized by increased susceptibility to fatigue.

Astrocyte: A large nonnervous cellular element of the central nervous system.

Ataxia: A loss of muscular coordination.

Attenuated: A reduction or weakening of virulence (in a microorganism) obtained through selection of mutants that occur naturally or are obtained experimentally.

A-type virus: A morphologic classification of the oncornaviruses. The immature form of B-type oncornaviruses.

Australia antigen: A virus-like antigen associated with serum hepatitis (hepatitis B); the antigen was originally discovered in an Australian aborigine, hence the name.

Autoantibodies: Antibodies produced by an animal that react with the animal's own antigens. The stimulus is usually not known but could be the animal's own antigens or cross-reacting foreign antigens.

Autoimmune disease (autoallergic disease, autoantibody disease): A disease which by appropriate criteria is judged to result from the reaction of antibodies or from cellular immunity against antigens of the affected individual.

B-cells: Refers to bone-marrow-derived lymphocytes.

Bradykinesia: A condition characterized by extreme slow movement.

B-type virus: A morphologic classification of the oncornaviruses. The mature form of mouse mammary tumor virus.

Burkitt's lymphoma: A cancer of the lymphoid system associated with a herpesvirus (Epstein-Barr virus) first described in children living in certain areas of Africa.

Capsid: The protein coat that surrounds the nucleic acid of the virus.

Capsomeres: Substructures of virus particles composed of aggregates of polypeptide chains that interact to form the basic structural units of the capsid.

Cell-mediated immunity (cellular immunity): A state of immunity mediated by specifically immune lymphocytes (T-lymphocytes) coupled with lymphokine-directed participation of macrophages. It can be transferred with living immune lymphocytes but not by immune serum.

Cell strain: A cell culture derived from a primary culture by selection or cloning of cells having specific markers or properties.

Chlamydia: Bacteria belonging to the family Chlamydiaceae that cause the diseases psittacosis, lymphogranuloma venereum, trachoma, and inclusion conjunctivitis.

Choroid plexus cells: Cells that are derived from a network or interjoining of nerves and blood vessels.

Communicable: A property that relates to the ease with which infection is transmitted from one individual to another.

Complement: A multifactorial system (11 components) of normal serum; these components are characterized by their capacity to participate in certain antigen–antibody reactions.

Complement fixation (CF): The orderly fixation or participation of complement components with an antigen–antibody complex; some complex molecules (e.g., endotoxin) can fix complement by the alternate pathway from C3 to C9 in the absence of antibody.

Continuous cell line: A cell culture that possesses the potential of being subcultured indefinitely *in vitro*.

Coproantibodies: Antibodies occurring in the intestinal tract. They consist primarily of the IgA class.

Coryza: Inflammation of the nasal mucosa characterized by nasal discharge and watery eyes.

Councilman bodies: Inclusion bodies, found in hepatic cells, that are of diagnostic importance in yellow fever.

C-type virus: A morphologic classification of the oncornaviruses. The mature form of leukosis-sarcoma oncornaviruses.

Cytomegalic cell: A large swollen cell that is pathognomonic for cytomegalic inclusion disease (salivary inclusion disease).

Cytopathogenic effect (CPE):   This effect consists of morphologic alterations of host cells that usually result in cell death.

Delayed hypersensitivity: A specific sensitive state characterized by a delay of many hours in onset time of reaction following antigen administration; it peaks 24 to 36 hr after elicitation with antigen. It is transferable with specifically sensitive T-cells but not with serum.

Dementia: A general mental deterioration due to organic or psychological factors.

Demyelination: Destruction or loss of myelin from the medullary sheath of Schwann cells.

Deoxyribovirus: A term employed to designate those viruses that possess a DNA genome.

Dermatotropism: See *Tropism*.

Desquamation: The shedding of cells from the outer layer of the epidermis.

Diploid cell: A cell having the 2X number of gametic chromosomes.

Down's syndrome: The concurrence of symptoms related to mongolism.

Dysarthria: Disturbance of speech due to paralysis, uncoordination, or spasticity of the muscles used for speaking.

Dyspnea: Labored breathing, "shortness of breath," usually associated with serious diseases of the heart or lungs.

Endemic: The continuous presence of a disease in a community, usually with low incidence.

Endosymbiotic: A mutually advantageous association between two or more organisms and a host.

Envelope: A host-cell-derived membrane, containing virus specific antigens, that is acquired during virus maturation.

Epidemic: An outbreak of a disease that simultaneously affects a significant number of individuals in a community.

Erythema: An eruption of reddish patches in the skin.

"Fixed" virus: An attenuated variant of the virulent "street" rabies virus.

Gamma globulin: A fraction of serum based on electrophoretic mobility, composed of a number of molecular classes and subclasses of immunoglobulins and other nonantibody globulins.

Genome: A set of genes.

Giant cells: See *Syncytium*.

Gliosis: A condition marked by overgrowth of the neuroglia (nonnervous cellular elements of nervous tissue).

Guarnieri bodies: Acidophilic intracytoplasmic inclusion bodies in epidermal cells infected with smallpox virus.

Hemadsorption (HAd): The attachment of red blood cells to the surface of host cells.

Hemagglutination (HA): Aggregation of red blood cells.

Hemagglutinin (viral hemagglutinin): A nonantibody protein on the outer surface of some viruses (e.g., orthomyxoviruses) which reacts with a surface determinant(s) on red cells to cause agglutination of the red cells (hemagglutination).

Herpangina: Vesiculopapular lesions about 1 to 2 mm in diameter that are present above the pharynx. These lesions are associated with coxsackievirus infections.

Heterophil antibody: An antibody having heterogenetic distribution.

Heteroploid: Denotes chromosome numbers deviating from the normal chromosome number.

Hyperplasia: An increase in the size of a tissue or organ due to increase in cell numbers.

Hypoxia: A condition characterized by reduced levels of oxygen in the blood.

Icosahedron: A geometric figure composed of 12 vertices, 20 triangular faces and 30 edges.

Icterus (jaundice): A condition characterized by excess of bile pigments in the blood and tissues that leads to a yellow color of the surface integuments.

Immune complex disease: A vasculitis mediated by antigen–antibody complexes, complement, and neutrophils.

Immunity: The state of being able to resist and/or overcome harmful agents or influences.

    Active: Immunity acquired as the result of a natural experience with an infectious agent or due to vaccination.

    Passive: Immunity due to acquisition of maternal antibody or injection of preformed antibody.

Immunogen: An antigen that stimulates the production of protective antibodies.

Immunoglobulins (Ig): Classes of globulins to which antibodies belong, e.g., IgG, IgM, IgA, IgD, and IgE.

Inclusion body: Acidophilic or basophilic heterogenous masses of new material in the nucleus or cytoplasm of cells that are associated with some virus infections.

Infection: The presence of microorganisms in parenteral tissues.

Viral infection: The presence of a virus particle or its genome inside a host cell.

Infectious dose (ID_{50}; $TCID_{50}$): That amount of virus required to cause a demonstrable infection in 50% of the inoculated animals or tissue culture cells.

Inflammation: The vascular and tissue responses to injury; these are important in host defense and healing.

Insidious onset of infection: Onset of infection without readily apparent symptoms.

Kupffer cells: Macrophages lining the hepatic sinusoids.

Latent infection: A persistent infection with intermittent acute episodes of disease. The virus is not detectable between episodes.

Leukemic cell: The malignant cell of leukemia; may arise from monocytic, lymphocytic, or granulocytic stem cells.

Leukocytosis: An abnormally large number of leukocytes in the circulating blood.

Leukopenia: A condition associated with a smaller than normal number of circulating leukocytes.

Lymphadenopathy: Any disease process affecting a lymph node or lymph nodes.

Lymphatic leukemia: A malignant disease characterized by uncontrolled proliferation of malignant lymphocytes and conspicuous enlargement of lymphoid tissue (e.g., lymph nodes, spleen).

Lymphokines: Biologically active substances elaborated by stimulated lymphocytes.

Lymphoma: A neoplastic disease of lymphoid tissue, e.g., lymphosarcoma, lymphocytic leukemia, Hodgkin's disease.

Maturation: The final step in the production of new virus particles.

Molluscum bodies: Large eosinophilic inclusion bodies found in epidermal cells infected with molluscum contagiosum virus.

Morbidity: The ratio of sick to well individuals in a community.

Mortality: The ratio of the number of deaths to a given population in a defined situation.

Mutation: Heritable changes in the genome that do not result from the incorporation of genetic material from another organism.

Myalgia: Muscular pain.

Necrosis: The death of cells or tissues resulting from irreversible damage.

Negri bodies: Intracytoplasmic inclusion bodies in nerve cells associated with rabies virus infections.

Neoplasm: An abnormal collection of cells characterized by more rapid cellular proliferation than the surrounding normal tissue.

> *Benign:* A neoplasm that remains localized and does not spread to other parts of the body.
>
> *Malignant:* An invasive type of neoplasm that spreads to other parts of the body.

Neuraminidase: An enzyme on the outer surface of some viruses (e.g., orthomyxoviruses) that splits off the terminal N-acetylneuraminic acid on the mucoprotein receptors on cells (e.g., red blood cells).

Neurotropism: See *Tropism*.

Nosocomial infection: An infection acquired in a hospital.

Nucleocapsid: The virus structure composed of the nucleic acid surrounded by the capsid.

Nystagmus: The rhythmic oscillation of the eyeballs in a horizontal, rotary, or vertical motion.

Oncogenes: That portion of the virogene (RNA genome of oncornaviruses) responsible for cell transformation as proposed in the "Oncogene Theory of Viral Oncogenesis" (see p. 319).

Oncogenesis: The mode of development of a neoplasm.

Opsonin: A serum substance, usually an antibody, that adsorbs to the surface of microorganisms and promotes their phagocytosis.

Orchitis: Inflammation of the testis.

Pandemic: A disease attacking the population of a large geographic area(s); may be worldwide.

Parenchymal cells: The specific cells of a gland or organ that are supported by and contained in the connective tissue framework or stroma.

Pathogenesis: The mode of development of a disease or morbid process.

Paul-Bunnell test: A serologic test used in the laboratory diagnosis of infectious mononucleosis. The test measures the titer of heterophil antibodies that will react with antigens on the surface of sheep red blood cells.

Penetration: The entrance of the virion or virus nucleic acid into host cells.

Peplomeres: See *Spikes*. Projections extending from the outer surface of a virus envelope.

Peplos: See *Envelope*.

Phagosome: A cell vacuole resulting from phagocytosis of particulate materials.

Plaque: A defined area of cell destruction resulting from *in vitro* virus infection.

Plaque-forming unit (PFU): A fundamental measure of infectious virus particles. One infectious virus particle is equivalent to one plaque-forming unit.

Pleomorphism: The potential for morphologic variation.

Pleurodynia: A painful affection of the tendinous attachments of the thoracic muscles.

Pock: A discrete pustular lesion found on the chorioallantoic membrane or skin following infection with certain viruses.

Polyvalent vaccine: A vaccine that contains more than one immunogen.

Postinfectious encephalitis: Disease invoked by an allergic reaction following recovery from an acute virus infection.

Preicteric: See *Icterus*. Before the onset of jaundice.

Primary cell culture: A culture started from cells, tissues, or organs taken directly from living tissue.

Prodromal: Relates to an early sign or symptom that precedes overt signs of disease.

Prognosis: A forecast of the course and final outcome of a disease.

Provirus: The integrated or latent form of some viruses; e.g., the integrated DNA form of oncornaviruses.

Receptor sites: Specific areas on the surface of host cells that serve as points of attachment for viruses.

Repressors: A special group of molecules coded by DNA that block the synthesis of one or more proteins.

Rhabdomyosarcoma: A malignant neoplasm derived from skeletal muscle.

Rhinitis: Inflammation of the nasal mucous membrane.

Riboviruses: A term used to group together those viruses that possess an RNA genome.

RNA-dependent RNA polymerase: An enzyme that catalyzes the formation of RNA from an RNA template.

RNA-directed DNA polymerase (reverse transcriptase): An enzyme(s) associated with leukosis viruses that catalyzes the synthesis of DNA from an RNA template.

Sarcoma: A solid tumor growing from derivatives of embryonal mesoderm such as connective tissue, bone, muscle, and fat.

Sequela: A morbid (abnormal) condition that develops as a consequence of a disease.

Secretory IgA: A special molecular form of the IgA Ab composed of 2 Ab molecules plus a secretory piece; it is found in secretions and functions against microorganisms that colonize on mucosal surfaces.

Serum: The fluid portion of the blood obtained after removal of the fibrin clot and blood cells.

Acute phase serum: Serum recovered during the early stage of a disease.

Convalescent phase serum: Serum recovered during the recovery stage of a disease.

"Slow" virus: A virus that causes subacute or chronic diseases having long incubation periods lasting several weeks to years before the onset of clinical symptoms.

Spikes: Surface projections of varying lengths spaced at regular intervals on the virus envelope.

Status spongiosus: A condition in which multiple cavities are formed in the white matter of the brain due to degeneration of axons.

"Street" virus: See *"Fixed" virus.* Used to describe the virulent type of rabies virus isolated in nature from domestic or wild animals.

Structural units of a virus: The repeating polypeptide chain(s) that comprise the morphologic unit or capsomere of viruses.

Syncytium: A multinucleated protoplasmic mass formed by the fusion of originally separate cells.

Syngeneic: Relates to tissue transplant between identical twins or individuals who are identical with respect to histocompatibility genes.

T-cells: Lymphocytes processed through the thymus.

Tachycardia: A condition characterized by rapid beating of the heart.

Teratogen: Any agent that may induce abnormal development of the fetus.

Thrombosis: The formation of a blood clot in the blood circulatory system.

Titer: The assay value of an unknown measured by volumetric means.

TMV: Tobacco mosaic virus. A single-stranded RNA virus that infects and multiplies in tobacco leaf cells.

Transformation, viral: A permanent heritable change induced in a cell by an oncogenic virus or foreign nucleic acid.

Tropism, infection: Infection preferentially supported by a particular cell, tissue, or organ.

Neurotropism: Infection preferentially supported by the cells of the CNS.

Dermatotropism: Infection preferentially supported by cells of the skin.

Tumorigenicity: Capacity to induce tumors in a susceptible animal.

Uncoating, virus: An intracellular event in which all or part of the virus capsid is removed from the virus nucleic acid; this process allows the viral genome to be transcribed and replicated.

Vaccination: The administration of a protective (immunogenic) antigen(s).

Vaccine: A suspension of dead or living microorganisms or their products administered for the purpose of producing active immunity.

Viral interference: A phenomenon whereby one intracellular virus inhibits the replication of a second virus.

Viremia: Presence of virus particles in the blood.

Virion: The mature infectious virus particle.

Virogene: See *Oncogene*. The complete RNA genome of oncornaviruses.

Viroid: Infectious subviral particles consisting of nucleic acid without a protein capsid.

Viruria: Presence of virus particles in the urine.

Virus: A small obligate intracellular parasite that depends on a living host cell for energy, precursors, enzymes, and ribosomes to multiply. It consists of a single type of nucleic acid, either DNA or RNA, and a protein coat surrounding the nucleic acid.

Index